Orthodontic Management of Class II Malocclusion

Martyn T. Cobourne
Editor

Orthodontic Management of Class II Malocclusion

An Evidence-Based Guide

Springer

Editor
Martyn T. Cobourne
Faculty of Dentistry, Oral & Craniofacial Sciences
King's College London
London, UK

ISBN 978-3-031-57529-7 ISBN 978-3-031-57530-3 (eBook)
https://doi.org/10.1007/978-3-031-57530-3

This Springer imprint is published by the registered company Springer Nature Switzerland AG
The registered company address is: Gewerbestrasse 11, 6330 Cham, Switzerland

Preface

Class II malocclusion represents a significant component of the day-to-day case load for most working orthodontists. It manifests with a wide range of clinical variation and can represent something of a challenge to achieve consistently successful outcomes. This textbook has been written as an evidence-based guide to the clinical management of class II malocclusion and will serve as a useful reference for all clinicians interested in managing this wide-ranging malocclusion.

The chapters have been written by an international group of orthodontists with considerable experience and expertise in the theoretical and practical aspects of class II management. The first section of the book contains a brief overview of the clinical and epidemiological characteristics of class II malocclusion, followed by a discussion of treatment timing and then an extensive overview of the contemporary evidence base relating to outcomes for class II treatment. The second section deals with the practical aspects of managing class II treatment in children and adults and includes chapters on the use of removable and fixed functional appliances, molar distalisation, fixed appliances, and an outline of current aspects relating to aligner-based treatment. These chapters are followed by a separate overview of class II division 2 treatment and a final chapter on orthodontic-surgical management of class II cases.

This text will be of interest to specialist trainees in orthodontics, newly graduated orthodontic practitioners, and those with more experience in managing class II cases. It provides a succinct and definitive overview of strategies aimed at correcting this type of malocclusion with multiple clinical examples and reference to the contemporary evidence base. We hope it will be of relevance to the global orthodontic community and will find its place on their bookshelves.

London, UK — Martyn T. Cobourne

Contents

1 Epidemiological and Clinical Features of Class II Malocclusion

Jadbinder Seehra

1.1 Introduction

A Class II occlusion has been recognised since the 1900s [1]. In the antero-posterior dimension, this malocclusion is subdivided into three categories. A Class II Division 1 incisor relationship is defined as when the lower incisor edges lie palatal to the cingulum plateau of the upper incisors. Typically, the upper incisors are proclined or of an average inclination with an increased overjet (Fig. 1.1). In a Class II intermediate incisor relationship, the upper incisors are upright or slightly retroclined with an increased overjet present. In contrast, in a Class II Division 2 incisor relationship, the upper incisors are retroclined with a minimal overjet (Fig. 1.2). However, in this category, the lower incisors can also be retroclined and the overjet maybe increased [2].

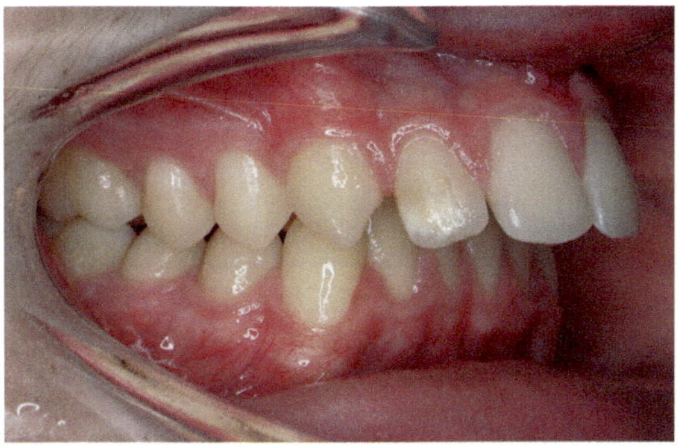

Fig. 1.1 Class II Division 1 incisor relationship

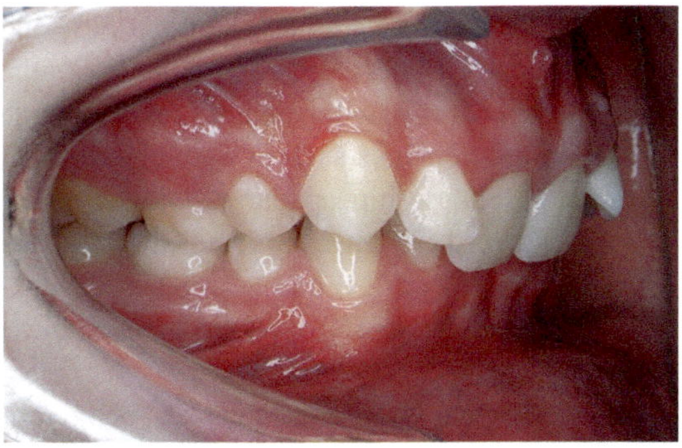

Fig. 1.2 Class II Division 2 incisor relationship

Based on molar relationship, within a Caucasian sample the prevalence of Class II Division 1 and Class II Division 2 malocclusions were reported at 19% and 4% respectively [1]. More contemporary prevalence studies have reported variation in the prevalence of a Class II malocclusion within different genders and ethnicities (Table 1.1).

J. Seehra (✉)
Department of Orthodontics, Faculty of Dentistry,
Oral & Craniofacial Sciences, Kings College London,
London, UK
e-mail: Jadbinderpal.seehra@kcl.ac.uk

M. T. Cobourne (ed.), *Orthodontic Management of Class II Malocclusion*,
https://doi.org/10.1007/978-3-031-57530-3_1

Table 1.1 Prevalence of Class II malocclusion

Study	Ethnicity	Sample size	Age (Years)	Prevalence (%)	Sub-division (%)
Silva and Kang 2001 [3]	Latino	507	12-18	21.5	II Div 1 (91.5%) II Div 2 (8.5%)
El-Mangoury and Mostafa 1990 [4]	Egyptian	501	18-24	21.0	II Div 1 (16.2%) II Div 2 (4.8%)
Horowitz 1970 [5]	White	718	10-12	22.5	
Helm 1968 [6]	Danish	3842	6-18	24.5	
Lew et al. 1993 [7]	Chinese	1050		21.5	
Garner and Butt 1985 [8]	American (Afro-carribean)	445	13-15	16.0	
Garner and Butt 1985 [8]	African	505	13-14	7.9	II Div 1 (7.9%) II Div 2 (0.0%)
Grewe et al. 1968 [9]	Indian	651	9-14	9.6	
Salzmann 1977 [10]	American	7514	12-17	32.0	

1.2 Aetiology of Class II Malocclusion

As with many malocclusions, a multifactorial model consisting of both environmental and genetic factors has been proposed in the aetiology of a Class II malocclusion. Both exposure to alcohol during embryonic development [11] and preterm births [12] have been associated with the development of retrognathic mandibles. Although inter-arch relationships such as overjet, overbite, and molar relationship appear not to be under genetic control [13], environmental factors such as caries experience [14] and non-nutritive sucking behaviours (NNSB) can influence these occlusal traits.

The term non-nutritive sucking behaviour (NNSB) describes habitual sucking of digits, pacifiers, and objects by a child in order to source comfort, a sense of security, and calmness [15]. Although this may be viewed as a normal process of a child's growth and development, depending on the age of the child, the presence of NNSB can result in occlusal disturbance and contribute to the development of a malocclusion which exhibits Class II features [16] [17]. Historically, in the vertical dimension, as a result of reduced alveolar growth [18], an anterior open bite with an associated tongue thrust swallowing pattern can manifest. The horizontal component of forces generated by NNSB can increase the maxillary arch length with concomitant proclination of the maxillary incisors [16]. The size of the resultant increased overjet can be exacerbated by retroinclination of the mandibular incisors [16]. Finally, in the transverse dimension, more commonly in the primary dentition, a posterior crossbite can develop [16]. Systematic evidence has also reported variations in the impact on the occlusion depending on if the NNSB involves the use of a pacifier or sucking of digits. For instance, an increased overjet in the primary dentition is less likely to occur if a pacifier is used. However, the use of a pacifier is associated with an increased risk of developing a Class II canine relationship and posterior crossbite. In contrast, in the mixed dentition, the risk of developing a posterior crossbite and anterior open bite is greater with digit sucking [19]. The vertical and antero-posterior effects on the occlusion tend to diminish once the NNSB has been ceased [16]. However, the more the NNSB persists the greater the risk of developing a malocclusion [19].

Support for the genetic basis of a Class II malocclusion stems from the observation of retrognathic mandibles in patients with congenital craniofacial abnormalities such as Pierre Robin sequence and Treacher Collins [20]. Additionally, dental anomalies such as ectopic maxillary canines [21] and microdontia [22] which have been proposed to have a genetic aetiology are commonly associated with a Class II Division 2 malocclusion leading to some authors to propose a shared genetic basis for the development of the maxillomandibular discrepancy. More recent studies have provided further insight into the development of a Class II malocclusion [20]. Polygenic inheritance and autosomal dominance models, with incomplete penetrance and variable expressivity, have been proposed for both Class II Division 1 and Class II Division 2 [22, 23, 24]. At a genetic level, a Class II malocclusion characterised by mandibular hypoplasia was detected in four families in which the affected individuals were homozygous for the rare allele of the polymorphism rs1348322 within the NOGGIN gene [25] which has been shown to be involved in mandibular formation in a mice model [26].

1.3 Clinical Features of Class II Malocclusion

1.3.1 Dentoskeletal

Within the literature, longitudinal growth studies have reported great variability in the dentoskeletal components of a Class II malocclusion. These studies tended to employ serial lateral cephalograms to assess the growth and development of the Class II skeletal and dental complex against a sample of "normal occlusions." However, inconsistent use of different cephalometric analyses may explain the observed variability in the reported dentoskeletal components of a Class II malocclusion.

Between the ages of 3 and 7 years, the cranial base and the maxilla are normal. The mandibular corpus and lower facial height are reduced, the gonial angle is large, and the dentoalveolar position of the mandible is in a retruded position. Both the height of the ramus and the skeletal position of the mandible are normal. However, the chin becomes slightly retruded after 5 years of age. In the transverse dimension, the maxilla is deficient. Importantly, the skeletal component of a Class II does not appear to be established during the deciduous dentition [27]. However, this observation is not universal, as mandibular retrusion and a short mandibular length have been reported in a sample of 5–8-year-olds [28]. In contrast, the occlusal features of a Class II are established during this age range. These include distal terminal plane of the second deciduous molars, Class II canine relationship, increased overjet and overbite and both a narrow upper dental arch and maxillary base [27, 28].

Between 8 and 10 years of age, the skeletal components of the Class II malocclusion seem to establish. However, variability exists in both the antero-posterior and vertical dimensions [29]. In the majority of cases, the maxilla is in the normal position. When it deviates from this position it is more likely to be retrusive rather than protrusive. A more protrusive maxilla as a key component of the Class II malocclusion has been reported [30]. However, overall, mandibular retrusion appears to be a common feature of Class II malocclusions [29] which is exacerbated by a shorter total mandibular length [28]. Indeed, in addition to a reduced lower face height proportion, a degree of mandibular retrusion appears to be a key characteristic in both Class II Division I and Class II Division II malocclusions [31]. Dentally, the maxillary incisors can be average, proclined, or of a more retroclined position which is particular to Class II Division II malocclusions [31]. The lower incisors can have an average, retroclined, or proclined inclination [29]. The position of both the upper and lower incisors can be reflective of the degree of dentoalveolar compensation for the underlying skeletal discrepancy. Rather than reporting features from a cohort of radiographs and comparing them to a control group, statistical modelling has been employed to identify dentoskeletal predicators or distinct facial patterns of a Class II malocclusion. Using this method, five vertical and six horizontal (A-F) morphological features of a Class II malocclusion have been described [32] (Table 1.2). As highlighted previously, even with this classification, different features in both the vertical and

Table 1.2 Morphological features of a Class II malocclusion as classified by Moyers et al. [32]

Feature	Type	Dentoskeletal component
Horizontal	A	Normal skeletal profile. Maxillary dentition is protracted resulting in Class II molar relationship, increased overjet and overbite.
	B	Midface prominence with normal mandible size.
	C	Marked Class II profile characterized by retrusion of the maxilla and mandible. Proclined lower incisors. Upper incisors upright or proclined.
	D	Retrognathic profile characterized by a small mandible. Midface is normal or slightly retruded. Mandibular incisors are upright or retroclined. Upper incisors proclined.
	E	Maxillary protrusion with normal or protruded mandible. Maxillary and mandibular incisor proclination.
	F	Milder Class II profile with mandibular retrusion.
Vertical	1	Steep mandibular plane (High angle). Anterior face height greater than posterior face height.
	2	Mandibular, functional occlusal and palatal plane are flatter than normal. Increased overbite present. "Square face" appearance.
	3	Palatal plane tipped upward anteriorly. Steep mandibular plane (High angle) with skeletal open-bite.
	4	Mandibular, functional occlusal and palatal plane are tipped downwards.
	5	Mandibular and functional occlusal plane are normal. Palatal plane is tipped downwards. Skeletal deep-bite.

horizontal dimensions can contribute to the Class II dentoskeletal features.

In a Class II malocclusion, it is unlikely that the dentoskeletal discrepancy will improve or "self-correct" with further growth [33, 34]. A greater skeletal facial convexity with a retruded mandibular position is maintained into adulthood [35]. However, in adolescence, a reduction in this facial convexity characterised by a decrease in ANB angle has been reported resulting in a marginal improvement in the overjet [36].

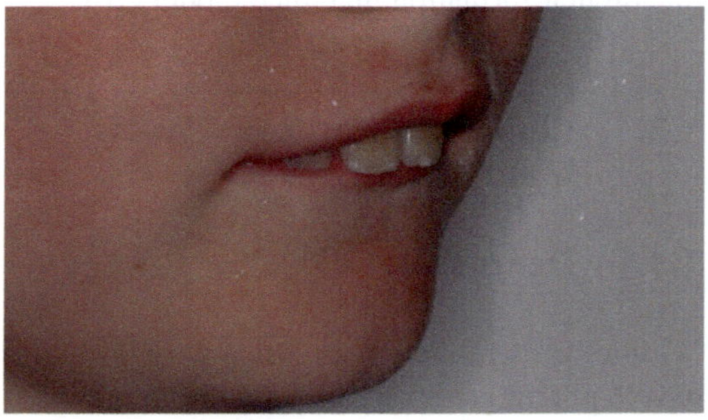

Fig. 1.3 Class II Division 1 incisor relationship complicated by a lower lip trap

1.3.2 Soft Tissues

The position of the lower lip relative to the labial surface of upper and lower incisors plays a role in the aetiology of a Class II Division 1 and Class II Division 2 malocclusion. In a sample of patients with a Class II Division 1 incisor relationship, the presence of a complete lower lip trap has been reported to result in more mandibular incisor retroclination and an increased overjet compared to a matched sample of patients without a lower lip trap [37]. The proclination of the upper incisors in a Class II Division 1 malocclusion can also be exacerbated by a short upper lip and a low lip level with flaccid tone which exerts less lip pressure allowing the upper incisors to "escape control" of the lower lip [38] (Fig. 1.3).

The role of resting pressure exerted from the lower lip and the resultant position of the maxillary incisors is also pertinent in the aetiology of Class II Division 2 incisor relationship. This is clinically described as a high lip level and in this situation the lip has a thicker lip shape but is not hypertonic in nature [39]. However, compared to Class I patients, a higher lip pressure was recorded in patients with a Class II Division 2 malocclusion. Clinically, the resultant effect on the maxillary incisors is a more extruded and retroclined incisor position [40]. This observation was further confirmed in a cephalometric evaluation which suggests that a high lip-line level is a primary aetiological factor in the development of Class II Division 2 malocclusion [41].

References

1. Angle EH. Malocclusions of the teeth. 7th ed. Philadelphia, PA: S.S White Mig. Co.; 1907.
2. British Standards Institutes. Glossary of Dental Terms (BS4492). London: BSI; 1983.
3. Silva RG, Kang DS. Prevalence of malocclusion among Latino adolescents. Am J Orthod Dentofacial Orthop. 2001;119(3):313–5. https://doi.org/10.1067/mod.2001.110985.
4. El-Mangoury NH, Mostafa YA. Epidemiologic panorama of dental occlusion. Angle Orthod. 1990;60(3):207–14. https://doi.org/10.1043/0003-3219(1990)060<0207:EPODO>2.0.CO;2.
5. Horowitz HS. A study of occlusal relations in 10 to 12 year old Caucasian and Negro children summary report. Int Dent J. 1970;20(4):593–605.
6. Helm S. Malocclusion in Danish children with adolescent dentition: an epidemiologic study. Am J Orthod. 1968;54(5):352–66. https://doi.org/10.1016/0002-9416(68)90304-7.
7. Lew KK, Foong WC, Loh E. Malocclusion prevalence in an ethnic Chinese population. Aust Dent J. 1993;38(6):442–9. https://doi.org/10.1111/j.1834-7819.1993.tb04759.x.
8. Garner LD, Butt MH. Malocclusion in black Americans and Nyeri Kenyans. An epidemiologic study. Angle Orthod. 1985;55(2):139–46. https://doi.org/10.1043/0003-3219(1985)055<0139:MIBAAN>2.0.CO;2.
9. Grewe JM, Cervenka J, Shapiro BL, Witkop CJ Jr. Prevalence of malocclusion in Chippewa Indian children. J Dent Res. 1968;47(2):302–305. https://doi.org/10.1177/00220345680470021701.
10. Salzmann JA. Malocclusion and treatment need in United States youths 12 to 17 years of age. Am J Orthod. 1977;72(5):579–81. https://doi.org/10.1016/0002-9416(77)90027-6.
11. Naidoo S, Harris A, Swanevelder S, Lombard C. Foetal alcohol syndrome: a cephalometric analysis of patients and controls. Eur J Orthod. 2006;28:254–61.
12. Rythén M, Thilander B, Robertson A. Dento-alveolar characteristics in adolescents born extremely preterm. Eur J Orthod. 2013;35:475–82.
13. Santana LG, Flores-Mir C, Iglesias-Linares A, Pithon MM, Marques LS. Influence of heritability on occlusal traits: a systematic review of studies in twins. Prog Orthod. 2020;21(1):29.
14. Mtaya M, Brudvik P, Astrøm AN. Prevalence of malocclusion and its relationship with socio-demographic factors, dental caries, and oral hygiene in 12- to 14-year-old Tanzanian schoolchildren. Eur J Orthod. 2009;31:467–76.
15. Newson J, Newson E, Mahalski PA. Persistent infant comfort habits and their sequelae at 11 and 16 years. J Child Psychol Psychiatry. 1982;23:421–36.
16. Larsson E. The effect of finger-sucking on the occlusion: a review. Eur J Orthod. 1987;9:279–82.
17. Mistry P, Moles DR, O'Neill J, Noar J. The occlusal effects of digit sucking habits amongst school children in Northamptonshire (UK). J Orthod. 2010;37:87–92.
18. Larsson E, Rönnerman A. Clinical crown length in 9-, 11- and 13-year-old children with and without finger-sucking habit. Br J Orthod. 1981;8:171–3.
19. Doğramacı EJ, Rossi-Fedele G. Establishing the association between nonnutritive sucking behavior and malocclusions: a systematic review and meta-analysis. J Am Dent Assoc. 2016;147:926–34.
20. Moreno Uribe LM, Miller SF. Genetics of the dentofacial variation in human malocclusion. Orthod Craniofac Res. 2015;18 Suppl 1(0 1):91–99. https://doi.org/10.1111/ocr.12083.
21. Pereira PM, Ferreira AP, Tavares P, Braga AC. Different manifestations of class II division 2 incisor retroclination and their association with dental anomalies. J Orthod. 2013;40:299–306.
22. Peck S, Peck L, Kataja M. Class II division 2 malocclusion: a heritable pattern of small teeth in well-developed jaws. Angle Orthod. 1998;68:9–20.
23. Harris JE. Genetic factors in the growth of the head. Inheritance of the craniofacial complex and malocclusion. Dent Clin N Am. 1975;19:151–60.
24. Morrison MW. Relative risk of Class II division 2 malocclusion in first- degree relatives of probands with Class II division 2 malocclusion. 2008.
25. Gutiérrez SJ, Gómez M, Rey JA, Ochoa M, Gutiérrez SM, Prieto JC. Polymorphisms of the noggin gene and mandibular micrognathia: a first approximation. Acta Odontol Latinoam. 2010;23:13–9.
26. Stottmann RW, Anderson RM, Klingensmith J. The BMP antagonists chordin and noggin have essential but redundant roles in mouse mandibular outgrowth. Dev Biol. 2001;240:457–73.
27. Varrela J. Early developmental traits in class II malocclusion. Acta Odontol Scand. 1998;56:375–7.
28. Baccetti T, Franchi L, McNamara JA Jr, Tollaro I. Early dentofacial features of Class II malocclusion: a longitudinal study from the deciduous through the mixed dentition. Am J Orthod Dentofacial Orthop. 1997;111:502–9.
29. McNamara JA Jr. Components of class II malocclusion in children 8-10 years of age. Angle Orthod. 1981;51:177–202.
30. Rosenblum RE. Class II malocclusion: mandibular retrusion or maxillary protrusion? Angle Orthod. 1995;65:49–62.
31. Pancherz H, Zieber K, Hoyer B. Cephalometric characteristics of Class II division 1 and Class II division

2 malocclusions: a comparative study in children. Angle Orthod. 1997;67:111–20.
32. Moyers RE, Riolo ML, Guire KE, Wainright RL, Bookstein FL. Differential diagnosis of class II malocclusions. Part 1. Facial types associated with class II malocclusions. Am J Orthod. 1980;78:477–94.
33. Stahl F, Baccetti T, Franchi L, McNamara JA Jr. Longitudinal growth changes in untreated subjects with Class II division 1 malocclusion. Am J Orthod Dentofacial Orthop. 2008;134:125–37.
34. Bishara SE, Jakobsen JR, Vorhies B, Bayati P. Changes in dentofacial structures in untreated Class II division 1 and normal subjects: a longitudinal study. Angle Orthod. 1997;67:55–66.
35. Bishara SE. Mandibular changes in persons with untreated and treated Class II division 1 malocclusion. Am J Orthod Dentofacial Orthop. 1998;113:661–73.
36. Taloumtzi M, Padashi-Fard M, Pandis N, Fleming PS. Skeletal growth in class II malocclusion from childhood to adolescence: does the profile straighten? Prog Orthod. 2020;21:13.
37. Lew KK. Lower incisor angulation differences in Class II division 1 malocclusions with and without full 'lip trap'. Aust Orthod J. 1991;12:29–32.
38. Lambrechts H, De Baets E, Fieuws S, Willems G. Lip and tongue pressure in orthodontic patients. Eur J Orthod. 2010;32:466–71.
39. McIntyre GT, Millett DT. Lip shape and position in Class II division 2 malocclusion. Angle Orthod. 2006;76:739–44.
40. Lapatki BG, Mager AS, Schulte-Moenting J, Jonas IE. The importance of the level of the lip line and resting lip pressure in Class II, division 2 malocclusion. J Dent Res. 2002;81:323–8.
41. Lapatki BG, Klatt A, Schulte-Mönting J, Jonas IE. Dentofacial parameters explaining variability in retroclination of the maxillary central incisors. J Orofac Orthop. 2007;68:109–23.

2 Treatment Timing in the Management of Class II Malocclusion

Martyn T. Cobourne

2.1 Background

Class II malocclusion is characterized by a discrepancy in the sagittal relationship, which leads to a post-normal occlusion. This is often associated with an increased overjet in class II division 1 cases; but if the upper incisors are retroclined, then a class II division 2 occlusion will exist. The extent of the skeletal discrepancy will influence the severity of the post-normal relationship and complexity of potential treatment; and whilst dentoalveolar disproportion often plays a role in the etiology of class II malocclusion, it is the skeletal discrepancy that usually represents the main contributing factor. The maxilla can be too far forward within the facial complex, the mandible can be too far back, or some combination of maxillary prognathia and mandibular retrognathia may co-exist. In many cases, mandibular retrognathia is the defining feature. These discrepancies can also be seen in association with a vertical component, either increased vertical proportions and a reduced overbite or open bite; or reduced vertical proportions and an increased overbite.

M. T. Cobourne (✉)
Centre for Craniofacial Development & Regeneration, Faculty of Dentistry, Oral & Craniofacial Sciences, King's College London, London, UK
e-mail: martyn.cobourne@kcl.ac.uk

In the growing child with a class II skeletal discrepancy, a common treatment approach is to attempt growth modification: most commonly, encouraging upward and forward growth of the mandible and restriction of forward maxillary growth, or some combination of the two. In this chapter we will briefly review the data relating to how the jaws grow within the context of overall body growth, and how successful growth modification strategies can be in the management of class II skeletal discrepancies. Finally, we will discuss the evidence relating to how the timing of class II growth modification strategies can potentially influence treatment outcomes.

2.2 Mandibular Growth and Growth in Stature

The relationship between height versus chronological age or height-distance curve for a developing child will demonstrate a relatively constant approximate three-fold increase in height from birth through to the age of around 18–19 years (Fig. 2.1, left panel). However, an incremental plot of height change versus chronological age or height-velocity curve will show significant fluctuations in rates of growth. There is rapid growth at birth, progressively decelerating until around 3 years of age; then a more slowly decelerating phase that lasts until puberty, albeit punctuated by a short acceleration of juvenile growth around the

M. T. Cobourne (ed.), *Orthodontic Management of Class II Malocclusion*,
https://doi.org/10.1007/978-3-031-57530-3_2

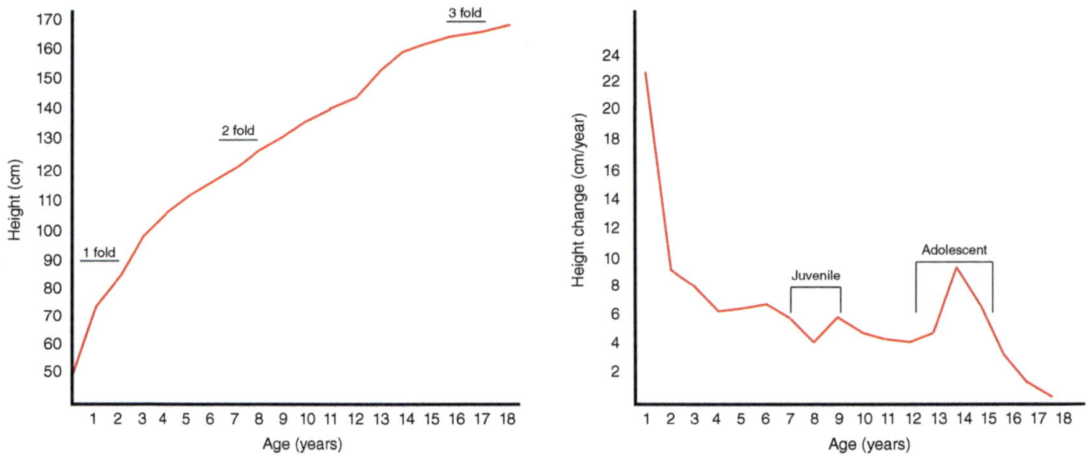

Fig. 2.1 Schematic representation of height-distance (left panel) and height-velocity curves (right panel) for a male from birth to 18 years of age. There is an approximately three-fold increase in height (left panel) and two growth spurts, both juvenile and adolescent—with the adolescent growth spurt being associated with significant changes in height-velocity

age of 6–8 years, followed by the adolescent growth spurt around the ages of 12–14 years, which varies in timing between males and females, and different individuals, and is followed by a progressive deceleration in growth velocity until adulthood (Fig. 2.1, right panel). Thus, height-velocity change does not have a constant relationship with chronological age and will reach a maximum during the pubertal growth spurt.

The mandibular condyle is a key driver of postnatal mandibular growth, and it is known that condylar growth is not constant during development—following a broadly similar pattern to that observed for somatic growth. A correlation between the condylar growth curve and pubertal growth spurt has also been reported [1–3] although this is not a precise relationship and condylar peak velocity does not seem to absolutely coincide with peak height-velocity [4] (Fig. 2.2). In terms of stature, peak height-velocity generally occurs around 12 years of age in females and 14 years in males, with the onset of this growth period generally occurring around 2 years prior to the peak [5]. However, these figures are associated with wide individual variation and there is no universally accepted method of reliably predicting skeletal age or the point of onset associated with an individual's pubertal growth spurt (or more specifically for the orthodontist—mandibular growth spurt). A number of techniques have been described, which can broadly be classified as those associated with clinical evaluation, including chronological age [6], sexual maturity [7], and monitoring of height changes [8]; or more direct

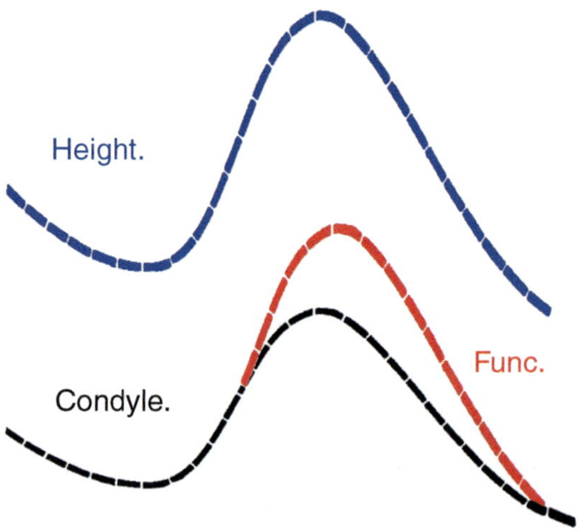

Fig. 2.2 Evidence exists to suggest that there is a correlation between the adolescent growth spurt (height-velocity; blue hatched line) and condylar growth-velocity (black hatched line). There is less evidence that the use of a functional appliance during the pubertal growth spurt can produce accelerated condylar growth (red hatched line). The x-axis represents chronological age spanning the pubertal growth spurt (increasing age from left to right); the y-axis represents height-velocity (blue) and mandibular condylar growth-velocity (black)

assessment of skeletal maturity based upon radiographic investigation, which has included development of the dentition [9], maturation of bones in the hand-wrist [10], or cervical vertebrae [11]. Orthodontists have investigated the relative merits of these techniques for many years and the literature is replete with conflicting data [3, 12–14]. The use of individual hand-wrist radiographs (or indeed, serial radiographs) to predict the pubertal growth spurt is not sufficiently accurate for use in clinical orthodontics [15, 16] and does not seem to afford any meaningful correlation with growth increases in mandibular length [17]. The additional radiation associated with the taking of hand-wrist radiographs as a method of estimating skeletal age in relation to orthodontic treatment cannot be justified. The cervical vertebral maturation (CVM) method has been described as a useful alternative to the hand-wrist radiograph for growth rate estimation [11]. The method is based upon morphological characteristics of the second to fourth cervical vertebrae, which are identifiable on a collimated lateral skull radiograph and therefore do not require any additional exposure to radiation beyond that for a normal pre-treatment examination (assuming of course, that assessment of CVM is not the specific reason for taking the lateral skull radiograph). There is conflicting data within the current literature that CVM represents a more accurate assessment than the hand-wrist method in predicting skeletal maturation—although on balance, the weight of evidence would suggest that it does [18–21]. However, there do not seem to be any significant advantages of CVM in assessing skeletal age or predicting the pubertal growth spurt in comparison to chronological age [12].

2.3 Treatment Changes Induced by Class II Growth Modification

Classic dentofacial orthopedic treatment in class II cases aims to maximize forward growth of the mandible whilst restraining growth of the maxilla. This can be achieved with the use of a functional appliance and/or the application of extra-oral force through headgear. The essential philosophy relating to these approaches is that condylar growth can potentially be accelerated through stimulation of the condylar cartilage, whilst maxillary sutural growth can be restrained through the class II forces established by a postured mandible and certainly through the application of headgear directly to the maxilla. In relation to the condyle, acceleration of growth may then ultimately lead to a larger mandible (and by inference although not necessarily by logic) correction of the class II skeletal pattern (Fig. 2.3).

Animal studies have shown evidence of molecular, cellular, and dimensional changes accompanied by growth and remodeling of the condyle (and glenoid fossa) when the mandible is habitually postured forward with a fixed intra-oral appliance [22, 23]. However, human clinical studies investigating clinically relevant growth changes related to functional appliance treatment are less convincing. The evidence base is generally low-level—being composed predominantly of retrospective case-control studies, some prospective

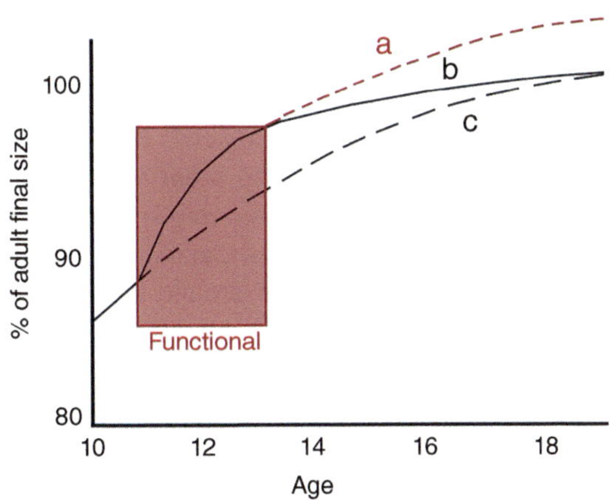

Fig. 2.3 (**a**) Growth stimulation with a functional appliance—growth is accelerated with the functional appliance during treatment (red rectangle) and continues at the expected rate after completion of treatment to produce a larger jaw; (**b**) Growth acceleration with a functional appliance—growth is accelerated with the functional appliance treatment but continues at a reduced rate after completion of treatment to produce a jaw that is ultimately the same size as that achieved with no treatment; (**c**) Normal mandibular growth in the absence of treatment. (Redrawn from Proffit, WR, Fields, HW, Larsson, BE, Sarver, DM. Contemporary Orthodontics, Sixth Edition, Elsevier, ISBN 978-0-323-54387-3)

controlled studies, and only a few randomized clinical trials. Moreover, these investigations rely primarily upon cephalometric analysis to measure growth changes and often focus on mandibular unit length (which often does not correlate with meaningful class II correction in the sagittal plane). These methodological problems notwithstanding, early orthopedic treatment with headgear will provide a posterior translation of the anterior maxilla through an annualized mean reduction in SNA of around 1.6 degrees [24]; whilst analysis of removable functional appliance data has suggested that this treatment can achieve an increase in mandibular unit length of around 2 mm, but this figure is based primarily upon retrospective data and analysis of RCTs alone shows less difference [25]. This is not to say that functional appliances are not effective at correcting a sagittal discrepancy associated with a class II malocclusion, but this seems to be achieved predominantly through dentoalveolar rather than skeletal change [26]. There is some evidence to suggest that they can also have a slight inhibitory effect on sagittal growth of the maxilla over the short term, but this represents less than 1 mm per year [27]. In relation to fixed functional appliances, there is little high-quality evidence that these devices can significantly influence craniofacial growth [28] and dentoalveolar effects also seem to predominate [29] although again, when retrospective data is incorporated into the analysis, maximal changes in mandibular unit length of around 2 mm have also been reported in pubertal patients [30].

Overall, it would seem that the effectiveness of functional appliances is mostly due to early correction of the buccal occlusion and overjet reduction through differential tooth movement, allowing the establishment of a class I relationship that is maintained whilst normal condylar growth catches up [31].

2.4 Do We Get a Better Response with Early Treatment?

Historically, there has been considerable interest amongst orthodontists regarding the relative advantages and disadvantages of early class II treatment. In the broadest sense, some early studies suggested that treating a young child with a class II skeletal discrepancy in the early mixed dentition with a functional appliance and/or headgear could produce significant skeletal changes [32]. This led the advocates of early intervention to claim that starting at this time maximized the success of treatment through enhanced orthopedic change, simplifying any subsequent treatment with fixed appliances in the permanent dentition, and reducing any reliance on dental compensation and extractions. Moreover, it has been argued that early correction of an increased overjet can improve a child's self-esteem and reduce the risk of trauma to the maxillary incisor dentition. However, the data supporting many of these claims was retrospective, and there had been more than a suspicion from some of these studies that the enhanced skeletal growth afforded by early treatment was often lost over the longer term [33].

Recognizing this lack of high-quality evidence, three landmark randomized clinical trials (RCTs) were conducted over a period of around a decade in the late 1990s and early 2000s, two in the United States of America and one in the United Kingdom [34–39]. These trials compared early mixed dentition treatment of class II malocclusion with either a functional appliance (bionator or twin-block) and/or headgear followed by any further treatment required in the permanent dentition, to a single course of comprehensive treatment carried out in early adolescence. The American studies were interested primarily in whether growth could be significantly influenced by early treatment, whilst the UK-based study was more invested in understanding differences in the process of treatment for class II cases, depending upon whether you started early or late. Interestingly, the findings were remarkably similar—early treatment was effective in correcting a class II malocclusion and reducing an increased overjet; however, later treatment achieved this very effectively as well. There were few differences in extraction rates between early and late treatment strategies, but a single course of later treatment did require less appointments and take slightly less time overall—although the period of treatment during adolescence was slightly shorter if an early phase of treatment had previously been undertaken. Importantly, at the end of the overall evaluation period, no clinically significant skeletal or dental differences were apparent between children treated early or late [40].

One further argument for early treatment of class II malocclusion has been to help prevent maxillary incisor trauma [41]. It is well known that an increased overjet is a risk factor for incisor trauma and it is intuitive to conclude that the earlier an overjet is reduced, the less potential risk there is for the child traumatizing their upper front teeth. These RCTs [34–39, 42] and a more recent one based in Sweden [43] did investigate trauma incidence in their samples and collectively found a reduction in the early treatment groups. However, there was much heterogeneity in how trauma was recorded and none of the trials were powered to detect trauma. Interestingly, in all of these trials, a significant number of children had experienced trauma before embarking on early treatment—meaning that as a trauma prevention strategy early overjet reduction needs to be started very early. However, in selected cases with high vulnerability to possible trauma, early overjet reduction might represent a reasonable strategy [44].

2.5 Is Orthopedic Correction of Mandibular Deficiency with a Functional Appliance Enhanced When Treatment Coincides with the Pubertal Growth Spurt?

Those who advocate an orthopedic approach to the management of class II malocclusion argue that the condylar cartilage has a primary role in directing growth of the mandible and will respond positively to forward posture with a functional appliance. Given the known (albeit poorly understood) association between increased mandibular growth and the pubertal growth spurt (see Fig. 2.2), the natural conclusion of this philosophy is that orthopedic functional appliance treatment undertaken during the pubertal growth spurt will be more successful than that carried out either in the pre- or post-pubertal periods. This theory makes a number of assumptions; not least, that the significant gross growth-related changes observed in the condylar cartilages of various juvenile animal models subjected to a variety of mandibular advancement appliances can be extrapolated to humans treated with functional appliances; that the pubertal growth spurt can be predicted with any degree of accuracy in different individuals; that the minimal long-term differences in overall mandibular growth observed between children treated with and without functional appliances is fundamentally wrong (i.e., functional appliances can make the mandible grow larger to a clinically significant degree) and that any accelerated growth beyond what might be achieved without intervention will be essentially linear and contribute to meaningful sagittal correction.

It is difficult to institute high-quality prospective RCTs investigating the influence of treatment timing on orthopedic outcomes in the management of class II malocclusion. Indeed, the accuracy of different methods available to identify whether a child has even entered the growth spurt is questionable—and even if these methods were definitive, the ethics of denying treatment to a child about to undergo their growth spurt as part of an RCT make this area of clinical research challenging. Unfortunately, because of this, the evidence base and therefore appropriate systematic review is problematic [45]. The data relating to removable functional appliances is populated by retrospective studies [46], those using historical growth studies for control groups [47] and indeed, studies that have only investigated either pre-pubertal or post-pubertal subjects in isolation [48]. Current data would suggest an annualized increase in total mandibular length of no more than 2 mm in children treated during the pubertal growth spurt in comparison to those treated before [45]. However, the meta-analysis relating to these data is dominated by one study with a significant risk of bias [47] and if this study is excluded from the analysis there is little difference between groups. Overall, the data to suggest that timing functional appliance treatment to coincide with the growth spurt will result in any clinically significant difference in mandibular dimensions is weak.

2.6 Conclusions

It would seem sensible when treating class II cases with growth modification to accept that the treatment effects will be essentially dentoalveolar. The evidence that this treatment strategy can elicit clinically significant skeletal change is weak. On this basis, a reasonable strategy would be to start treatment in the late mixed dentition with the expectation that the "growth modification" phase would be complete by the early permanent dentition, facilitating a seamless transition into fixed appliances. Advocating early treatment or treatment during the pubertal growth spurt to encourage clinically significant additional mandibular growth is not supported by the evidence.

References

1. Bergersen EO. The male adolescent facial growth spurt: its prediction and relation to skeletal maturation. Angle Orthod. 1972;42(4):319–38.
2. Hunter CJ. The correlation of facial growth with body height and skeletal maturation at adolescence. Angle Orthod. 1966;36(1):44–54.
3. Mellion ZJ, Behrents RG, Johnston LE Jr. The pattern of facial skeletal growth and its relationship to various common indexes of maturation. Am J Orthod Dentofacial Orthop. 2013;143(6):845–54.
4. Patcas R, Herzog G, Peltomaki T, Markic G. New perspectives on the relationship between mandibular and statural growth. Eur J Orthod. 2016;38(1):13–21.
5. Tanner JM, Whitehouse RH, Marubini E, Resele LF. The adolescent growth spurt of boys and girls of the Harpenden growth study. Ann Hum Biol. 1976;3(2):109–26.
6. Fishman LS. Chronological versus skeletal age, an evaluation of craniofacial growth. Angle Orthod. 1979;49(3):181–9.
7. Hagg U, Taranger J. Menarche and voice change as indicators of the pubertal growth spurt. Acta Odontol Scand. 1980;38(3):179–86.
8. Sullivan PG. Prediction of the pubertal growth spurt by measurement of standing height. Eur J Orthod. 1983;5(3):189–97.
9. Demirjian A, Buschang PH, Tanguay R, Patterson DK. Interrelationships among measures of somatic, skeletal, dental, and sexual maturity. Am J Orthod. 1985;88(5):433–8.
10. Hagg U, Taranger J. Skeletal stages of the hand and wrist as indicators of the pubertal growth spurt. Acta Odontol Scand. 1980;38(3):187–200.
11. Baccetti T, Franchi L, McNamara JA Jr. An improved version of the cervical vertebral maturation (CVM) method for the assessment of mandibular growth. Angle Orthod. 2002;72(4):316–23.
12. Beit P, Peltomaki T, Schatzle M, Signorelli L, Patcas R. Evaluating the agreement of skeletal age assessment based on hand-wrist and cervical vertebrae radiography. Am J Orthod Dentofacial Orthop. 2013;144(6):838–47.
13. Perinetti G, Contardo L, Primozic J. Diagnostic accuracy of the cervical vertebral maturation method. Eur J Orthod. 2018;40(4):453–4.
14. Perinetti G, Primozic J, Sharma B, Cioffi I, Contardo L. Cervical vertebral maturation method and mandibular growth peak: a longitudinal study of diagnostic reliability. Eur J Orthod. 2018;40(6):666–72.
15. Flores-Mir C, Nebbe B, Major PW. Use of skeletal maturation based on hand-wrist radiographic analysis as a predictor of facial growth: a systematic review. Angle Orthod. 2004;74(1):118–24.
16. Houston WJ, Miller JC, Tanner JM. Prediction of the timing of the adolescent growth spurt from ossification events in hand-wrist films. Br J Orthod. 1979;6(3):145–52.
17. Verma D, Peltomaki T, Jager A. Reliability of growth prediction with hand-wrist radiographs. Eur J Orthod. 2009;31(4):438–42.
18. Cericato GO, Bittencourt MA, Paranhos LR. Validity of the assessment method of skeletal maturation by cervical vertebrae: a systematic review and meta-analysis. Dentomaxillofac Radiol. 2015;44(4):20140270.
19. Ferrillo M, Curci C, Roccuzzo A, Migliario M, Invernizzi M, de Sire A. Reliability of cervical vertebral maturation compared to hand-wrist for skeletal maturation assessment in growing subjects: a systematic review. J Back Musculoskelet Rehabil. 2021;34(6):925–36.
20. Santiago RC, de Miranda Costa LF, Vitral RW, Fraga MR, Bolognese AM, Maia LC. Cervical vertebral maturation as a biologic indicator of skeletal maturity. Angle Orthod. 2012;82(6):1123–31.
21. Szemraj A, Wojtaszek-Slominska A, Racka-Pilszak B. Is the cervical vertebral maturation (CVM) method effective enough to replace the hand-wrist maturation (HWM) method in determining skeletal maturation? A systematic review. Eur J Radiol. 2018;102:125–8.
22. McNamara JA Jr, Bryan FA. Long-term mandibular adaptations to protrusive function: an experimental study in Macaca mulatta. Am J Orthod Dentofacial Orthop. 1987;92(2):98–108.

23. Tang GH, Rabie AB, Hagg U. Indian hedgehog: a mechanotransduction mediator in condylar cartilage. J Dent Res. 2004;83(5):434–8.
24. Papageorgiou SN, Kutschera E, Memmert S, Golz L, Jager A, Bourauel C, et al. Effectiveness of early orthopaedic treatment with headgear: a systematic review and meta-analysis. Eur J Orthod. 2017;39(2):176–87.
25. Cozza P, Baccetti T, Franchi L, De Toffol L, McNamara JA Jr. Mandibular changes produced by functional appliances in class II malocclusion: a systematic review. Am J Orthod Dentofacial Orthop. 2006;129(5):599 e1–12; discussion e1–6
26. Koretsi V, Zymperdikas VF, Papageorgiou SN, Papadopoulos MA. Treatment effects of removable functional appliances in patients with class II malocclusion: a systematic review and meta-analysis. Eur J Orthod. 2015;37(4):418–34.
27. Nucera R, Lo Giudice A, Rustico L, Matarese G, Papadopoulos MA, Cordasco G. Effectiveness of orthodontic treatment with functional appliances on maxillary growth in the short term: a systematic review and meta-analysis. Am J Orthod Dentofacial Orthop. 2016;149(5):600–11 e3.
28. Ishaq RA, AlHammadi MS, Fayed MM, El-Ezz AA, Mostafa Y. Fixed functional appliances with multibracket appliances have no skeletal effect on the mandible: a systematic review and meta-analysis. Am J Orthod Dentofacial Orthop. 2016;149(5):612–24.
29. Zymperdikas VF, Koretsi V, Papageorgiou SN, Papadopoulos MA. Treatment effects of fixed functional appliances in patients with class II malocclusion: a systematic review and meta-analysis. Eur J Orthod. 2016;38(2):113–26.
30. Perinetti G, Primozic J, Furlani G, Franchi L, Contardo L. Treatment effects of fixed functional appliances alone or in combination with multibracket appliances: a systematic review and meta-analysis. Angle Orthod. 2015;85(3):480–92.
31. Johnston LE. If wishes were horses: functional appliances and growth modification. Prog Orthod. 2005;6(1):36–47.
32. Wieslander L. Intensive treatment of severe class II malocclusions with a headgear-Herbst appliance in the early mixed dentition. Am J Orthod. 1984;86(1):1–13.
33. Wieslander L. Long-term effect of treatment with the headgear-Herbst appliance in the early mixed dentition. Stability or relapse? Am J Orthod Dentofacial Orthop. 1993;104(4):319–29.
34. Keeling SD, Wheeler TT, King GJ, Garvan CW, Cohen DA, Cabassa S, et al. Anteroposterior skeletal and dental changes after early class II treatment with bionators and headgear. Am J Orthod Dentofacial Orthop. 1998;113(1):40–50.
35. O'Brien K, Wright J, Conboy F, Appelbe P, Davies L, Connolly I, et al. Early treatment for class II division 1 malocclusion with the twin-block appliance: a multi-center, randomized, controlled trial. Am J Orthod Dentofacial Orthop. 2009;135(5):573–9.
36. O'Brien K, Wright J, Conboy F, Sanjie Y, Mandall N, Chadwick S, et al. Effectiveness of early orthodontic treatment with the twin-block appliance: a multicenter, randomized, controlled trial. Part 1: dental and skeletal effects. Am J Orthod Dentofacial Orthop. 2003;124(3):234–43. quiz 339
37. Tulloch JF, Phillips C, Koch G, Proffit WR. The effect of early intervention on skeletal pattern in class II malocclusion: a randomized clinical trial. Am J Orthod Dentofacial Orthop. 1997;111(4):391–400.
38. Tulloch JF, Proffit WR, Phillips C. Outcomes in a 2-phase randomized clinical trial of early class II treatment. Am J Orthod Dentofacial Orthop. 2004;125(6):657–67.
39. Wheeler TT, McGorray SP, Dolce C, Taylor MG, King GJ. Effectiveness of early treatment of class II malocclusion. Am J Orthod Dentofacial Orthop. 2002;121(1):9–17.
40. Batista KB, Thiruvenkatachari B, Harrison JE, O'Brien KD. Orthodontic treatment for prominent upper front teeth (class II malocclusion) in children and adolescents. Cochrane Database Syst Rev. 2018;3:CD003452.
41. Thiruvenkatachari B, Harrison J, Worthington H, O'Brien K. Early orthodontic treatment for class II malocclusion reduces the chance of incisal trauma: results of a Cochrane systematic review. Am J Orthod Dentofacial Orthop. 2015;148(1):47–59.
42. Chen DR, McGorray SP, Dolce C, Wheeler TT. Effect of early class II treatment on the incidence of incisor trauma. Am J Orthod Dentofacial Orthop. 2011;140(4):e155–60.
43. Kallunki J, Bondemark L, Paulsson L. Early headgear activator treatment of class II malocclusion with excessive overjet: a randomized controlled trial. Eur J Orthod. 2021;43(6):639–47.
44. Cobourne MT, DiBiase AT, Seehra J, Papageorgiou SN. Should we recommend early overjet reduction to prevent dental trauma? Br Dent J. 2022;233(5):387–90.
45. Perinetti G, Primozic J, Franchi L, Contardo L. Treatment effects of removable functional appliances in pre-pubertal and pubertal class II patients: a systematic review and meta-analysis of controlled studies. PLoS One. 2015;10(10):e0141198.
46. Faltin KJ, Faltin RM, Baccetti T, Franchi L, Ghiozzi B, McNamara JA Jr. Long-term effectiveness and treatment timing for Bionator therapy. Angle Orthod. 2003;73(3):221–30.
47. Baccetti T, Franchi L, Toth LR, McNamara JA Jr. Treatment timing for twin-block therapy. Am J Orthod Dentofacial Orthop. 2000;118(2):159–70.
48. Perillo L, Femiano A, Palumbo S, Contardo L, Perinetti G. Skeletal and dental effects produced by functional regulator-2 in pre-pubertal class II patients: a controlled study. Prog Orthod. 2013;14:18.

An Evidence Base of Treatment Outcome for Class II Malocclusion

3

Spyridon N. Papageorgiou

3.1 Introduction

Class II malocclusion is the most prevalent type of malocclusion seen and comprises a big part of patients seeking orthodontic treatment globally [1–3]. Several factors contribute to the development of Class II malocclusion, and differentiating among its different morphological characteristics can heavily influence the decision to treat a Class II patient with a specific treatment approach. Among the various Class II phenotypes, mandibular retrognathism is often present [4, 5], either alone or together with other sagittal, transverse, or vertical discrepancies. Treatment of Class II malocclusion entails a very wide spectrum of therapeutic approaches, including among others removable appliances in the mixed dentition, comprehensive treatment with fixed appliances, and combined orthodontic-surgical approaches, depending on case complexity, treatment goals, and personal preferences. Likewise, the optimal timing to treat a Class II malocclusion can vary considerably, from the early mixed dentition of pre-adolescent children up to the permanent dentition or even late adulthood. Although clinical decision-making is also based on personal preferences of both the treating orthodontist and the patient (or the patient's parents), the aim of this chapter is to provide a critical overview of scientific evidence that supports each treatment approach, in terms of efficacy and potential adverse effects.

3.2 Methodology

An effort was made for this chapter to provide clinical recommendations for the various aspects of Class II malocclusion treatment based on robust scientific evidence—i.e., study designs with inherently high internal validity and low risk of bias. As in most instances treatment efficacy (how well does each treatment alternative work?) or adverse effects (which treatment alternative is associated with less adverse effects?) is being questioned, randomized clinical trials (RCTs) or non-randomized long-term comparative before-and-after clinical (cohort) studies might be considered to be the most appropriate study design to provide a clinically relevant answer, even though the latter might present higher risk of bias than RCTs [6–10]. Therefore, efforts have been made to base this chapter's conclusions on either (i) ideally only RCTs, or (ii) meta-analysis (statistical quantitative synthesis) of multiple RCTs. In instances where adverse effects are mainly concerned or few RCTs exist, non-randomized clini-

S. N. Papageorgiou (✉)
Clinic of Orthodontics and Pediatric Dentistry, Center for Dental Medicine, University of Zurich, Zurich, Switzerland

M. T. Cobourne (ed.), *Orthodontic Management of Class II Malocclusion*,
https://doi.org/10.1007/978-3-031-57530-3_3

cal studies (non-RCT) have also been included to maximize data output, but separate analyses according to study design are provided, whenever possible, as suggested in the Cochrane Handbook for Systematic Reviews of Interventions [11]. In some cases, existing systematic reviews and their meta-analyses have been identified and, where deemed necessary, updated with more recently published clinical studies or their data re-analyzed with more advanced statistical methods (random-effects model with a residual maximum likelihood variance estimator and utilizing the Hartung-Knapp correction) that have been shown to outperform other approaches [12, 13]. Results of meta-analyses or single trials are reported ideally with mean differences (MD) for continuous outcomes (or standardized mean differences [SMD] in selected cases where different scales measure the same outcome) and odds ratios (OR) with the corresponding 95% confidence intervals (CI). Additional meta-analysis metrics (tau^2/I^2 for absolute/relative inconsistency; uncertainty around heterogeneity estimates; and 95% random-effects predictions) are sometimes reported but not overly discussed here for ease of interpretation. Selected meta-analyses are visualized on forest plots, which have been augmented with contours of effect magnitude to put them in the context of study imprecision and clinical relevance (using the cut-offs of half, one, and two standard deviations [SD] of the baseline outcome measurement in the control group) [14]. In selected cases, random-effects subgroup analyses and meta-regressions are also provided to identify clinically relevant differences between various treatment approaches. All analyses were run in R (version 4.0.4) and the dataset is openly available [15]. All *P* values are 2-sided, and the significance level (alpha) is set at 5%—except for tests of heterogeneity between study subgroups, where alpha is set at 10%. It is important however to keep in mind that this chapter is not based on multiple up-to-date properly conducted systematic reviews with meta-analyses, but relies on the author's best efforts to provide an up-to-date honest summary of currently existing studies.

3.3 Orthopedic Mandibular Advancement with Functional Appliances

Functional appliances are traditionally considered one of the most commonly used alternatives for the early treatment of Class II malocclusions—especially those associated with a retrognathic mandible and a hypodivergent or normodivergent skeletal configuration. Treatment with such mostly removable appliances is based on the notion of either advancing anteriorly the mandible through bite-jumping (with appliances such as the Monobloc, Activator, Bionator, Twin Block falling into this category) or periosteal pull (with the Fränkel-II appliance being a good example) or a combination thereof. There exist countless appliances of different designs, but all of them are rooted in the basic principles from Melvin Moss' functional matrix theory [16], according to which mandibular growth can be altered through a change in the postural activity of the craniofacial musculature. Traditional allegations about the modus operandi of functional appliances include primarily increasing the natural growth of the mandible or alternatively restructuring the temporo-mandibular joint and secondarily having a restrictive effect on the growth and position of the maxilla [17]. Additionally, fixed "functional appliances" have also been used as an alternative for non-compliant or older children that work through bite-jumping and incorporate mostly some kind of dentally anchored inter-arch spring mechanism that forces the mandible anteriorly when the patient bites down (with the Herbst appliance being the most characteristic example of this category).

Although early studies on animals indicated a proof-of-concept stimulation of mandibular growth with functional appliances [18–20], subsequent studies on humans failed to unanimously agree on this. Even though favorable mandibular growth effects, in terms of increased mandibular length [21–23] or condylar growth [24, 25], have been reported, other studies fail to report any clinically relevant benefits [26, 27]. The effects of functional appliances on the maxilla are similarly debated, with some finding an inhibitory effect on maxillary growth (termed "headgear effect" [28–30]) and others disputing this [31, 32].

Systematic evaluations of the morphological treatment-induced changes of the maxillomandibular complex after functional appliance treatment led to the conclusion that the dentoalveolar components of functional appliances might in the end be equal or even greater than any skeletal effects seen [33, 34]. Skeletal and dentoalveolar components of functional appliance treatment all contribute towards achieving a successful treatment outcome for Class II malocclusion. However, it is important to accurately describe the modus operandi of functional appliances, in order to better select which patients might be the best candidates to profit best from them and since Class II correction through mainly dental effects might be more prone to long-term relapse [35]. Assessment of treatment-induced changes of such appliances is mostly based on combining data from two published systematic reviews: one on removable functional appliances [36] and one on fixed functional appliances [37]. Both reviews included RCTs and non-RCTs published up to 2014 comparing Class II patients treated with functional appliances with untreated Class II control groups followed through natural growth and reported annualized changes on lateral cephalograms.

Overall, compared to normal craniofacial growth of untreated Class II patients, Class II treatment with any kind of functional appliances was characterized by a statistically significant ($P < 0.001$) reduction of the ANB angle (MD −1.59 °; 95% CI −2.26 to −0.91 °; Fig. 3.1), which was attributed more to an increase of the SNB angle (MD 0.71 °; 95% CI 0.43 to 0.99 °) and less to a reduction of the SNA angle (MD −0.46 °; 95% CI −0.71 to −0.21 °) (Table 3.1). At the same time, functional appliance treatment was associated with a slight posterior rotation (opening) of the mandibular plane (MD 0.62 °; 95% CI 0.35 to 0.90 °) and considerable proclination of the mandibular incisors (MD 5.52 °; 95% CI 2.47 to 8.57 °; Fig. 3.2), both of which can be considered as potentially unwanted adverse effects in the correction of a sagittal apical base discrepancy. Extraorally, functional appliance treatment was associated with a considerable improvement (increase) of the mentolabial angle (MD 19.43 °; 95% CI 14.66 to 24.19 °) compared to untreated patients, but no consistent improvement of the nasolabial angle ($P > 0.05$), which is more related to potential retraction of proclined incisors [38].

When the effects of removable and fixed functional appliances are assessed separately, removable appliances are associated with significantly smaller reduction of the SNA angle compared to fixed appliances (MDs of −0.30 ° and −0.74 °, respectively). Additionally, removable functional appliances are associated with less proclination of the mandibular incisors than fixed functional appliances (MDs of 2.36 ° and 9.58 °, respectively) and greater improvement of the mentolabial angle (MDs of 22.06 ° and 14.99 °, respectively).

Among the various removable functional appliances, existing evidence indicated that the Twin Block was significantly more effective in the improvement of the ANB, SNA, and SNB angles compared to the Activator, Bionator, and Fränkel-II appliances [36]. Bite-jumping appliances were more effective in improving the SNB and the ANB angle than appliances based on periosteal pull, while two-piece appliances were more effective than one-piece appliances. Finally, a separate RCT comparing Class II treatment with Twin Block activated either in a single maximum bite advancement or an incremental advancement [39] found no significant differences in produced skeletal or dentoalveolar effects.

As far as fixed functional appliances are concerned, potential differences in their effectiveness to improve anteroposterior jaw relationship were identified but could not be precisely evaluated due to the limited number of controlled studies available for each appliance [38]. Class

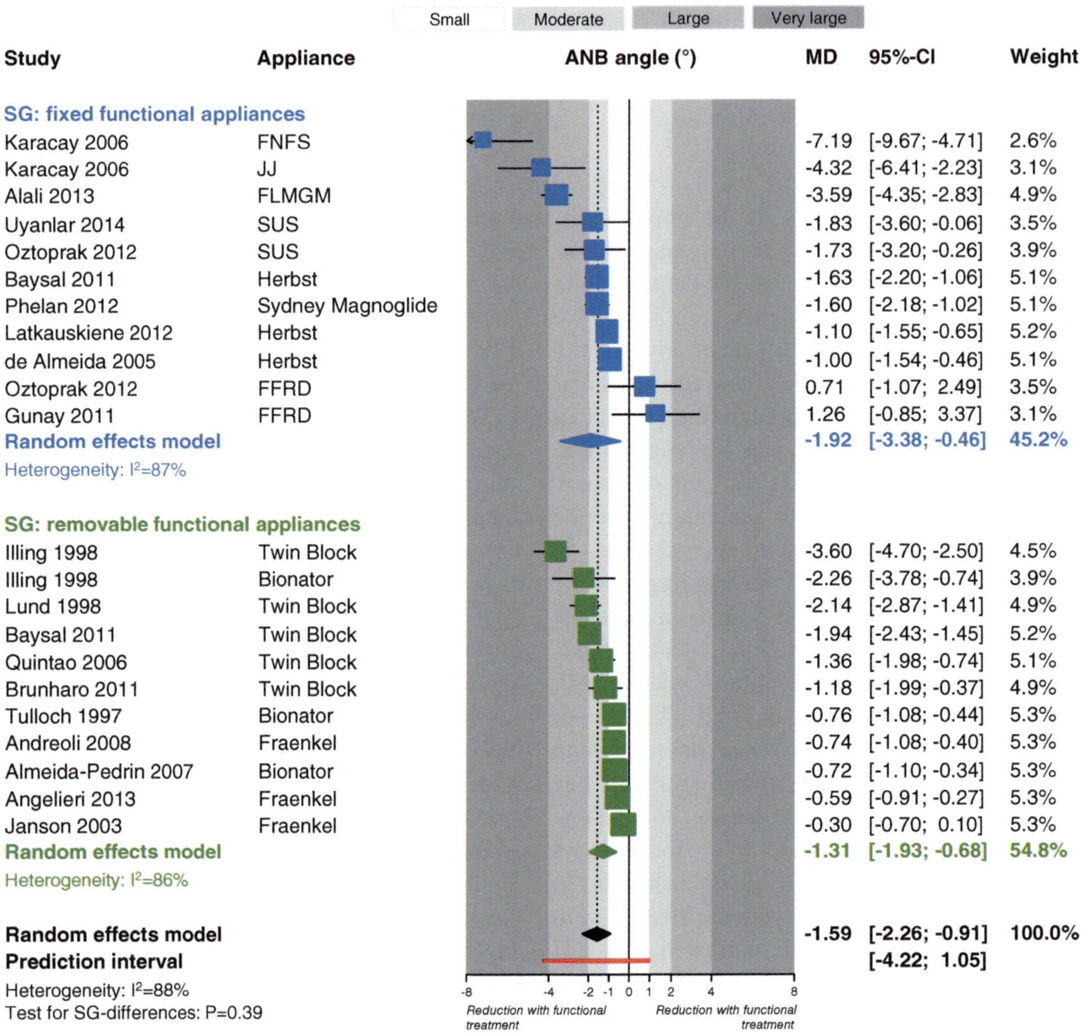

Fig. 3.1 Contour-enhanced forest plot of annualized ANB changes for functional appliance treatment compared to untreated Class II controls (subset by study design). *CI* confidence interval, *FFRD* Forsus fatigue resistant device, *FLMGM* fixed lingual mandibular growth modificator, *FNFS* Forsus Nitinol Flat Spring, *JJ* Jasper jumper, *MD* mean difference, SG subgroup, *SUS* Sabbagh universal spring

II treatment at the post-pubertal phase was associated with significantly more pronounced mandibular plane opening and dental effects (including lower incisor proclination) compared with treatment performed at the pre-pubertal or pubertal phases, which might indicate that choice of the appropriate time to initiate treatment might influence its outcome. Finally, another RCT comparing the Functional Mandibular Advancer appliance activated either in a single step or in a stepwise manner indicated that stepwise activation was more beneficial than single-step in terms of improvement in SNB (additional improvement by 0.66 °), ANB (additional improvement by 0.55 °), horizontal Pg position (additional improvement by 0.74 mm), effective mandibular length (Co-Gn; additional improvement by 1.05 mm), and in terms of less proclination of the mandibular incisors (less proclination by 1.92 °) [40].

Table 3.1 Meta-analyses comparing functional with control groups (annualized changes). Data from the systematic reviews of Koretsi et al. [36] and Zymperdikas et al. [37]

	Overall			RFA		FFA		
Outcome	*n*	MD (95% CI)	*P*	*n*	MD (95% CI)	*n*	MD (95% CI)	P_{SG}
SNA (°)	24	−0.46 (−0.71, −0.21)	0.001	13	−0.30 (−0.54, −0.06)	11	−0.74 (−1.26, −0.22)	0.09[a]
SNB (°)	24	0.71 (0.43, 0.99)	<0.001	13	0.61 (0.31, 0.91)	11	0.87 (0.25, 1.49)	0.40
ANB (°)	22	−1.59 (−2.26, −0.91)	<0.001	11	−1.31 (−1.93, −0.68)	11	−1.92 (−3.38, −0.46)	0.39
SN-ML (°)	19	0.62 (0.35, 0.90)	<0.001	9	0.67 (0.19, 1.16)	10	0.48 (0.22, 0.74)	0.43
1i-ML (°)	25	5.52 (2.47, 8.57)	0.001	14	2.36 (0.89, 3.84)	11	9.58 (2.99, 16.18)	0.02[a]
Nasolabial angle (°)	13	1.63 (−0.69, 3.95)	0.15	7	2.73 (−1.03, 6.50)	6	−0.08 (−3.36, 3.19)	0.16
Mentolabial angle (°)	7	19.43 (14.66, 24.19)	<0.001	5	22.06 (17.51, 26.62)	2	14.99 (−29.73, 59.70)	0.07[a]

CI confidence interval, *FFA* fixed functional appliance, *MD* mean difference, *n* number of studies, P_{SG} *p* value for subgroup differences, *RFA* removable functional appliance
[a] Statistically significant subgroup differences ($P < 0.10$)

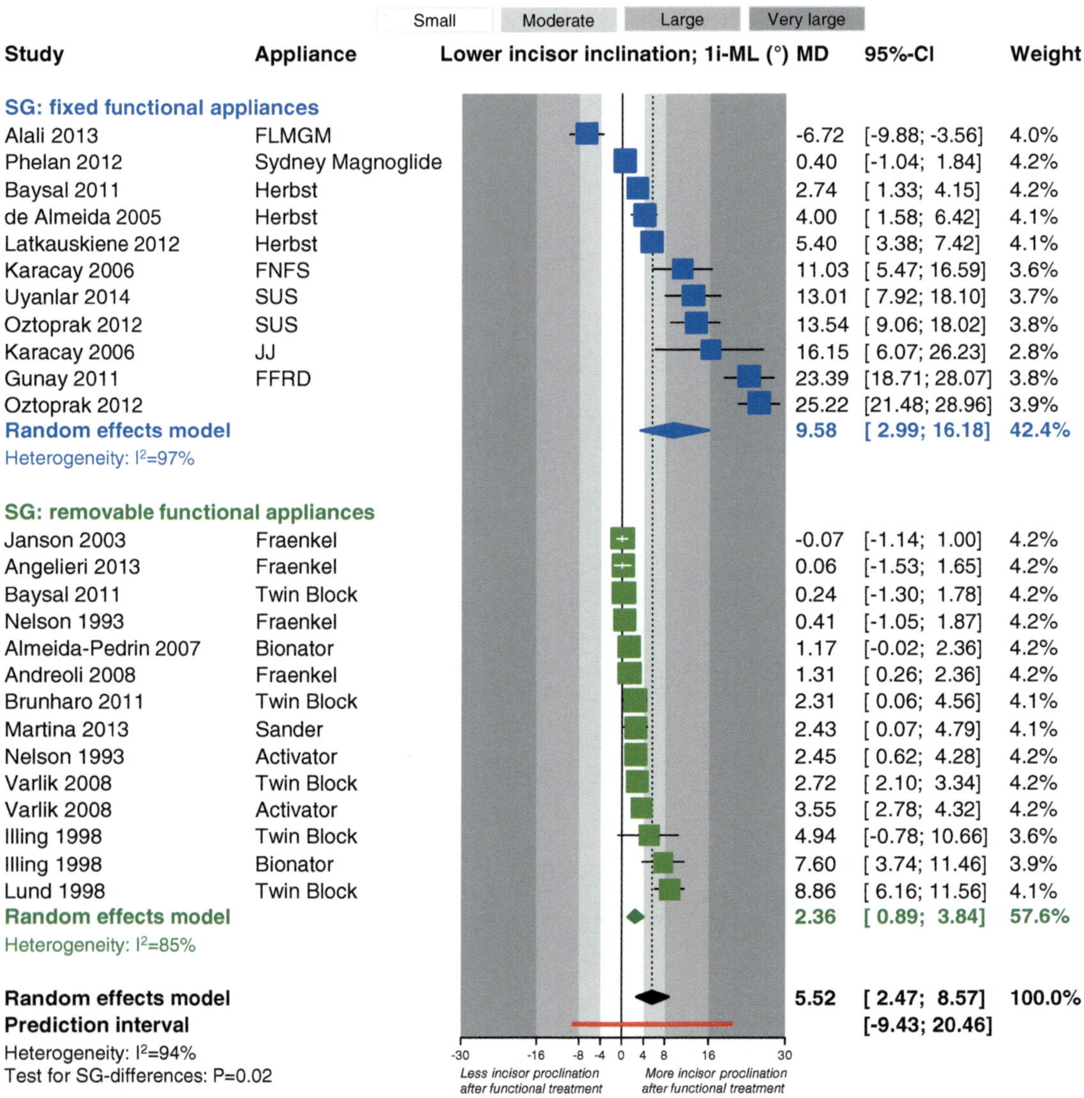

Fig. 3.2 Contour-enhanced forest plot of annualized lower incisor inclination (1i-ML) changes for functional appliance treatment compared to untreated Class II controls (subset by study design). *CI* confidence interval, *FFRD* Forsus fatigue resistant device, *FLMGM* fixed lingual mandibular growth modificator, *FNFS* Forsus Nitinol Flat Spring, *JJ* Jasper jumper, *MD* mean difference, *SG* subgroup, *SUS* Sabbagh universal spring

3.4 Benefits of Skeletal Anchorage Reinforcement for Functional Appliances

There is a vast plethora of scientific publications spanning across several decades documenting the successful treatment of Class II malocclusions in growing patients with various functional appliances. The most commonly reported clinical observations that might be considered as adverse effects from this kind of treatment are the proclination of the lower incisors and the increase in face height due to posterior mandibular rotation. After the successful introduction of temporary anchorage devices (miniscrew implants, palatal implants, and miniplates) as a means of anchorage reinforcement for space closure, mesialization, or distalization of teeth within a single arch

Table 3.2 Meta-analyses comparing skeletally anchored with conventional functional appliances. Data from pooling of existing clinical studies [45–50]

	Overall			RCT		Non-RCT		
Outcome	*n*	MD (95% CI)	*P*	*n*	MD (95% CI)	*n*	MD (95% CI)	P_{SG}
SNA (°)	6	−0.22 (−0.65, 0.21)	0.24	3	−0.26 (−0.52, −0.01)	3	−0.15 (−1.87, 1.57)	0.78
SNB (°)	6	0.77 (−0.39, 1.92)	0.15	3	0.18 (−0.93, 1.30)	3	1.44 (−1.86, 4.75)	0.12
ANB (°)	6	−0.91 (−2.32, 0.50)	0.16	3	−0.22 (−0.32, −0.12)	3	−1.65 (−5.99, 2.70)	0.16
1i-ML (°)	5	−7.69 (−14.72, −0.67)	0.04	2	−8.23 (−39.93, 23.46)	3	−7.40 (−26.34, 11.54)	0.87
Mandibular length[a]	5	1.46 (−0.72, 3.64)	0.14	3	1.38 (−4.23, 6.99)	2	1.61 (−11.30, 14.52)	0.89
SN-ML	6	0.17 (−1.38, 1.71)	0.79	3	0.51 (−2.60, 3.61)	3	−0.30 (−5.12, 4.53)	0.55

CI confidence interval, *MD* mean difference, *n* number of studies, P_{SG} *p* value for subgroup differences, *RCT* randomized clinical trial

[a]Standardized mean difference used instead of MD to pool Co-Gn (from lateral cephs or cone-beam computerized tomographies) and Ar-Pg

[41–44], such temporary anchorage devices were also suggested as successful adjuncts in Class II treatment with fixed functional appliances. The underlying philosophy is that anchoring the Class II corrector skeletally would minimize any dental side-effects (like proclination of lower incisors) and enhance any skeletal effects (like advancement of supramentale or pogonion).

There are currently 6 published clinical studies that compare Class II treatment with a skeletally anchored fixed functional appliance (variations of the Forsus or the Herbst appliance) with a conventional (dentally anchored) version of the same appliance—three RCTs [45–47] and three non-RCTs [48–50], including a total of 164 patients (median 30 patients/study). As can be shown in Table 3.2, reinforcing the Class II fixed functional appliance with skeletal anchorage had no statistically significant effect on treatment-induced changes in the SNA angle (MD −0.22 °; 95% CI −0.65 to 0.21 °), SNB angle (MD 0.77 °; 95% CI −0.39 to 1.92 °), the ANB angle (MD −0.91 °; 95% CI −2.32 to 0.50 °), mandibular length (measured through Co-Gn or Ar-Pg; SMD 1.46; 95% CI −0.72 to 3.64), or mandibular plane inclination (MD 0.17 °; 95% CI −1.38 to 14.49 °; Fig. 3.3) ($P > 0.05$ in all instances). The only benefit observed by skeletal anchorage reinforcement was a significant reduction of mandibular incisor proclination (through the 1i-ML angle) on average by −7.69 ° (95% CI −14.72 to −0.67 °; $P = 0.04$) compared to the conventionally anchored appliance and this effect was consistent among RCTs and non-RCTs (reductions of −8.23 ° and − 7.40 °, respectively; $P > 0.10$). This can be considered a moderate to large effect and could potentially be useful for Class II patients with already proclined mandibular incisors prior to treatment. However, a considerable variation was seen in the inclination control of skeletally anchored appliances among the included studies, with reported effects ranging from small retroclination (−2.9 °) to small proclination (+1.6 °) during treatment—something that reflects the different options for the orthodontist to actively or passively connect the temporary anchorage devices to the fixed appliances. Further studies are needed to identify which is the optimal anchorage reinforcement protocol and describe potential side-effects (like root damage during miniscrew insertion or potentially greater root resorption through treatment) before strong clinical recommendations can be formulated.

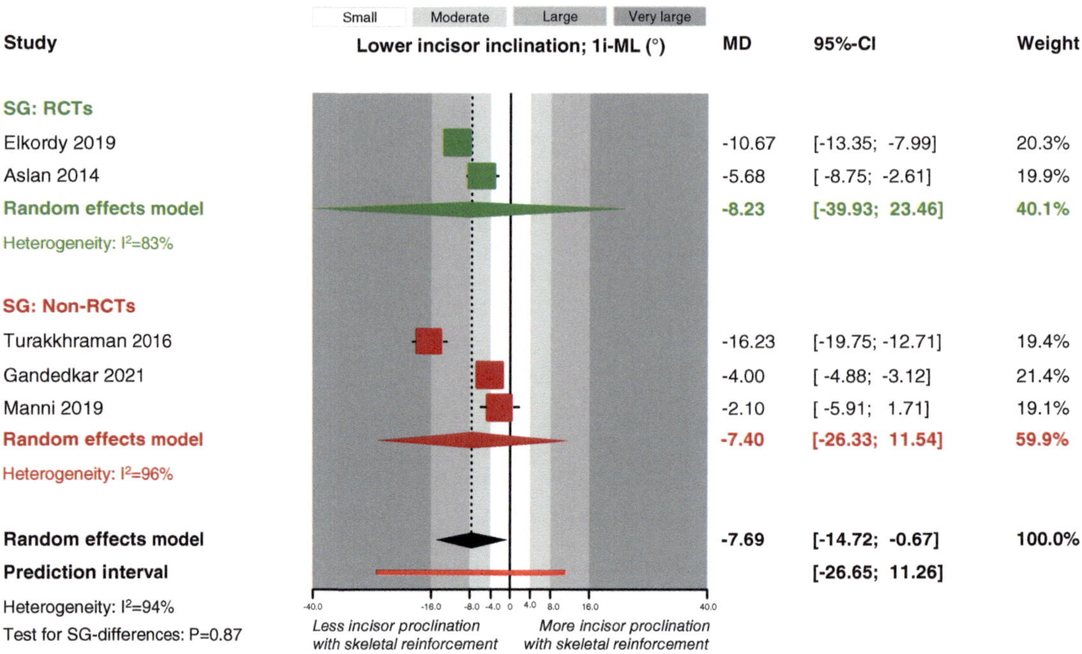

Fig. 3.3 Contour-enhanced forest plot of lower incisor inclination (1i-ML) changes for skeletally anchored functional appliances compared to conventional (dentoalveolarly anchored) functional appliances for Class II (subset by study design). *CI* confidence interval, *MD* mean difference, *RCT* randomized clinical trial, *SG* subgroup

3.5 Prefabricated Myofunctional Appliances for Class II Correction

It's been over half a century since Melvin Moss described an interaction between the soft tissue pressure by the lips or the tongue, children's habits, or breathing disturbances and the development of the craniofacial complex [51]. Therefore, it was postulated that in cases of oral dysfunction, attention has to be paid to the early re-establishment of muscular balance and problem-free function in an effort to normalize dentofacial growth [52]. In this direction, oral myofunctional therapy, consisting of manual exercises of the orofacial muscles, has been introduced, even though there still is a profound lack of robust evidence to support their effectiveness [53]. It is important however to stress out that such exercises were initially thought as an adjunct to proper treatment of the deviant morphology and to promote post-treatment stability [54]—not as a standalone treatment for malocclusions.

In the last decade, and especially among areas of Scandinavian countries with limited specialist resources, myofunctional protocols have also included treatment with pre-fabricated removable "myofunctional" appliances such as the oral shield [55], the double oral screen [56], the Eruption Guidance Appliance [57], LM-Activator™, Myobrace®, Trainer for Kids™, and Occluso-Guide®. Most therapeutic protocols additionally propagate that treatment with such prefabricated appliances should be accompanied by orofacial exercises [58] but can generally be an effective and cost-efficient alternative for the early correction of Class II malocclusion.

Several reports of anecdotal evidence or clinical studies with low internal validity propose that such early therapeutic protocols among pre-adolescent children are associated with effects on oral muscle activity, reduced overjet, increases in

SNB angle, and increased facial height. It remains, however, unclear if such claims actually do hold true under the light of evidence-based medicine.

This chapter presents data from a recent systematic review [59] that included three RCTs up to 2019 [60–62], updated here with a more recently published RCT [63]. Compared to treatment with functional appliances (which can be considered a gold standard for early Class II treatment), no difference was found with myofunctional appliance treatment for SNA (MD −0.12 °; 95% CI −0.88 to 0.65 °), SN-ML (MD 1.47 °; 95% CI −4.55 to 7.49 °), NL-ML (MD 0.53 °; 95% CI −0.39 to 1.45 °), N-Me (MD −1.73 mm; 95% CI −4.91 to 1.46 mm), overbite (MD 0.64 mm; 95% CI −0.08 to 1.36 mm), 1 s-NL (MD −2.48 °; 95% CI −13.82 to 8.86 °), 1i-ML (MD 3.19 °; 95% CI −11.92 to 18.30 °), and 1 s–1i (MD −4.23 °; 95% CI −18.82 to 10.36 °; Fig. 3.4; Table 3.4). However, prefabricated myofunctional appliances performed significantly worse than functional appliances in terms of SNB increase (MD −1.16 °; 95% CI −2.13 to −0.18 °; $P = 0.04$), ANB reduction (MD 0.94 °; 95% CI 0.57 to 1.30 °; $P = 0.008$), and overjet reduction (MD 1.50 mm; 95% CI 0.88 to 2.11 mm; $P < 0.001$). Furthermore, custom-made functional appliances were associated with greater increase in lower anterior face height (measured through the ANS-Me distance) than prefabricated myofunctional appliances (MD

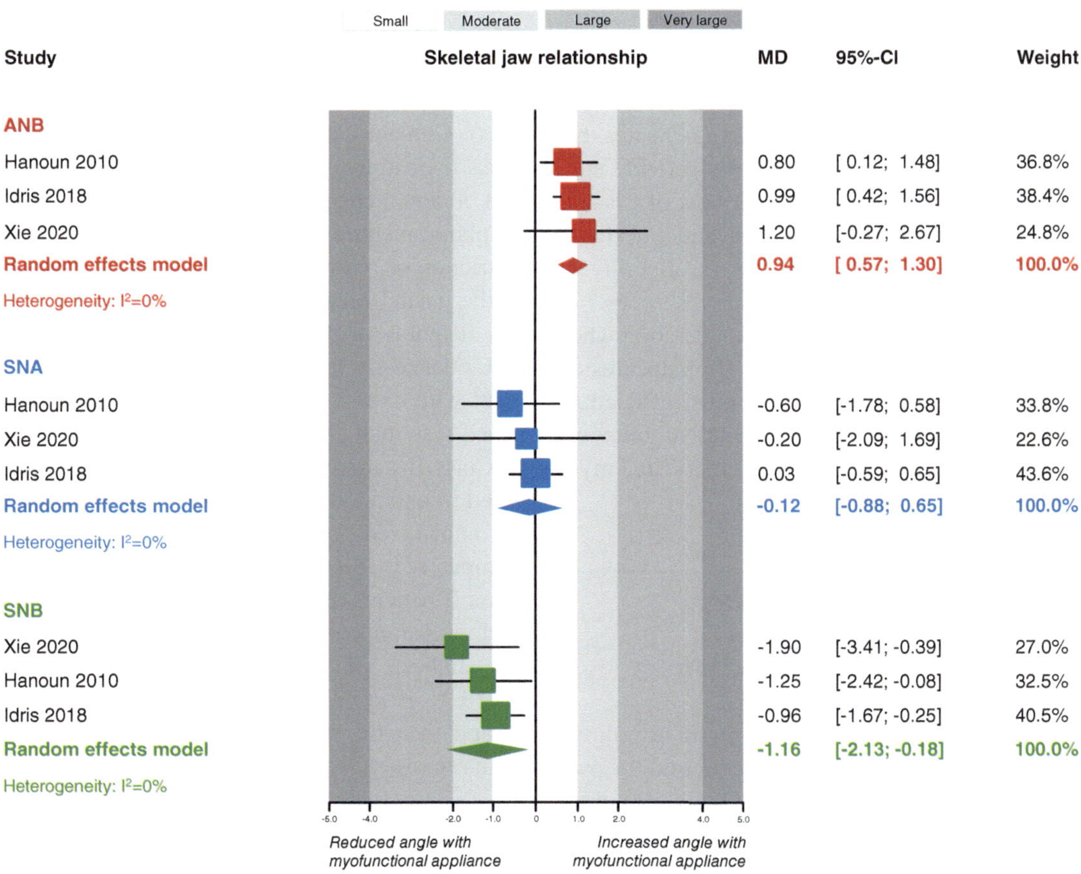

Fig. 3.4 Contour-enhanced forest plot of skeletal jaw relationship (SNA/SNB/ANB) changes for prefabricated myofunctional appliances compared to functional appliances for Class II. *CI* confidence interval, *MD* mean difference

Table 3.4 Meta-analyses comparing prefabricated myofunctional appliances with functional appliances. Data from the systematic review of Papageorgiou et al. [59], including another trial published afterward [63]

Outcome	Trials	MD (95% CI)	*P*	I^2 (95% CI)	tau² (95%CI)	95% prediction
Overjet (mm)	3	1.50 (0.88, 2.11)	<0.001	0% (0%, 94%)	0 (0, 4.53)	−2.48, 5.47
Overbite (mm)	2	0.64 (−0.08, 1.36)	0.08	0% (0%, 98%)	0 (0, 17.43)	Not applicable
SNA (°)	3	−0.12 (−0.88, 0.65)	0.58	0% (0%, 90%)	0 (0, 3.75)	−3.54, 3.31
SNB (°)	3	−1.16 (−2.13, −0.18)	0.04	0% (0%, 90%)	0 (0, 8.74)	−4.79, 2.48
ANB (°)	3	0.94 (0.57, 1.30)	0.008	0% (0, 90%)	0 (0, 1.24)	−1.78, 3.65
SN-ML (°)	3	1.47 (−4.55, 7.49)	0.40	87% (62%, 95%)	5.06 (0.83, >100)	−32.05, 34.98
NL-ML (°)	2	0.53 (−0.39 to 1.45)	0.26	0% (0–98)	0 (0–20.69)	Not applicable
N-Me	2	−1.73 (−4.91 to 1.46)	0.29	77% (0–100)	4.04 (0–662.35)	Not applicable
ANS-Me	2	−1.39 (−2.50 to −0.28)	0.01	0% (0–98)	0 (0–33.04)	Not applicable
1 s-NL (°)	3	−2.48 (−13.82, 8.86)	0.45	96% (91%, 98%)	19.77 (4.64, >100)	−68.08, 63.12
1i-ML (°)	3	3.19 (−11.92, 18.30)	0.46	96% (91%, 98%)	35.30 (8.42, >100)	−84.41, 90.80
1 s–1i (°)	3	−4.23 (−18.82, 10.36)	0.34	91% (77%, 97%)	31.45 (6.27, >100)	−87.55, 79.09

CI confidence interval, *MD* mean difference

−1.39 mm; 95% CI −2.50 to −0.28 mm; $P = 0.01$), which is a common side-effect of successful Class II treatment with functional appliances. Therefore, existing evidence indicates that prefabricated appliances generally provide sub-optimal results for the early treatment of Class II malocclusion compared to conventional functional appliances. Other reasons (availability of specialized providers, financial resources, or logistics) might be taken into consideration when choosing how to treat Class II malocclusion among the general population most efficiently, but assessment of optimal treatment outcome does not favor the use of such prefabricated myofunctional appliances.

3.6 Orthopedic Maxillary Growth Restriction with Extraoral Traction

The use of extraoral forces to restrain or redirect skeletal growth of the jaw has been used for over a century [64] and has been also implemented for the treatment of Class II patients, especially those with maxillary excess [65]. This is implemented in the headgear appliance, which should exert an inhibitory effect on maxillary anterior displacement, and can be divided into three categories, based on the direction of the applied force: high-pull headgear (anchored at the upper back of the head), cervical headgear (anchored at the back of the neck), and combi-headgear (anchored at both sites). Clinical data indicates that the effects of Class II treatment with headgear are a combination of dental changes in the sagittal or the vertical plane and pure skeletal changes due to growth restriction or redirection [66, 67], while rotation of the palatal plane and changes in the anterior face height have also been reported [66, 68].

Evidence on the effects of orthopedic treatment with extraoral traction is based on a published systematic review of RCTs and non-RCTs of Class II patients treated with headgear compared to untreated Class II controls and reported as annualized cephalometric changes [69]. Compared to the natural growth of untreated Class II patients, headgear treatment was associated with significant reduction in the SNA angle (12 studies; MD −1.66 °; 95% CI −2.21 to −1.10 °; $P < 0.001$), which was significantly greater than the restrictive effect on SNA seen from removable/fixed functional appliances (MD of −0.46 °; Table 3.1). On the other side, headgear treatment had no significant effect on the SNB angle (11 studies; MD −0.19 °; 95% CI −0.51 to 0.12 °; $P = 0.20$), contrary to the significant improvement seen with removable/fixed functional appliances (MD of 0.71 °; Table 3.1). Additionally, orthopedic headgear treatment for

Class II malocclusion was associated with posterior (downward) rotation of the palatal plane (12 studies; SMD 0.54; 95% CI 0.09 to 1.00; $P = 0.02$) and posterior displacement of the anterior border of the maxilla (A point; 8 studies; SMD −0.61; 95% CI −0.95 to −0.26; $P = 0.001$) [69]. The restrictive effect of headgear treatment on the SNA angle was independent of the rotation of the palatal plane and the inclination of the upper incisors, which can potentially influence measurements using the A point. Overall, clear differences were identified between the observed treatment effects of headgear and functional appliances, which indicate that choice between these two options should preferably be based on the phenotype of the patient in question.

3.7 Sagittal Effects of Maxillary Expansion

Interestingly, another intervention that has been proposed through the years for the treatment of mild Class II malocclusions of patients in the mixed dentition is the transverse development of the maxillary arch, usually manifested as a rapid maxillary expansion appliance fitted on maxillary posterior teeth. This idea had been initially proposed by Norman Kingsley in 1880 in the States [70], who proposed that transverse expansion can favor mandibular advancement, and was later supported by Alfred Körbitz in 1914 in Germany [71]. This idea was further adopted later by other renowned orthodontists like Jim McNamara [72] and Tony Gianelly [73] based mostly on anecdotal evidence.

The real-life example often given to simulate the Class II effects of maxillary expansion is that of a foot not fitting a narrow shoe, while the foot moves spontaneously forward once the shoe has been widened. The theoretical background lies with the theory that orthopedic expansion removes occlusal interferences and allows the mandible to posture forward, thus improving the inter-arch sagittal relationship. One implication of this view is that the mandible, in centric occlusion, is in a distal position relative to centric relation because the "constricted" maxilla prevents it from assuming the centric relation position. This analysis suggests that the condyles are in a distal position and is similar to the belief that the conversion of a Class II Division 2 malocclusion to a Class II Division 1 will result in forward movement of the mandible and, at times, in a Class II molar relationship [74, 75].

Anecdotal findings might be useful for the birth of a scientific theory, but clinical recommendations in the modern era need to be substantiated by robust experimental clinical evidence. Unfortunately, more than a century after the introduction of this idea, only two RCTs have been published: one comparing bonded or banded rapid maxillary expansion to proper concurrent Class II untreated controls [76] and another comparing two different palatal wire expanders connected to the first molar bands to an existing historical control group [77]. Statistical pooling of these two small RCTs (Table 3.3) found no statistically significant improvements in SNA (MD 0.10 °; 95% CI −0.13 to 0.33 °), SNB (MD 0.43 °; 95% CI −2.44 to 3.29 °), ANB (MD −0.42; 95% CI −2.45 to 1.61 °), mandibular length (Co-Gn distance; MD 0.01 mm; 95% CI −0.69 to 0.72 mm), and sagittal position of the mandible (Pg-N perpendicular; MD −0.24 mm; 95% CI −8.81 to 8.34 mm) (Fig. 3.5; $P > 0.05$). One of the trials [77] reported that patients treated with maxillary expansion showed greater Wits reduction than untreated patients (MD −0.75 mm; 95% CI −1.01 to −0.49 mm; $P < 0.001$). However, as this great benefit was seen only for one of the two similar expanders and a historical control group was used (which is more prone to

Table 3.3 Meta-analyses of sagittal effects between Class II patients treated with rapid maxillary expansion and untreated controls. Data from pooling existing randomized clinical trials [76, 77]

Outcome	*n*	MD (95% CI)	*P*
SNA (°)	2	0.10 (−0.13, 0.33)	0.11
SNB (°)	2	0.43 (−2.44, 3.29)	0.31
ANB (°)	2	−0.42 (−2.45, 1.61)	0.23
Co-Gn (mm)	2	0.01 (−0.69, 0.72)	0.85
Wits (mm)	1	−0.75 (−1.01, −0.49)	<0.001
Pg-Nperp	2	−0.24 (−8.81, 8.34)	0.78

CI confidence interval, *MD* mean difference, *n* number of studies

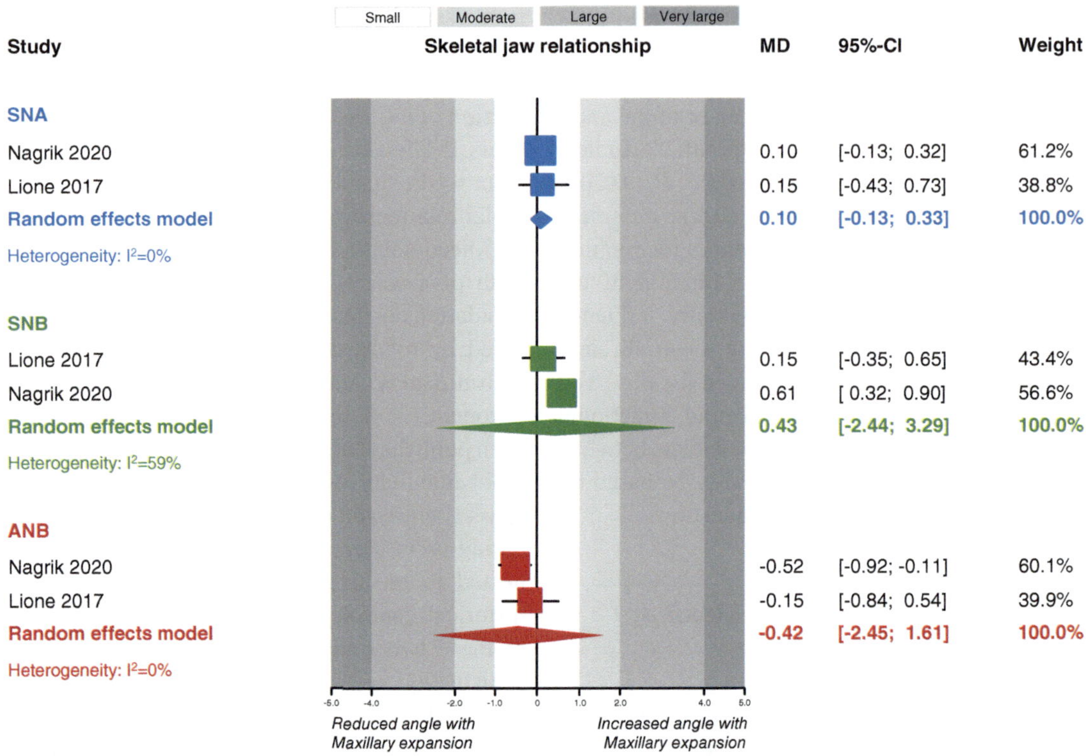

Fig. 3.5 Contour-enhanced forest plot of skeletal jaw relationship (SNA/SNB/ANB) changes for rapid maxillary expansion compared to untreated Class II controls. *CI* confidence interval, *MD* mean difference

bias than concurrent controls [8]), caution is warranted by the interpretation of this finding. In any case, no claims for consistent spontaneous correction of Class II malocclusion after maxillary expansion can be robustly supported by existent evidence.

3.8 Dentoalveolar Class II Correction with Camouflage Treatment

Correction of Class II malocclusions that include skeletal sagittal discrepancies (maxillary prognathism, mandibular retrognathism, or a combination thereof) among patients past the pubertal growth spurt can usually be achieved with two treatment approaches: either a combined orthodontic-orthognathic treatment aiming to harmonize skeletal and dental relationships or a purely dentoalveolar correction that aims to "mask" the underlying skeletal discrepancy (a so-called "camouflage" treatment). There are several factors that need to be appraised when deciding between the two approaches, including among others the extent of the skeletal discrepancy, the esthetic/functional needs of the patient, and the costs, duration, and risks of each treatment approach.

Orthodontic camouflage treatment sometimes includes the extraction of permanent teeth (usually upper and/or lower premolars), in order to create the space to retract the anterior teeth and establish an appropriate relationship between the dental arches. At the same time, the choice to extract teeth for a camouflage treatment might have substantial impact on various outcomes, such as the face's vertical dimensions [78], the long-term stability of treatment outcomes [79], the width of the dental arch [80], as well as the perioral soft tissues and the convexity of the face [81]. A previously published systematic review of RCTs and comparative non-RCTs comparing extraction and non-extraction treatment of any kind of malocclusion was taken as basis [82], and from it only studies reporting on Class II malocclusions were selected for this chapter. Its results indicated that extraction-based treatment was associated with significantly more retruded lower lip relative to Rickett's esthetic plane (11 studies; MD −1.45 mm; 95% CI −2.57 to −0.34 mm; $P = 0.02$), more retruded upper lip (11 studies; MD −1.13 mm; 95% CI −2.21 to −0.05 mm; $P = 0.04$), and greater nasolabial angle (11 studies; MD 2.76 °; 95% CI 1.70 to 3.81 °; $P < 0.001$) compared to non-extraction treatment. When comparing patients having 4 premolars extracted and those having only 2 premolars extracted, the former showed a tendency from greater differences from non-extraction treatment than the latter for the lower lip (−1.98 and −1.13 mm for 4- and 2-premolars, respectively), the upper lip (−2.21 and −0.81 mm for 4- and 2-premolars, respectively), and the nasolabial angle (3.49 and 2.43 ° for 4- and 2-premolars, respectively). However, additional meta-regression analyses showed that the difference between extraction and non-extraction patients in terms of upper and lower lip prominence was significantly associated with the baseline (pre-treatment) similarity of the two groups in lip prominence ($P < 0.001$ in both cases). In other words, among studies with borderline extraction and non-extraction patients who had similar lip profiles, there was a significantly smaller influence of extractions on the soft-tissue profile. When limiting the meta-analyses only to studies that had pre-treatment similar upper/lower lip prominences between extraction and non-extraction patients (i.e., "borderline samples"), extraction-based treatment had no significant effect in upper lip prominence ($P = 0.07$) or lower lip prominence ($P = 0.18$). Essentially, this means that cases where extraction treatment led to significant changes in the patient's lip prominence could be patients with originally more protruded lips, presumably supported by more protruded incisors that were more retracted through treatment. Previous studies [83–85] have reported that upper lip retraction in premolar extraction cases is significantly correlated to the actual amount of upper incisor retraction during orthodontic treatment, even though different amounts of lip retraction per mm of incisor retraction have been reported (0.26, 0.59, and 0.75 mm), and this seems to be highly unpredictable. Other factors such as pre-treatment lip thickness, lip seal, and lip strain might influence the lips' reaction to orthodontic retraction [82, 84] and therefore, each case should be assessed separately. Generally, however, it seems that the facial effects of extraction and non-extraction treatment are of little clinical significance for the average patient, besides some limited changes in the nasolabial angle [86].

Even though orthodontic camouflage treatment might be an effective treatment alternative for skeletal Class II malocclusion, especially for patients not willing to undergo the risks associated with orthognathic surgery, this doesn't mean that camouflage treatment is objectively the best approach. Focusing solely on treatment effects, evidence from a small RCT confirms what is only logical—that a combined orthodontic-surgical approach allows for a better correction of the skeletal discrepancy, more optimal dental occlusion, and a more harmonic soft tissue profile compared to camouflage treatment (enhanced with temporary anchorage devices), while being also significantly shorter in duration [87]. This confirms data from a previous systematic review of non-RCTs [88] reporting significant differences in the effects of camouflage and orthodontic-orthognathic treatment in terms of changes in SNB, ANB, overjet, and face convexity. These scientific facts need to be explained in detail to the patients when analyzing their treatment alternatives, so they can make an adequately informed decision, based on their orthodontic problem, available solutions, and personal preferences.

3.9 Maxillary Arch Distalization for Class II Treatment

Correction of a Class II malocclusion, especially in cases with mesial drift of the maxillary dentition, crowding, and a protruded upper lip, might include the distalization of maxillary posterior teeth. This has been traditionally done with the application of extraoral traction on banded upper first molars of compliant patients. This has been for many patients an effective and cost-efficient approach with acceptable outcomes over a treatment period of several months. Caution, however, must be exercised, since early distalization of the upper molars is associated with a distalizing effect and a transitory slowing down effect on the eruption of the upper second molar buds, which does not however necessarily lead to malposition or impaction [89]. In any case, when early molar distalization is undertaken to correct a Class II malocclusion, it is important that an adequate follow-up period is included to ensure the unimpeded eruption of the permanent second molars in the correct position.

However, in patients who are not willing to comply with the orthodontist's instructions or are unable to wear headgear, several non-compliant approaches with fixed appliances incorporating some kind of spring mechanism exist. Dental- (or dentoalveolar-) anchored non-compliance distalization approaches take several months to correct the Class II molar relationship but are sometimes associated with unwanted adverse effects (like anchorage loss, overjet increase, distal rotation and distal tipping of the upper first molars, and mesial rotation of the premolars [90, 91]) that are seen less often with headgear [90, 92].

Skeletal anchorage reinforcement using temporary anchorage devices (miniscrew implants, mini-plates, or palatal implants) has penetrated everyday clinical orthodontic practice for a wide spectrum of indications, aims, and treatment phases, including also Class II correction through maxillary arch distalization. Compared to traditional extraoral traction (headgear), a small RCT found that skeletally anchored intraoral appliances were effective in increasing the rate of first molar distalization, reducing overall needed time from 6.4 months to 5.2 months [93]. Compared to conventionally anchored intraoral appliances, there is some evidence from RCTs that skeletally anchored distal-jet-type distalization appliances are associated with greater molar distalization, less anchorage loss (in terms of anterior displacement and tipping of premolars or incisors), and less extrusion compared to conventional dentally anchored appliances [94, 95]. It seems, therefore, that incorporating temporary anchorage devices in maxillary distalization protocols confers several benefits in terms of effective distalization and reduction of unwanted side effects on the neighboring teeth compared to conventional protocols. As far as distalization efficacy relative to the eruption phase of the second molar is concerned, a small observational study found no difference in distalization speed or amount of bodily molar movement but suggested that higher forces might be needed to compensate for potentially higher resistance caused by second molars [96]. Another point to consider for these kinds of Class II protocols is that total arch distalization causes the third molars (if existent) to move backward and upward, instead of downward and forward [97], which might potentially increase their risk for impaction, and warrants prolonged follow-up periods.

Finally, another treatment option for motivated patients, who can comply with the instructions of wearing them at least 20–22 h/day, is the use of orthodontic aligners that sequentially distalize the posterior teeth. Limited evidence from an RCT indicates that aligners are equally effective (if not more) to a pendulum-type appliance in molar distalization, while also providing better control of vertical dimension, occlusal plane rotation, and molar extrusion [76]. However, more studies on this will help reduce uncertainty about this treatment approach.

3.10 Orthodontic Aligners for Class II Correction

Since their introduction in the late 1990s as a comprehensive treatment alternative to move teeth, orthodontic aligners have gained considerable popularity, in part due to aggressive marketing, but also due to obvious advantages in terms of improved aesthetics, oral hygiene, patient comfort, and shorter chair time. Although orthodontic aligners are mostly used to correct mild to moderate malocclusions through purely dental movements, the spectrum of malocclusions treated with aligners has been extended to include more complex cases, including extractions, orthognathic surgery, ectopic eruptions, and open bites. Systematic reviews [98, 99] and single studies [100–106] published in the early 2020s indicated that compared to fixed appliances, aligners are associated with worse objective occlusal outcomes, while the predictability for many planned movements is moderate to poor, leading to multiple mid-course adjustments ("refinements") needed for almost all patients.

During the couple past years, one of the biggest aligner providers introduced the incorporation of plastic wings on aligners to advance the mandible and produce a Class II correction for children 8–15 years of age with a retrognathic mandible. As is unfortunately often the case for novel treatment approaches in orthodontics, there exists a lack of high-quality studies to support this approach. At the time this chapter was written, only four published studies could be located [107–110] that compare mandibular advancement using aligners with removable functional appliances for growing children with Class II malocclusion. Unfortunately, all of these studies are retrospective non-randomized before-and-after (cohort) studies, some with historical control groups, with very limited sample sizes (10–23 patients per group), considerable baseline imbalances between the compared groups, and different treatment durations—all of which can introduce significant bias in their results and potentially produce misleading conclusions.

Nevertheless, eyeballing the results of these studies seems to find common ground for some key outcomes that all studies agree. All four existing studies reported that mandibular advancement with aligners was associated with smaller reduction in SNA (0.07–1.21 ° smaller), smaller improvement in SNB (0.15–1.53 ° smaller), smaller reduction in ANB (0.16–1.21 ° smaller), greater opening of the mandibular plane (SN-ML; 0.27–0.40 ° greater), greater proclination of the lower incisors (1i-ML; 0.54–3.78 ° greater), and smaller reduction in overjet (0.79–2.99 ° smaller) compared to removable functional appliances (Twin-Block or Van Beek Activator). Additionally, traditional functional appliances seemed to produce greater advancement of the chin (2.1 mm more) [109] compared to aligner-based mandibular advancement. Even though these results tend to support the use of conventional functional appliances over aligners for early Class II correction, it is important to note that the existing studies are of very poor internal validity (quality) and proper prospective, ideally randomized, studies are needed for a verdict to be drawn on the subject.

3.11 Effect of Class II Malocclusion and Its Correction on Airways

There has long been a debate in orthodontics as to whether certain kinds of malocclusions, especially those with a skeletal discrepancy, might be linked to breathing disorders among children or adults. The same debate is being held in reverse, as to whether certain therapeutic approaches in orthodontics or dentofacial orthopedics can have a positive (or negative) impact on breathing.

As basis for the theoretical link between certain skeletal malocclusions and breathing disorders is usually taken the fact that obstructive sleep apnea among adults seems to be associated with certain craniofacial anatomical characteristics, namely: small length of the maxilla and/or mandible, retrognathic mandible, increased lower anterior face height, a vertical skeletal pattern, inferior hyoid bone position, and decreased pharyngeal airway dimensions [111]. Obstructive sleep apnea among children seems to be associated with mandibular retrognathia, reduced anteroposterior linear dimensions of the bony nasopharynx (decreased pharyngeal diameters at the levels of the adenoids), longer facial profile, and narrower intercanine widths compared to healthy children [112]. Further support to this notion can be theoretically provided by three-dimensional volumetric assessments of the upper airways indicating that patients with Class II malocclusion have significantly smaller airway volumes at the level of the nasal cavity ($-3.478\ mm^3$), the palatopharynx ($-1996\ mm^3$), the glosopharynx ($-1101\ mm^3$), the oropharynx ($-2818\ mm^3$), and the total pharynx (−2256 mm^3) compared to Class I patients—regardless of whether they presented sleep apnea or not [113].

Reversely, there are certain orthopedic or surgical treatment approaches that are known to alleviate at least in part the symptoms of obstructive sleep apnea. There is ample evidence indicating that mandibular advancement devices [114] and possibly also orthognathic surgical advancement of both jaws [115] are associated with significant improvements among adults with obstructive sleep apnea. Although evidence for the latter is extremely limited (only one RCT), evidence on the latter indicates that mandibular advancement devices can be for many sleep apnea patients equally effective as the objective gold standard of ventilation masks [114].

These treatment approaches have at the same time been shown to have a positive effect on the airways of most patients. A systematic review of children with Class II malocclusion treated early with removable/fixed functional appliances indicated that compared to the normal growth of untreated children, functional appliances led to increases in various airway compartments, be it linear (supero-posterior. Middle, and inferior airway space; McNamara's lower pharynx, lower adenoid thickness; epiglottis-posterior pharyngeal wall base; bony nasopharynx depth; airway minimum axial area) or volumetric (nasopharynx and oropharynx volume) [116] (Table 3.5; Fig. 3.6). It is however crucial to note here that patient selection among the analyzed patient cohorts was based solely on a diagnosis of Class II malocclusion (presumably with a retrognathic mandible), which does not constitute diagnosis of any kind of breathing disorders. Even if some part of these Class II patients had initially any undiagnosed breathing problems, arbitrary increases in the airway dimensions do not necessarily correlate with functional improvements for these patients. Patients with suspicion of a breathing disorder, including sleep apnea, should be referred to a pulmonary medicine specialist that can make a formal diagnosis and, if needed, consult with the orthodontist for any potential treatment concepts that might benefit the patient.

Finally, to our knowledge, there is only a single RCT that has ever assessed the effect of early Class II treatment with headgear on airway dimensions [117]. A recent moderately sized RCT from Finland analyzing lateral cephalograms reported that early headgear treatment had

Table 3.5 Meta-analyses of airway changes comparing airway measurements with functional appliances or untreated controls. Data from the Bidjan et al. [116] systematic review

Outcome	*n*	MD (95% CI)	*P*
Superoposterior airway space (mm)	8	1.63 (1.03, 2.23)	<0.001
Posterior airway space (mm)	8	0.52 (−0.20, 1.24)	0.15
Middle airway space (mm)	11	1.25 (0.53, 1.98)	0.001
Inferior airway space (mm)	10	1.32 (0.26, 2.38)	0.02
McNamara's upper pharynx (mm)	3	1.35 (−0.57, 3.27)	0.17
McNamara's lower pharynx (mm)	3	2.31 (0.79, 3.82)	0.003
Upper adenoid thickness (AD2-H; mm)	2	0.24 (−2.10, 2.58)	0.84
Lower adenoid thickness (AD1-Ba; mm)	2	1.16 (0.46, 1.86)	0.001
Upper airway thickness (PNS-AD2; mm)	5	0.38 (−0.18, 0.94)	0.19
Nasopharynx height (PNS-BaN; mm)	2	0.13 (−0.77, 1.02)	0.78
Upper pharyngeal airway passage (Ptm-UPW; mm)	2	−0.37 (−1.73, 0.99)	0.60
Base of epiglottis-posterior pharyngeal wall (V-LPW; mm)	4	0.70 (0.11, 1.29)	0.02
Sagittal depth of bony nasopharynx (Ba-PNS; mm)	2	1.25 (0.06, 2.43)	0.04
Minimum axial area (mm^2)	2	59.91 (41.46, 78.35)	<0.001
Oropharynx sagittal dimension (mm)	2	1.20 (−2.12, 4.52)	0.48
Oropharynx area (units)	2	556.10 (−279.88, 1392.08)	0.19
Nasopharynx volume (mm^3)	3	0.95[a] (0.36, 1.54)	0.002
Oropharynx volume (mm^3)	4	2356.14 (1276.36, 3435.92)	<0.001

CI confidence interval, *MD* mean difference, *n* number of studies
[a] SMD used instead of MD due to big differences in the control group baseline measurements

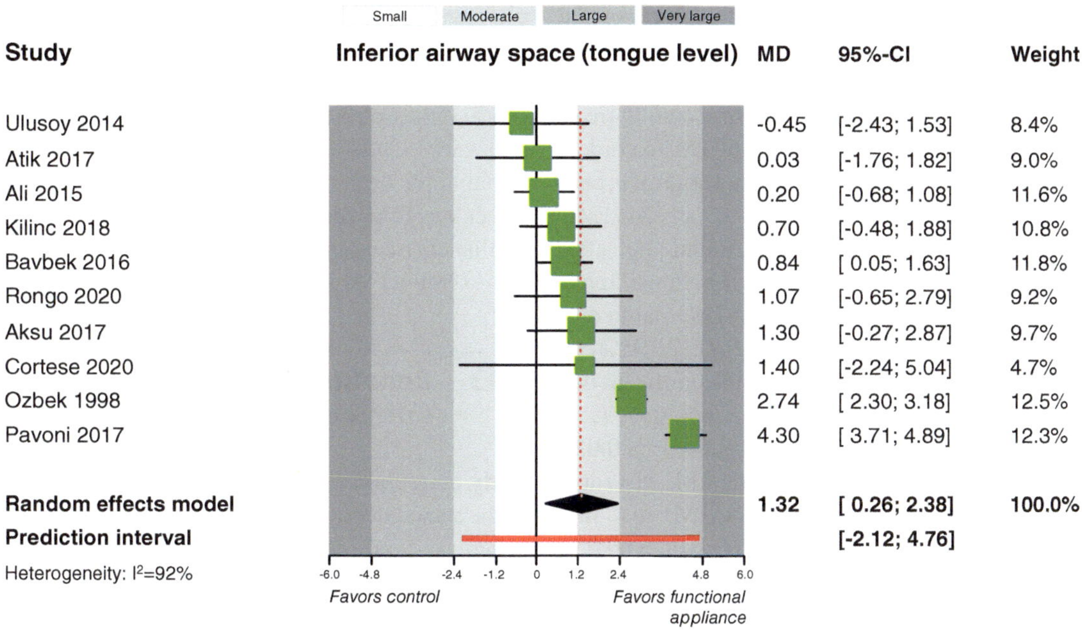

Fig. 3.6 Contour-enhanced forest plot of inferior airway space (at the level of the tongue) changes for functional appliance treatment compared to untreated Class II controls. *CI* confidence interval, *MD* mean difference

no effect on the depth of the nasopharynx, the soft palate thickness/length, and the upper oropharynx. On the contrary, patients treated early with headgear showed in the short term (directly after treatment) a statistically significant increase in the lower oropharynx depth at the level of the tongue's base (MD 1.9 mm; 95% CI 0.2 to 3.6 mm) and in the hypopharynx at the level of the epiglottis (MD 1.7 mm; 95% CI 0.2 to 3.2 mm). These increases were seen specifically among boys rather than girls, both at the oropharynx (+3.0 and +0.3 mm for boys and girls, respectively) and at the hypopharynx (+2.0 mm and 1.2 mm for boys and girls, respectively). A possible explanation for this might be that headgear wear is associated with increased pressure exerted from the tongue on the lower incisors' lingual surface, which might result in patency of the lower airways [118], as reflected to the increased airway dimensions at the level of the tongue. However, these beneficial effects seen specifically for boys are of limited clinical relevance, since the observed effects were of moderate magnitude (between half and one SD of these airway compartments).

3.12 Effect of Class II Treatment on the Temporomandibular Joint

Contrary to initial proof-of-concept studies on animals and early human trials indicating considerable benefits in terms of increased mandibular length, the current consensus is that the actual sagittal position of the anterior border of the mandible is only slightly affected by functional appliance treatment [119–121]. However, initial claims of condylar growth and remodeling [19, 20, 25] have been confirmed by subsequent studies. A recent systematic review of RCTs and non-RCTs indicated that compared to normal growth of Class II children, early functional appliance treatment is associated with anterior and inferior repositioning of the condyle, vertical displacement of the glenoid fossa, and increased condylar growth [122]. However, the clinical relevance of these alterations of the temporo-mandibular joint (TMJ) in the long term remains unclear, while at the same time, another question is raised. If functional appliance treatment can influence the position and form of the TMJ, could it theoretically also be associated with detrimental effects on the TMJ?

Only a handful of published studies have longitudinally assessed the effect of Class II treatment on any signs or symptoms of TMJ disorders and compared them to an untreated control group: one RCT [123] and three non-RCTs [124–126]. The single RCT from Florida found that after treatment, patients treated with functional appliances reported significantly less TMJ pain compared to untreated patients (OR 0.32; 95% CI 0.14 to 0.76; $P = 0.009$), while no significant differences were found for TMJ sounds (OR 1.16; $P > 0.05$) and muscle pain (OR 0.54; $P > 0.05$). The non-RCTs found no effect on TMJ disorders (1 study; OR 1.00; $P > 0.05$) or TMJ disc displacement (2 studies; OR 0.69; $P > 0.05$). Looking solely at the treated Class II patients before-and-after Class II treatment, no significant differences were found in the existence of TMJ sounds, muscle pain, or disc displacement. The only difference was seen for TMJ pain, where significantly less TMJ sounds were seen after functional appliance treatment (17%) compared to before treatment (40%).

The single existing RCT from Florida [123] also reported that, compared to untreated controls, early headgear treatment had no effect on TMJ pain (OR 0.59; $P > 0.05$), TMJ sounds (OR 1.10; $P > 0.05$), or muscle pain (OR 0.65; $P > 0.05$).

However, existence of signs and symptoms of TMJ disorders before treatment plays a significant role as to whether such symptoms are seen after treatment. The authors of the same RCT [123] concluded that patients without any signs or symptoms before treatment had no increased risk to develop any TMJ problems and the only variable associated with emergence of TMJ symptoms was increasing patient age. Patients with initial TMJ pain were significantly less likely to report TMJ pains after treatment with functional appliances (13% versus 55%). Similarly, patients with TMJ sound before treatment were less likely to report TMJ sounds afterward if they had been treated with functional appliances (25% versus 75%) or with headgear (40% versus 75%). Little effect was seen on muscle pain however, since patients with such pains initially were only slightly less likely to report pains after treatment with functional appliances (45% versus 65%). Overall, it can be concluded that early Class II treatment with either functional appliances or headgear has no detrimental effect on TMJ function, while early functional appliance treatment might even alleviate some pre-existing TMJ symptoms.

3.13 Benefits of Early Class II Correction

Early correction of a Class II malocclusion (i.e., in the mixed dentition) has been traditionally proposed and administered by orthodontists for many decades. However, such an early correction is associated with potential disadvantages, including among others an increased overall treatment duration, the need for a prolonged retention period for the early corrected overjet, and the potential for loss of compliance from the patient when the time for the definite (fixed-appliance) treatment comes. As far as benefits of an early Class II correction are concerned, a Cochrane review [127] found that early treatment during adolescence followed by a definitive fixed appliance treatment (two-phase treatment) did not convey any additional benefits in terms of final overjet, final ANB, quality of occlusal outcome (through the Peer Assessment Rating [PAR] score), or self-concept compared to a single-phase treatment with fixed appliances at a later stage. Moreover, meta-analysis of the three large RCTs on the subject [119–121] indicated that early Class II correction was not associated with lower extraction rate at the subsequent fixed appliance treatment (OR 0.83; 95% CI 0.49 to 1.43; $P = 0.51$). On the other hand, excessively prominent upper front teeth (increased overjet) among schoolchildren have been associated with lower oral health-related quality of life and a greater potential for the child to be bullied or victimized [128, 129]. Even though early correction is not necessarily accompanied by an improved quality of life for the child [130], there are still some instances where early Class II correction

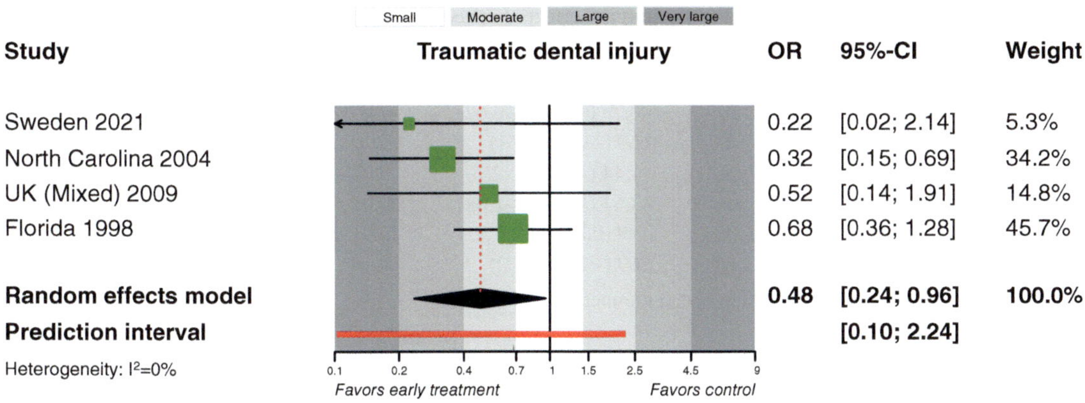

Fig. 3.7 Contour-enhanced forest plot of new traumatic dental injuries for early functional appliance/headgear treatment compared to untreated Class II controls (with/without subsequent phase II treatment). *CI* confidence interval, *OR* odds ratio, *UK* United Kingdom

might be considered for some children, who might benefit directly from it.

Increased overjet during adolescence (especially when the incisors are protruded and inadequately covered by the soft tissues) is associated with increased risk of traumatic dental injuries [131], which accounts for one-fifth of all dental injuries worldwide [132]. In such cases, meta-analysis of four RCTs on the subject [119–121, 130] indicated that early Class II correction with normalization of the anterior occlusion is associated with a significant reduction in dental trauma (OR 0.48; 95% CI 0.28 to 0.81; $P = 0.006$; Fig. 3.7). The possible benefits from such an early intervention range from small to large and additional risk factors for dental trauma should be taken into account, like patient sex, anterior open bite, participation in sports, certain medical disorders, social deprivation, obesity, inappropriate oral habits, previous dental injury and oral piercings [133]. Dental trauma is a well-known public health concern with considerable direct and indirect costs and, when permanent teeth are concerned, involves a long period of treatment that is seldom finished before the age of 20 [134]. Therefore, for such patients with increased overjet and increased risk for dental trauma, early correction of Class II malocclusion as a means to reduce trauma risk should be evaluated by both the patient and the orthodontist, alongside other objective and subjective factors.

3.14 Long-term Effects of Early Class II Correction

Correction of a Class II malocclusion includes a broad spectrum of set treatment goals, used appliances, and time-points of treatment initiation, while the specific treatment plan for each patient depends on existing clinical evidence, personal preferences of the orthodontist or the doctor, schools of thought, and even logistic reasons within a clinical setting. In many instances, early correction of Class II malocclusion is attempted during the mixed dentition stage and considerable changes due to residual growth of the jaws and physiological maturation of the dentition are expected after treatment. It is therefore important to evaluate what is the long-term stability of the outcomes of Class II treatment, as prolonged retention protocols or even renewed treatment might be needed in some cases.

Several studies have shown that several effects of functional appliance treatment are either small, transient, or pertain more to an acceleration of growth, rather than true growth stimulation. According to anecdotal evidence [135], functional appliances might result in an early period of accelerated mandibular growth, which is followed by a subsequent period of diminished mandibular growth rate compared to untreated patients [136], so that in the long-term any observed differences in mandibular length are

Table 3.6 Meta-analyses of long-term (>3 years) differences between patients treated with functional appliances and untreated controls. Re-analyzed data from the Cacciatore et al. [139] systematic review

Outcome	*n*	MD (95% CI)	*P*	95% prediction
SNA (°)	3	−0.73 (−0.83, −0.62)	0.001	−4.55, 3.09
SNB (°)	5	0.69 (−0.23, 1.61)	0.10	−1.29, 2.68
ANB (°)	3	−1.44 (−3.14, 0.26)	0.07	−10.31, 7.43
Wits (mm)	3	−3.61 (−6.15, −1.08)	0.03	−15.77, 8.55
Co-Gn (mm)	4	1.99 (0.85, 3.13)	0.01	0.28, 3.70
Co-Gn/Co-A difference (mm)	2	2.69 (−2.64, 8.02)	0.10	Not applicable

CI confidence interval, *MD* mean difference, *n* number of studies

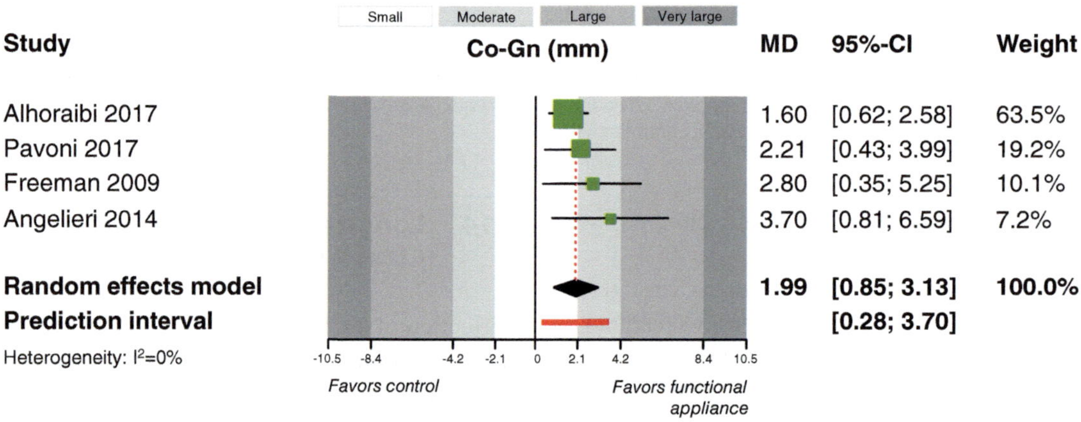

Fig. 3.8 Contour-enhanced forest plot of long-term (>3 years post-treatment) mandibular length (Co-Gn) changes for functional appliance treatment compared to untreated Class II controls. *CI* confidence interval, *MD* mean difference

very small. Similar findings are reported for so-called "catch-up growth" after an early restriction of maxillary anterior growth [137] or for a tendency of the increased lower anterior height to diminish with time [138].

The important question on the subject of treatment stability is "Do Class II patients treated with functional appliances during adolescent have morphologic differences in the long term from untreated Class II patients?." Evidence for this question is based on a published systematic review of RCTs and non-RCTs [139], the data of which has been re-analyzed (Table 3.6). After a post-retention period of at least 3 years after completion of Class II treatment, treated Class II patients seem to have significantly smaller SNA angle (MD −0.73 °; 95% CI −0.83 to −0.62 °), smaller Wits appraisal (MD −3.61 mm; 95% CI −6.15 to −1.08 mm), and significantly larger effective mandibular length (Co-Gn; MD 1.99 mm; 95% CI 0.85 to 3.13 mm; Fig. 3.8) compared to untreated Class II patients. On the other side, no statistically significant differences are seen for SNB angle, ANB angle, and Co-Gn/Co-A difference ($P > 0.05$). This indicates that although many initial treatment effects seem to be "blended out" by residual growth, there still exist some small morphological differences that can be attributed to the early intervention with functional appliances. However, whether these differences are of any clinical relevance to the patient in terms of improved esthetics, function, or quality of life remains questionable.

3.15 Conclusions

This chapter attempted to summarize existing high-quality evidence on the various treatment approaches for Class II malocclusion in the orthodontist's armamentarium. Two-phase Class II treatment with either headgear or functional appliances with a subsequent comprehensive fixed-appliance phase seems to be largely as effective as a single-phase later treatment, although some patients might benefit from an early intervention. In Class II treatment with removable appliances, conventional functional appliances seem to be preferable to either prefabricated myofunctional appliances or aligner-based alternatives. Skeletal anchorage might be beneficial for Class II correction in either reducing unwanted side effects in terms of anchorage loss or providing efficient alternative for maxillary distalization. For mild to moderate skeletal Class II malocclusions, a dentoalveolar correction to camouflage the underlying discrepancy might be attempted, but for severe cases a combined orthodontic-surgical approach might be needed for harmonious dental, skeletal, and soft-tissue outcomes. Finally, the results of Class II treatment seem to be stable in the long term for many patients. It is however worth noticing that even though several treatment approaches exist for several decades, the underlying evidence base is severely limited—both in terms of quantity and quality of clinical studies.

Conflicts of Interest None.

Funding None.

References

1. Goldstein MS, Lindsten FL. Various types of occlusion and amounts of overbite in normal and abnormal occlusion between two and twelve years. Int J Orthod Oral Surg. 1936;22(6):549–69.
2. Ast DB, Carlos JP, Cons NC. The prevalence and characteristics of malocclusion among senior high school students in upstate New York. Am J Orthod. 1965;51:437–45.
3. Josefsson E, Bjerklin K, Lindsten R. Malocclusion frequency in Swedish and immigrant adolescents--influence of origin on orthodontic treatment need. Eur J Orthod. 2007;29(1):79–87.
4. McNamara JA Jr. Components of class II malocclusion in children 8–10 years of age. Angle Orthod. 1981;51(3):177–202.
5. Pancherz H, Zieber K, Hoyer B. Cephalometric characteristics of class II division 1 and class II division 2 malocclusions: a comparative study in children. Angle Orthod. 1997;67(2):111–20.
6. Papageorgiou SN, Kloukos D, Petridis H, Pandis N. Publication of statistically significant research findings in prosthodontics and implant dentistry in the context of other dental specialties. J Dent. 2015;43(10):1195–202.
7. Papageorgiou SN, Xavier GM, Cobourne MT. Basic study design influences the results of orthodontic clinical investigations. J Clin Epidemiol. 2015;68(12):1512–22.
8. Papageorgiou SN, Koretsi V, Jäger A. Bias from historical control groups used in orthodontic research: a meta-epidemiological study. Eur J Orthod. 2017;39(1):98–105.
9. Papageorgiou SN, Antonoglou GN, Sándor GK, Eliades T. Randomized clinical trials in orthodontics are rarely registered a priori and often published late or not at all. PLoS One. 2017;12(8):e0182785.
10. Papageorgiou SN, Antonoglou GN, Martin C, Eliades T. Methods, transparency and reporting of clinical trials in orthodontics and periodontics. J Orthod. 2019;46(2):101–9.
11. Higgins JPT, Thomas J, Chandler J, Cumpston M, Li T, Page MJ, Welch VA. Cochrane handbook for systematic reviews of interventions version 6.3 (updated February 2022). Cochrane; 2022. www.training.cochrane.org/handbook.
12. Langan D, Higgins JPT, Jackson D, Bowden J, Veroniki AA, Kontopantelis E, Viechtbauer W, Simmonds M. A comparison of heterogeneity variance estimators in simulated random-effects meta-analyses. Res Synth Methods. 2019;10(1):83–98.
13. van Aert RCM, Jackson D. A new justification of the Hartung-Knapp method for random-effects meta-analysis based on weighted least squares regression. Res Synth Methods. 2019;10(4):515–27.
14. Papageorgiou SN. Meta-analysis for orthodontists: part II—Is all that glitters gold? J Orthod. 2014;41(4):327–36.
15. Papageorgiou SN. An evidence base of treatment outcome for class II malocclusion [Data set]. Zenodo. 2023; https://doi.org/10.5281/zenodo.7809839.
16. Moss ML, Salentijn L. The primary role of functional matrices in facial growth. Am J Orthod Dentofacial Orthop. 1969;55:566–77.
17. Mills JR. The effects of orthodontic treatment on the skeletal pattern. Br J Orthod. 1978;5(3):133–43.
18. Charlier JP, Petrovic A, Herrmann-Stutzmann J. Effects of mandibular hyperpropulsion on the prechondroblastic zone of young rat condyle. Am J Orthod. 1969;55(1):71–4.
19. Stöckli PW, Willert HG. Tissue reactions in the temporomandibular joint resulting from anterior displacement of the mandible in the monkey. Am J Orthod. 1971;60(2):142–55.
20. McNamara JA Jr, Bryan FA. Long-term mandibular adaptations to protrusive function: an experimental study in Macaca mulatta. Am J Orthod Dentofacial Orthop. 1987;92(2):98–108.

21. Toth LR, McNamara JA Jr. Treatment effects produced by the twin-block appliance and the FR-2 appliance of Fränkel compared with an untreated class II sample. Am J Orthod Dentofacial Orthop. 1999;116(6):597–609.
22. Janson GR, Toruño JL, Martins DR, Henriques JF, de Freitas MR. Class II treatment effects of the Fränkel appliance. Eur J Orthod. 2003;25(3):301–9.
23. Marsico E, Gatto E, Burrascano M, Matarese G, Cordasco G. Effectiveness of orthodontic treatment with functional appliances on mandibular growth in the short term. Am J Orthod Dentofacial Orthop. 2011;139(1):24–36.
24. Pancherz H, Ruf S, Kohlhas P. "Effective condylar growth" and chin position changes in Herbst treatment: a cephalometric roentgenographic long-term study. Am J Orthod Dentofacial Orthop. 1998;114(4):437–46.
25. Voudouris JC, Woodside DG, Altuna G, Angelopoulos G, Bourque PJ, Lacouture CY, Kuftinec MM. Condyle-fossa modifications and muscle interactions during Herbst treatment, part 2. Results and conclusions. Am J Orthod Dentofacial Orthop. 2003;124(1):13–29.
26. Gianelly AA, Brosnan P, Martignoni M, Bernstein L. Mandibular growth, condyle position and Fränkel appliance therapy. Angle Orthod. 1983;53(2):131–42.
27. Cozza P, Baccetti T, Franchi L, De Toffol L, McNamara JA Jr. Mandibular changes produced by functional appliances in class II malocclusion: a systematic review. Am J Orthod Dentofacial Orthop. 2006;129(5):599.e1–12.
28. Whitney EF, Sinclair PM. An evaluation of combination second molar extraction and functional appliance therapy. Am J Orthod Dentofacial Orthop. 1987;91(3):183–92.
29. Vargervik K, Harvold EP. Response to activator treatment in class II malocclusions. Am J Orthod. 1985;88(3):242–51.
30. Hashim HA. Analysis of activator treatment changes. Aust Orthod J. 1991;12(2):100–4.
31. McNamara JA Jr, Bookstein FL, Shaughnessy TG. Skeletal and dental changes following functional regulator therapy on class II patients. Am J Orthod. 1985;88(2):91–110.
32. Sidhu MS, Kharbanda OP, Sidhu SS. Cephalometric analysis of changes produced by a modified Herbst appliance in the treatment of class II division 1 malocclusion. Br J Orthod. 1995;22(1):1–12.
33. Johnston LE Jr. Answers in search of questioners. Am J Orthod Dentofacial Orthop. 2002;121:552–3.
34. Bowman SJ. All roads lead to Rome: new directions for class II. Semin Orthod. 2014;20(4):247–8.
35. Pancherz H. The nature of class II relapse after Herbst appliance treatment: a cephalometric long-term investigation. Am J Orthod Dentofacial Orthop. 1991;100(3):220–33.
36. Koretsi V, Zymperdikas VF, Papageorgiou SN, Papadopoulos MA. Treatment effects of removable functional appliances in patients with class II malocclusion: a systematic review and meta-analysis. Eur J Orthod. 2015;37(4):418–34.
37. Zymperdikas VF, Koretsi V, Papageorgiou SN, Papadopoulos MA. Treatment effects of fixed functional appliances in patients with class II malocclusion: a systematic review and meta-analysis. Eur J Orthod. 2016;38(2):113–26.
38. Lo FD, Hunter WS. Changes in nasolabial angle related to maxillary incisor retraction. Am J Orthod. 1982;82(5):384–91.
39. Banks P, Wright J, O'Brien K. Incremental versus maximum bite advancement during twin-block therapy: a randomized controlled clinical trial. Am J Orthod Dentofacial Orthop. 2004;126(5):583–8.
40. Aras I, Pasaoglu A, Olmez S, Unal I, Tuncer AV, Aras A. Comparison of stepwise vs single-step advancement with the functional mandibular advancer in class II division 1 treatment. Angle Orthod. 2017;87(1):82–7.
41. Papadopoulos MA, Papageorgiou SN, Zogakis IP. Clinical effectiveness of orthodontic mini-screw implants: a meta-analysis. J Dent Res. 2011;90(8):969–76.
42. Jambi S, Walsh T, Sandler J, Benson PE, Skeggs RM, O'Brien KD. Reinforcement of anchorage during orthodontic brace treatment with implants or other surgical methods. Cochrane Database Syst Rev. 2014;2014(8):CD005098.
43. Sandler J, Murray A, Thiruvenkatachari B, Gutierrez R, Speight P, O'Brien K. Effectiveness of 3 methods of anchorage reinforcement for maximum anchorage in adolescents: a 3-arm multicenter randomized clinical trial. Am J Orthod Dentofacial Orthop. 2014;146(1):10–20.
44. Bayome M, Park JH, Bay C, Kook YA. Distalization of maxillary molars using temporary skeletal anchorage devices: a systematic review and meta-analysis. Orthod Craniofac Res. 2021;24(Suppl 1):103–12.
45. Aslan BI, Kucukkaraca E, Turkoz C, Dincer M. Treatment effects of the Forsus fatigue resistant device used with miniscrew anchorage. Angle Orthod. 2014;84(1):76–87.
46. Eissa O, El-Shennawy M, Gaballah S, El-Meehy G, El Bialy T. Treatment outcomes of class II malocclusion cases treated with miniscrew-anchored Forsus fatigue resistant device: a randomized controlled trial. Angle Orthod. 2017;87(6):824–33.
47. Elkordy SA, Abouelezz AM, Fayed MMS, Aboulfotouh MH, Mostafa YA. Evaluation of the miniplate-anchored Forsus fatigue resistant device in skeletal class II growing subjects: a randomized controlled trial. Angle Orthod. 2019;89(3):391–403.
48. Turkkahraman H, Eliacik SK, Findik Y. Effects of miniplate anchored and conventional Forsus fatigue

resistant devices in the treatment of class II malocclusion. Angle Orthod. 2016;86(6):1026–32.
49. Gandedkar NH, Shrikantaiah S, Patil AK, Baseer MA, Chng CK, Ganeshkar SV, Kambalyal P. Influence of conventional and skeletal anchorage system supported fixed functional appliance on maxillo-mandibular complex and temporomandibular joint: a preliminary comparative cone beam computed tomography study. Int Orthod. 2019;17(2):256–68.
50. Manni A, Migliorati M, Calzolari C, Silvestrini-Biavati A. Herbst appliance anchored to miniscrews in the upper and lower arches vs standard Herbst: a pilot study. Am J Orthod Dentofacial Orthop. 2019;156(5):617–25.
51. Moss ML, Rankow RM. The role of the functional matrix in mandibular growth. Angle Orthod. 1968;38(2):95–103.
52. Owman-Moll P, Ingervall B. Effect of oral screen treatment on dentition, lip morphology, and function in children with incompetent lips. Am J Orthod. 1984;85(1):37–46.
53. Koletsi D, Makou M, Pandis N. Effect of orthodontic management and orofacial muscle training protocols on the correction of myofunctional and myoskeletal problems in developing dentition. A systematic review and meta-analysis. Orthod Craniofac Res. 2018;21(4):202–15.
54. Proffit WR, Mason RM. Myofunctional therapy for tongue-thrusting: background and recommendations. J Am Dent Assoc. 1975;90(2):403–11.
55. Cheney EA. Factors in the early treatment and interception of malocclusion. Am J Orthod. 1958;44(11):807–26.
56. Rossi R, Mortara MC, Boccaccio E. Preventive orthodontics and the use of oral screens. Parodonto Stomatol. 1984;(Nuova) 23(Suppl 3):191–2.
57. Bergersen EO. The eruption guidance myofunctional appliances: how it works, how to use it. Funct Orthod. 1984;1(3):28–9, 31-5
58. Tallgren A, Christiansen RL, Ash M Jr, Miller RL. Effects of a myofunctional appliance on orofacial muscle activity and structures. Angle Orthod. 1998;68(3):249–58.
59. Papageorgiou SN, Koletsi D, Eliades T. What evidence exists for myofunctional therapy with prefabricated appliances? A systematic review with meta-analyses of randomised trials. J Orthod. 2019;46(4):297–310.
60. Hanoun AA. The efficacy of the prefabricated T4FTM myofunctional appliance in comparison to twin block appliance for class II division 1 malocclusion treatment: a randomized clinical trial. MSc Thesis, University Sains Malaysia; 2010.
61. Čirgić E, Kjellberg H, Hansen K. Treatment of large overjet in angle class II: division 1 malocclusion with Andresen activators versus prefabricated functional appliances-a multicenter, randomized, controlled trial. Eur J Orthod. 2016;38(5):516–24.
62. Idris G, Hajeer MY, Al-Jundi A. Soft- and hard-tissue changes following treatment of class II division 1 malocclusion with activator versus trainer: a randomized controlled trial. Eur J Orthod. 2019;41(1):21–8.
63. Xie L, Wang P, Wu J. Soft and hard tissue changes following treatment of class II division 1 malocclusion with twin-block and Myofunctional appliance: a pilot study. Chinese J Plastic Reconstruct Surg. 2020;2(4):217–27.
64. Thompson WM Jr. Occipital anchorage. Angle Orthod. 1940;10(4):206–11.
65. Ricketts RM. The influence of orthodontic treatment on facial growth and development. Angle Orthod. 1960;30(3):103–33.
66. Brown P. A cephalometric evaluation of high-pull molar headgear and face-bow neck strap therapy. Am J Orthod. 1978;74(6):621–32.
67. Boecler PR, Riolo ML, Keeling SD, TenHave TR. Skeletal changes associated with extraoral appliance therapy: an evaluation of 200 consecutively treated cases. Angle Orthod. 1989;59(4):263–70.
68. Gianelly AA, Valentini V. The role of "orthopedics" and orthodontics in the treatment of class II, division 1 malocclusions. Am J Orthod. 1976;69(6):668–78.
69. Papageorgiou SN, Kutschera E, Memmert S, Gölz L, Jäger A, Bourauel C, Eliades T. Effectiveness of early orthopaedic treatment with headgear: a systematic review and meta-analysis. Eur J Orthod. 2017;39(2):176–87.
70. Kingsley N. A treatise on Oral deformities as a branch of mechanical surgery. New York, NY: Appleton and Co.; 1880.
71. Körbitz A. Kursus der systematischen Orthodontik. Ein Leitfaden für Studium und Praxis. 2nd ed. Leipzig: Hans Licht; 1914.
72. McNamara JA Jr. Orthodontic and orthopedic treatment in the mixed dentition. Ann Arbor, MI: NeedhamPress Inc.; 1993.
73. Gianelly A. Rapid palatal expansion in the absence of crossbites: added value? Am J Orthod Dentofacial Orthop. 2003;124:362–5.
74. Timmons LS. Induced change in the anteroposterior relationship of the jaws. Angle Orthod. 1972;42(3):245–51.
75. Cleall JF, BeGole EA. Diagnosis and treatment of class II division 2 malocclusion. Angle Orthod. 1982;52(1):38–60.
76. Lione R, Balboni A, Di Fazio V, Pavoni C, Cozza P. Effects of pendulum appliance versus clear aligners in the vertical dimension during class II malocclusion treatment: a randomized prospective clinical trial. BMC Oral Health. 2022;22(1):441.
77. Nagrik AP, Bhad WA, Chavan SJ, Doshi UH. A randomized clinical trial to assess the sagittal effects of Transforce transverse appliance (TTA) and NiTi palatal expander (NPE) on skeletal class II malocclusion in growing patients during retention phase—a cephalometric study using a historical control group. Int Orthod. 2020;18(4):722–31.

78. Kouvelis G, Dritsas K, Doulis I, Kloukos D, Gkantidis N. Effect of orthodontic treatment with 4 premolar extractions compared with nonextraction treatment on the vertical dimension of the face: a systematic review. Am J Orthod Dentofacial Orthop. 2018;154(2):175–87.
79. Angst C, Eliades T, Papageorgiou SN. Stability of occlusal outcome during long-term retention: the time-dependent variation of the American Board of Orthodontics index. Eur J Orthod. 2021;43(1):1–7.
80. Herzog C, Konstantonis D, Konstantoni N, Eliades T. Arch-width changes in extraction vs nonextraction treatments in matched class I borderline malocclusions. Am J Orthod Dentofacial Orthop. 2017;151(4):735–43.
81. Erdinc AE, Nanda RS, Dandajena TC. Profile changes of patients treated with and without premolar extractions. Am J Orthod Dentofacial Orthop. 2007;132(3):324–31.
82. Konstantonis D, Vasileiou D, Papageorgiou SN, Eliades T. Soft tissue changes following extraction vs. nonextraction orthodontic fixed appliance treatment: a systematic review and meta-analysis. Eur J Oral Sci. 20181;126(3):167–79.
83. Waldman BH. Change in lip contour with maxillary incisor retraction. Angle Orthod. 1982;52(2):129–34.
84. Ramos AL, Sakima MT, Pinto Ados S, Bowman SJ. Upper lip changes correlated to maxillary incisor retraction--a metallic implant study. Angle Orthod. 2005;75(4):499–505.
85. Kuhn M, Markic G, Doulis I, Göllner P, Patcas R, Hänggi MP. Effect of different incisor movements on the soft tissue profile measured in reference to a rough-surfaced palatal implant. Am J Orthod Dentofacial Orthop. 2016;149(3):349–57.
86. Rongo R, Nissen L, Leroy C, Michelotti A, Cattaneo PM, Cornelis MA. Three-dimensional soft tissue changes in orthodontic extraction and non-extraction patients: a prospective study. Orthod Craniofac Res. 2021;24(Suppl 2):181–92.
87. Kochar GD, Londhe S, Chopra SS, Kohli S, Kohli VS, Chakranarayan A, Kambojh A, Bhatt S. Treatment effects and lip profile changes following surgical mandibular advancement versus premolar extractions in class II div 1 malocclusion: a randomized controlled trial. J Craniofac Surg. 2022;33(1):81–6.
88. Raposo R, Peleteiro B, Paço M, Pinho T. Orthodontic camouflage versus orthodontic-orthognathic surgical treatment in class II malocclusion: a systematic review and meta-analysis. Int J Oral Maxillofac Surg. 2018;47(4):445–55.
89. Abed Y, Brin I. Early headgear effect on the eruption pattern of maxillary second molars. Angle Orthod. 2010;80(4):454–60.
90. Acar AG, Gürsoy S, Dinçer M. Molar distalization with a pendulum appliance K-loop combination. Eur J Orthod. 2010;32(4):459–65.
91. Papadopoulos MA, Melkos AB, Athanasiou AE. Noncompliance maxillary molar distalization with the first class appliance: a randomized controlled trial. Am J Orthod Dentofacial Orthop. 2010;137(5):586.e1–586.e13.
92. Toy E, Enacar A. The effects of the pendulum distalising appliance and cervical headgear on the dentofacial structures. Aust Orthod J. 2011;27(1):10–6.
93. Bondemark L, Karlsson I. Extraoral vs intraoral appliance for distal movement of maxillary first molars: a randomized controlled trial. Angle Orthod. 2005;75(5):699–706.
94. Cassetta M, Brandetti G, Altieri F. Miniscrew-supported distal jet versus conventional distal jet appliance: a pilot study. J Clin Exp Dent. 2019;11(7):e650–8.
95. Altieri F, Mezio M, Guarnieri R, Cassetta M. Comparing distal-jet with dental anchorage to distal-jet with skeletal anchorage: a prospective parallel cohort study. Dent J (Basel). 2022;10(10):179.
96. Nienkemper M, Wilmes B, Pauls A, Yamaguchi S, Ludwig B, Drescher D. Treatment efficiency of mini-implant-borne distalization depending on age and second-molar eruption. J Orofac Orthop. 2014;75(2):118–32.
97. Lee YJ, Kook YA, Park JH, Park J, Bayome M, Vaid NR, Kim Y. Short-term cone-beam computed tomography evaluation of maxillary third molar changes after total arch distalization in adolescents. Am J Orthod Dentofacial Orthop. 2019;155(2):191–7.
98. Papageorgiou SN, Koletsi D, Iliadi A, Peltomaki T, Eliades T. Treatment outcome with orthodontic aligners and fixed appliances: a systematic review with meta-analyses. Eur J Orthod. 2020;42(3):331–43.
99. Koletsi D, Iliadi A, Eliades T. Predictability of rotational tooth movement with orthodontic aligners comparing software-based and achieved data: a systematic review and meta-analysis of observational studies. J Orthod. 2021;48(3):277–87.
100. Blundell HL, Weir T, Kerr B, Freer E. Predictability of overbite control with the Invisalign appliance. Am J Orthod Dentofacial Orthop. 2021;160(5):725–31.
101. Goh S, Dreyer C, Weir T. The predictability of the mandibular curve of Spee leveling with the Invisalign appliance. Am J Orthod Dentofacial Orthop. 2022;162(2):193–200.
102. Kravitz ND, Dalloul B, Zaid YA, Shah C, Vaid NR. What percentage of patients switch from Invisalign to braces? A retrospective study evaluating the conversion rate, number of refinement scans, and length of treatment. Am J Orthod Dentofacial Orthop. 2022;S0889-5406(22):00773–9.
103. Maree A, Kerr B, Weir T, Freer E. Clinical expression of programmed rotation and uprighting of bilateral winged maxillary central incisors with the Invisalign appliance: a retrospective study. Am J Orthod Dentofacial Orthop. 2022;161(1):74–83.
104. Smith JM, Weir T, Kaang A, Farella M. Predictability of lower incisor tip using clear aligner therapy. Prog Orthod. 2022;23(1):37.

105. Bowman E, Bowman P, Weir T, Dreyer C, Meade MJ. Occlusal contacts and treatment with the Invisalign appliance: a retrospective analysis of predicted vs achieved outcomes. Angle Orthod. 2023;93:275. [Epub ahead of print]
106. Bowman E, Bowman P, Weir T, Dreyer CW, Meade MJ. Evaluation of the predicted vs. achieved occlusal outcomes with the Invisalign® appliance: a retrospective investigation of adult patients. Int Orthod. 2023;21(2):100746.
107. Caruso S, Nota A, Caruso S, Severino M, Gatto R, Meuli S, Mattei A, Tecco S. Mandibular advancement with clear aligners in the treatment of skeletal class II. A retrospective controlled study. Eur J Paediatr Dent. 2021;22(1):26–30.
108. Sun Z, Pan Y, Lin T, Lu H, Ai H, Mai Z. Comparison of cephalometric measurements of the twin block and A6 appliances in the treatment of class II malocclusion: a retrospective comparative cohort study. Ann Transl Med. 2022;10(16):876.
109. Lombardo EC, Lione R, Franchi L, Gaffuri F, Maspero C, Cozza P, Pavoni C. Dentoskeletal effects of clear aligner vs twin block-a short-term study of functional appliances. J Orofac Orthop. 2023; https://doi.org/10.1007/s00056-022-00443-1. [Epub ahead of print]
110. Wu Y, Yu Q, Xia Y, Wang B, Chen S, Gu K, Zhang B, Zhu M. Does mandibular advancement with clear aligners have the same skeletal and dentoalveolar effects as traditional functional appliances? BMC Oral Health. 2023;23(1):65.
111. Neelapu BC, Kharbanda OP, Sardana HK, Balachandran R, Sardana V, Kapoor P, Gupta A, Vasamsetti S. Craniofacial and upper airway morphology in adult obstructive sleep apnea patients: a systematic review and meta-analysis of cephalometric studies. Sleep Med Rev. 2017;31:79–90.
112. Fagundes NCF, Gianoni-Capenakas S, Heo G, Flores-Mir C. Craniofacial features in children with obstructive sleep apnea: a systematic review and meta-analysis. J Clin Sleep Med. 2022;18(7):1865–75.
113. Altheer C, Papageorgiou SN, Antonoarakis GS, Papadopoulou AK. Do patients of different craniofacial patterns have different volumes of the upper airways? A systematic review with network meta-analysis. Eur J Orthod. 2024;46(2):cjae010. https://doi.org/10.1093/ejo/cjae010.
114. Koretsi V, Eliades T, Papageorgiou SN. Oral interventions for obstructive sleep apnea. Dtsch Arztebl Int. 2018;115(12):200–7.
115. Vicini C, Dallan I, Campanini A, De Vito A, Barbanti F, Giorgiomarrano G, Bosi M, Plazzi G, Provini F, Lugaresi E. Surgery vs ventilation in adult severe obstructive sleep apnea syndrome. Am J Otolaryngol. 2010;31(1):14–20.
116. Bidjan D, Sallmann R, Eliades T, Papageorgiou SN. Orthopedic treatment for class II malocclusion with functional appliances and its effect on upper airways: a systematic review with meta-analysis. J Clin Med. 2020;9(12):3806.
117. Julku J, Pirilä-Parkkinen K, Pirttiniemi P. Airway and hard tissue dimensions in children treated with early and later timed cervical headgear-a randomized controlled trial. Eur J Orthod. 2018;40(3):285–95.
118. Takahashi S, Ono T, Ishiwata Y, Kuroda T. Effect of wearing cervical headgear on tongue pressure. J Orthod. 2000;27(2):163–7.
119. Tulloch JF, Proffit WR, Phillips C. Outcomes in a 2-phase randomized clinical trial of early class II treatment. Am J Orthod Dentofacial Orthop. 2004;125(6):657–67.
120. O'Brien K, Wright J, Conboy F, Appelbe P, Davies L, Connolly I, Mitchell L, Littlewood S, Mandall N, Lewis D, Sandler J, Hammond M, Chadwick S, O'Neill J, McDade C, Oskouei M, Thiruvenkatachari B, Read M, Robinson S, Birnie D, Murray A, Shaw I, Harradine N, Worthington H. Early treatment for class II division 1 malocclusion with the twin-block appliance: a multi-center, randomized, controlled trial. Am J Orthod Dentofacial Orthop. 2009;135(5):573–9.
121. King GJ, Wheeler TT, McGorray SP, Aiosa LS, Bloom RM, Taylor MG. Orthodontists' perceptions of the impact of phase 1 treatment for class II malocclusion on phase 2 needs. J Dent Res. 1999;78(11):1745–53.
122. Kyburz KS, Eliades T, Papageorgiou SN. What effect does functional appliance treatment have on the temporomandibular joint? A systematic review with meta-analysis. Prog Orthod. 2019;20(1):32.
123. Keeling SD, Garvan CW, King GJ, Wheeler TT, McGorray S. Temporomandibular disorders after early class II treatment with bionators and headgears: results from a randomized controlled trial. Semin Orthod. 1995;1(3):149–64.
124. Chintakanon K. A prospective study of twin block appliance therapy in children with class I division 1 malocclusions assessed by MRI, 3D-cephalometry and muscle testing. Doctoral Thesis, University of Adelaide; 1999.
125. Arat ZM, Gökalp H, Erdem D, Erden I. Changes in the TMJ disc-condyle-fossa relationship following functional treatment of skeletal class II division 1 malocclusion: a magnetic resonance imaging study. Am J Orthod Dentofacial Orthop. 2001;119(3):316–9.
126. Franco AA, Yamashita HK, Lederman HM, Cevidanes LH, Proffit WR, Vigorito JW. Fränkel appliance therapy and the temporomandibular disc: a prospective magnetic resonance imaging study. Am J Orthod Dentofacial Orthop. 2002;121(5):447–57.
127. Batista KB, Thiruvenkatachari B, Harrison JE, O'Brien KD. Orthodontic treatment for prominent upper front teeth (class II malocclusion) in children and adolescents. Cochrane Database Syst Rev. 2018;3(3):CD003452.

128. Seehra J, Fleming PS, Newton T, DiBiase AT. Bullying in orthodontic patients and its relationship to malocclusion, self-esteem and oral health-related quality of life. J Orthod. 2011;38:247–56.
129. Kallunki J, Sollenius O, Paulsson L, Petrén S, Dimberg L, Bondemark L. Oral health-related quality of life among children with excessive overjet or unilateral posterior crossbite with functional shift compared to children with no or mild orthodontic treatment need. Eur J Orthod. 2019;41:111–6.
130. Kallunki J, Bondemark L, Paulsson L. Early headgear activator treatment of class II malocclusion with excessive overjet: a randomized controlled trial. Eur J Orthod. 2021;43:639–47.
131. Cobourne MT, DiBiase AT, Seehra J, Papageorgiou SN. Should we recommend early overjet reduction to prevent dental trauma? Br Dent J. 2022;233(5):387–90.
132. Petti S. Over two hundred million injuries to anterior teeth attributable to large overjet: a meta-analysis. Dent Traumatol. 2015;31:1–8.
133. Magno MB, Nadelman P, Leite KLF, Ferreira DM, Pithon MM, Maia LC. Associations and risk factors for dental trauma: a systematic review of systematic reviews. Community Dent Oral Epidemiol. 2020;48(6):447–63.
134. Glendor U, Jonsson D, Halling A, Lindqvist K. Direct and indirect costs of dental trauma in Sweden: a 2-year prospective study of children and adolescents. Community Dent Oral Epidemiol. 2001;29(2):150–60.
135. De Clerck HJ, Proffit WR. Growth modification of the face: a current perspective with emphasis on class III treatment. Am J Orthod Dentofacial Orthop. 2015;148(1):37–46.
136. Pancherz H. The effect of continuous bite jumping on the dentofacial complex: a follow-up study after Herbst appliance treatment of class II malocclusions. Eur J Orthod. 1981;3(1):49–60.
137. Melsen B. Effects of cervical anchorage during and after treatment: an implant study. Am J Orthod. 1978;73(5):526–40.
138. Pancherz H. The Herbst appliance—its biologic effects and clinical use. Am J Orthod. 1985;87(1):1–20.
139. Cacciatore G, Ugolini A, Sforza C, Gbinigie O, Plüddemann A. Long-term effects of functional appliances in treated versus untreated patients with class II malocclusion: a systematic review and meta-analysis. PLoS One. 2019;14(9):e0221624.

4 Removable Functional Appliances in the Treatment of Class II Malocclusion

Andrew DiBiase and Jonathan Sandler

4.1 The Development of Removable Functional Appliances

The first recognisable functional appliance systems that were developed were monobloc appliances collectively referred to as activators. The earliest was developed in Norway by a Danish dentist Andresen. Apocryphally it was following treatment of his own daughter with fixed appliances that the original appliance was developed as a retention plate to be worn at night [1]. She still had Class II tendency at the end of active treatment that was resolved during this retention period as the vulcanite plate used, incorporated a postural element. With his colleague Häupl, Andresen developed what became known as the Norwegian system. This consisted of simple and robust monbloc appliance known as an activator that postured the mandible forward by the extension of the vulcanite into the lingual sulcus of the lower arch. The only wire work the appliance had was a labial bow. The vulcanite or acrylic could be trimmed to 'guide the eruption' of the posterior teeth to aid in the Class II correction.

The majority of subsequent removable appliance systems have in part been based on this original activator. Appliances such as the Bionator developed by Balters and the appliance developed by Bimler reduced the bulk of the original activator, replacing acrylic with wire work. Later activators, such as the Teuscher and Van Beek appliances, incorporated the use of headgear in an attempt to restrain the maxilla and optimise the antero-posterior growth of the mandible, whilst limiting the rotational and inevitable vertical effects of appliances.

One major deviation from the original activator design was the functional regulators developed by Fränkel in East Germany in the second half of the twentieth century [2]. A believer in the functional matrix theory of growth espoused by Van der Klaauw and Moss, Fränkel developed a series of appliances designed to change the activity of musculature and soft tissues that in turn would then affect the positions of the teeth and jaws called functional regulators. To do this the FRII appliance for Class II correction incorporates buccal or vestibular shields to allow expansion of the dental arches as the forces of the cheeks and buccinator are removed and labial pallots in the lower labial sulcus to remove the force of the mentalis muscle away from the lower incisors. They are however both bulky and fragile appliances making compliance and breakages a problem.

A. DiBiase (✉)
East Kent Hospitals University NHS Foundation Trust, Canterbury, UK

J. Sandler
Chesterfield Royal Hospital, Chesterfield, UK

M. T. Cobourne (ed.), *Orthodontic Management of Class II Malocclusion*,
https://doi.org/10.1007/978-3-031-57530-3_4

In the 1970s Clark in Kirkaldy, Scotland developed the Twin Block appliance that has largely superseded activator-type appliances in the UK [3]. This a major departure from the monobloc, as the appliance is in two parts, the forward posture being created by occlusal blocks that encourage the patient to bite in a protrusive position. The advantage of this is the appliance can technically be worn full time as it has significantly less limitation on function. It has become one of the most widely used and researched removable appliances, and has been shown to be clinically extremely effective. The rest of this chapter will therefore focus exclusively on the use of the Twin Block appliance.

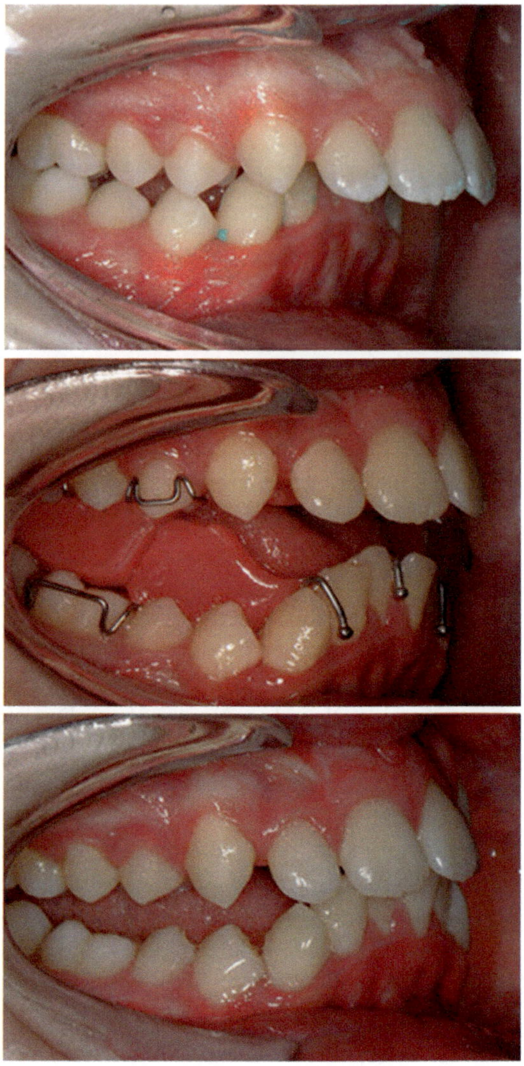

Fig. 4.1 Large overjet successfully reduced with a Twin Block functional appliance

4.2 Clinical Use of the Twin Block Appliance

When using a functional appliance to correct a Class II malocclusion it is imperative for the clinician to have explicit and specific aims of treatment, and in addition to understand all the effects that the appliance will have both on the jaws and the dentition, whether desirable or not. As such, embarking upon a course of Twin Block therapy can be likened to a journey and as with every journey, it is important to completely understand not only the starting point but also to have a clear view of the destination.

In a growing patient with a Class II Division I incisor relationship, on a skeletal II base, if an appropriately designed Twin Block is fitted to a reasonably cooperative patient, then we can reliably expect overjet and overbite correction, from a 10 mm overjet with an increased overbite down to an 'edge-to-edge' relationship, over an 8- or 9-month treatment period (Fig. 4.1) with a corresponding improvement in the facial profile (Fig. 4.2). One of the advantages of the Twin Block appliance compared to a monobloc such as an activator is the facility to simultaneously expand the upper arch to address any potential transverse discrepancy while addressing both the sagittal and the vertical discrepancies. This can be achieved using a midline expansion screw placed in the upper appliance that can be activated one-quarter of a turn per week, corresponding to approximately 0.2 mm of expansion.

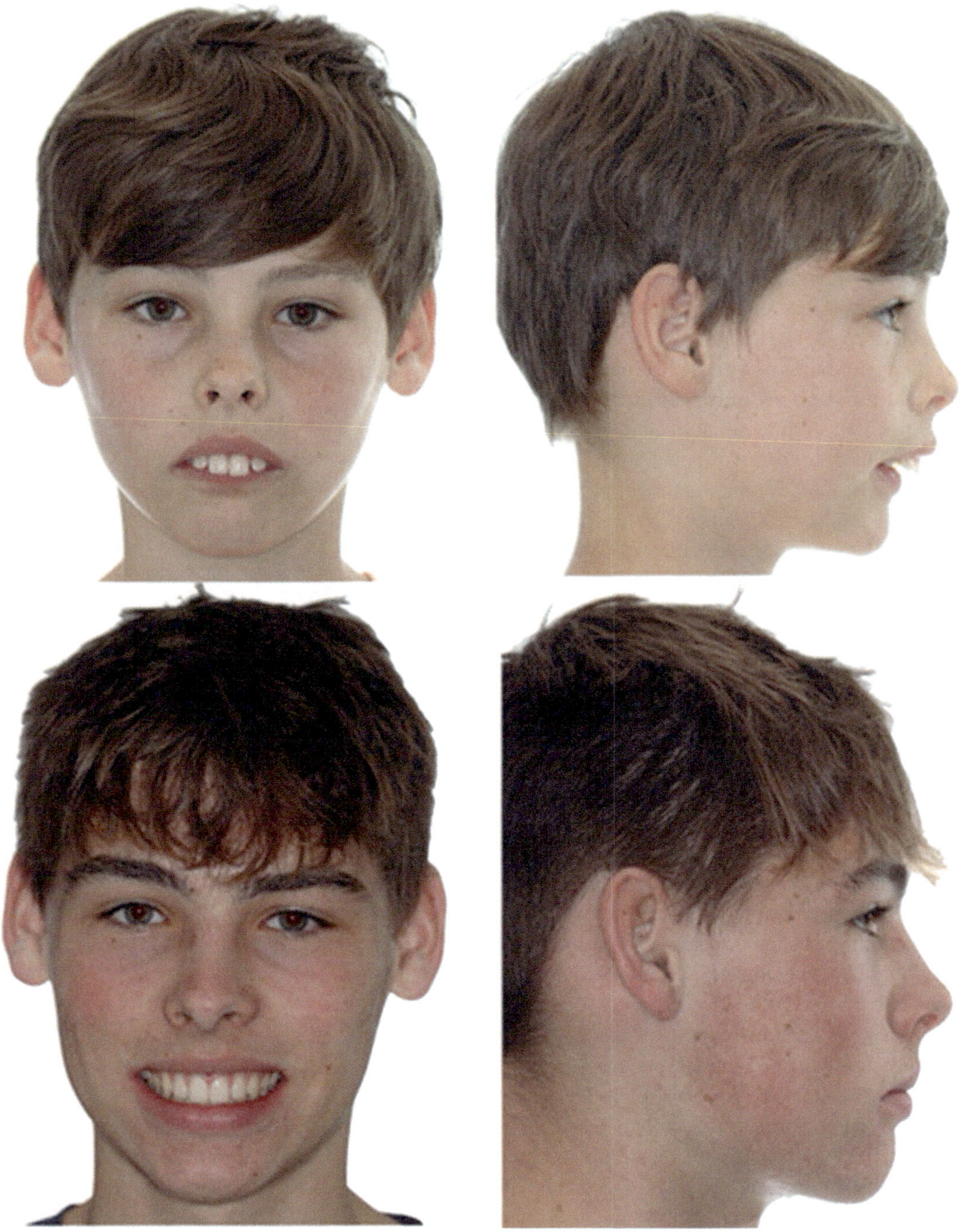

Fig. 4.2 Improvement in soft tissue profile following Twin Block appliance treatment

During the 9 months Twin Block treatment this would achieve a significant amount of upper arch expansion, which corrects the transverse discrepancy. The need for transverse expansion can be determined at the outset, merely by asking the patient to posture forwards in an edge-to-edge occlusion to allow reassessment of the transverse relationship between the upper and lower dentition.

Functional appliances have been shown to effect Class II correction primarily through dento-alveolar change. The Twin Block is no exception, and the upper incisors will, on average, retrocline 11 ° and the lower incisors will procline 8 ° [4]. This upper incisor retroclination and lower incisor proclination will generally occur whether or not this is one of the desirable treatment aims. These inevitable tooth movements will have to be factored into any future treatment plans when reassessing the space requirement at the end of the Twin Block phase of treatment. The benefit of carrying out the first 6–9 months of treatment with a Twin Block appliance is that all the 'heavy lifting' is performed during this period, converting a significant Class II malocclusion into a Class I malocclusion. In the vast majority of these cases, the functional appliance phase can then be seamlessly followed by a course of upper and lower fixed appliances for the next 12–15 months, aimed at consolidating the Class I occlusion, levelling and aligning the dentition and detailing the occlusion, including closing any lateral open bites that usually remain when treating a Class II malocclusion with an increased overbite and increased curve of Spee in the lower arch.

The beauty of the Twin Block is not only its effectiveness but also its versatility, in that it can be equally effective in correcting a Class II buccal segment relationship and increased overbite commonly seen in Class II Division 2 malocclusions [5]. At the same time as the sagittal correction of the malocclusion is being addressed, the upper incisors are actively advanced either by using a sectional fixed appliance on the upper anterior teeth, where there is sufficient crowding to 'keystone' the aligned teeth in a more anterior position, or alternatively adding T-springs palatal to the upper central incisors (Fig. 4.3). A labial bow can be added where T-springs are being used, adjusted to be 1 mm ahead of the upper central incisors at all times to allow their advancement under the effect of the springs. Sequential advancement of the labial bow and reactivation of the T-springs should occur at each six-weekly check-up visit, with the effect of converting the patient from having retroclined upper incisors to proclined upper incisors, but simultaneously correcting the sagittal discrepancy by sequential reactivation of the Twin Block.

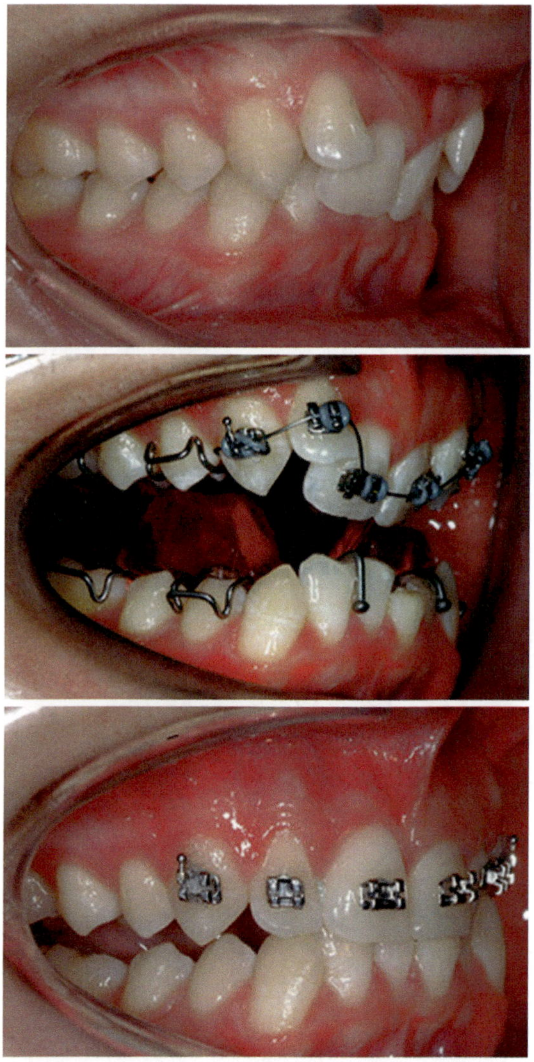

Fig. 4.3 Treatment of a Class II Division 2 malocclusion using a sectional upper fixed appliance to decompensate the upper labial segment and a Twin Block appliance for simultaneous sagittal correction

4.3 Design of the Twin Block Appliance

The single most important feature in the design of Twin Blocks is to ensure sufficient vertical opening of the blocks, which effect the success of Class II correction when the appliance is in place. As a 'rule of thumb' 7–8 mm vertical height of the blocks is recommended. This is because the success of treatment with a Twin Block appliance is solely dependent on having a sufficient amount of vertical opening in the buccal segments to ensure the patient occludes into the desired position, with the mandible postured forwards by a predetermined amount. Achieving sufficient vertical separation will ensure that for reasons of comfort, the patient actively chooses to slide their lower jaw forwards and keep their teeth together in the desired position, rather than occluding on the blocks in the retruded contact position, which will occur when the height of the bite blocks is too shallow, making the appliance less effective [6]. This is why these authors consider it vital the blocks should be between 7 and 8 mm in height rather than 5 mm or less as has been described [7].

Retention of the Twin Block is another reason for this appliance being adopted as the default functional appliance in the United Kingdom over the past 40 years. Whilst the original appliance design used Delta clasps, it has been found the use of Adams clasps on first molars and first premolars and ball clasps in the labial segment will in most cases provide the best retention. This is the simplest, most efficient and effective way to provide retention of the Twin Block, particularly during the first few weeks of use when the patient is initially getting used to the appliance, a period that is absolutely critical to the success of the treatment. The Adams clasps on the lower molar teeth may be cut away at subsequent visits if there is a need for differential eruption of the lower molar teeth to contribute to closure of the lateral open bites and overbite reduction. Eruption will occur when a small amount of acrylic is trimmed away from the upper block, however care must be taken to avoid reducing the inclined planes of the blocks which, if trimmed, would reduce the total height of the upper block. To allow this differential molar eruption the blocks must be positioned anteriorly enough so the anterior surface of the upper block sits mesially to the lower first permanent molar.

It is also important that the patient should not be overburdened with instructions at the Twin Block fit appointment, so generally it is advised that the midline screw should be turned one-quarter turn probably starting activation from the second visit after fitting the appliance, and continued until sufficient transverse correction has occurred. The labial bow, which was placed on the original Twin Block design, is no longer used routinely apart from the aforementioned Class II Division 2 modification. It adds little to retention, makes the appliance more unsightly and results in unfavourable dentoalveolar changes [8].

4.4 Bite Registration for Twin Block

The aim of bite registration in a typical Class II Division I patient is generally to correct the sagittal discrepancy in the canine and molar relationship, from Class II to a Class I or even a slight Class III tendency. There is no set rule on how far to advance the mandible when taking the bite, as this will vary in different patients. Usually, the overjet should be reduced by about 70–80% on the first bite registration, but of course this will be dependent upon the size of the original overjet. With very large overjets, over 15 mm, it would be unreasonable to expect an 80% reduction and the upper block may need to be reactivated sometimes two or even three times before the desired edge-to-edge position can be achieved. A much more important consideration when taking the jaw registration, as previously mentioned, is the amount of vertical opening in the buccal segments as irrespective of whatever advancement of the mandible is achieved, this can always be reactivated at a subsequent visit.

The authors recommend a full sheet of softened pink wax to be used for registration of the protruded bite, as opposed to pre-made bite registration fork. The problem with bite forks is that the thickness of plastic anteriorly determines the

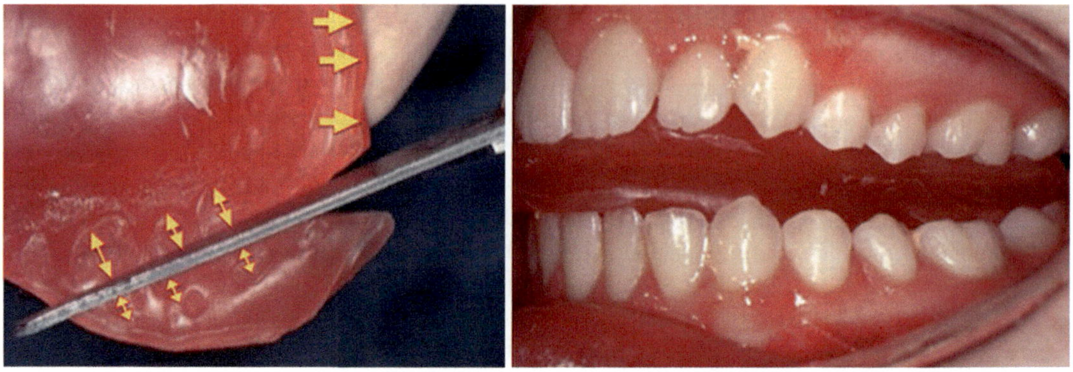

Fig. 4.4 Wax bite registration for a Twin Block appliance showing trimming of wax to allow accurate assessment of vertical clearance in buccal segments for the blocks

amount of vertical opening in the buccal segments. A carefully trimmed wax bite, that has been moulded into the palatal tissues and the palatal surfaces and lingual cusps of the upper teeth, allows the clinician to correctly assess and adjust this vertical separation (Fig. 4.4). Trimming of the wax bite is an important step in taking the postured bite registration before appliance construction. Wax should carefully be removed over the buccal half of the occlusal surface, so that the wax bite registers the palatal cusps of the premolar and molar teeth and also clearly shows some of the palatal surfaces of the anterior teeth. The buccal cusps should be completely clear of wax so that, when the wax bite is placed back in the patient's mouth, the amount of vertical separation of the teeth in the premolar area can be measured. It should also be removed from the labial surfaces of the incisors so the relative position of the dental centrelines can be assessed in the postured bite. If there is any skeletal asymmetry one of the aims of the functional phase of treatment maybe to attempt to correct this. The jaw registration must clearly register the lingual cusps and incisal edges of the lower teeth so that the technician can accurately locate the models on the simple hinge articulator in the laboratory.

4.5 Twin Block Fit

One of the main problems of any removable appliance including the Twin Block is non-compliance which will result in failed treatment. The fit visit is therefore extremely important. Simple explicit instructions must be given to the patient on the initial fit of the appliance. This involves engendering an enthusiastic and extremely positive approach which will help to get even the initially reluctant and nervous patients 'on-side.' If there are small design flaws, or issues of fit, they should be sorted out in a positive manner and the patient should not be unnecessarily alerted to any problems. This fit visit includes assessing the fit and design of the appliance, to make sure the patient can comfortably bite forward in front of the upper block. If the patient is really struggling to bite forward into the postured bite, or the blocks have been made too high, meaning the appliance will be very difficult to wear, the blocks will need adjusting. This may involve some careful chairside adjustment using a slow handpiece to reduce either the height or anteroposterior activation of the blocks or sending the appliance back to the laboratory for adjustment with a new postured bite. Once the patient has been shown how to insert and remove the upper and the lower blocks, how to bite together and how to speak with their teeth together this can then be explained by the patient to their parent or guardian. Again, a positive attitude is very important, and both the parent and patient should be reassured the initial issues with lisping and slurred speech and increased salivation will all improve with wear.

Some orthodontists advise a gradual increase in wear hours to allow patients to get used to the appliance. It is the authors' opinion that patients should be encouraged to wear full time from the start. Invariably patients will wear appliances for less hours than prescribed and despite this we still see remarkable results with the Twin Block appliance. The danger is that a prescription for part-time wear in reality becomes very part-time wear resulting in failure of treatment [9, 10]. This will result in the patient taking much longer to adapt to the appliance, slower Class II correction and ultimately the patient wearing the Twin Block appliance for significantly longer with a higher risk of treatment failure.

4.6 Twin Block Review and Monitoring Progress

The parent is told on the first visit that if their children are having problems with the Twin Blocks, they must keep wearing the blocks but return to the department as soon as possible to allow any necessary adjustments to be made. If the patients stop wearing the appliance, then any gains that have been hard won will be rapidly lost and the Twin Blocks will no longer fit comfortably. They must be given the opportunity to come back and be seen without delay if they are having problems. Ideally, the patient does not need to be seen following fit of the appliance for about 6–8 weeks as if the Twin Block has been well made, and the patient is wearing it as instructed, it will produce sagittal, vertical and transverse improvements.

At the first review, the most important thing is to listen to the patient speaking with the appliance in place. With a little experience with the Twin Block, just by listening to the patient it will be possible to estimate the degree of compliance. With good wear, the initial lisping should have all but resolved and the patient should be able to speak comfortably and intelligibly with the appliance in place. Any persistence of a lisp or difficulty speaking is a sign the appliance is not being worn as instructed. This will be evidenced by a lack of reduction in the overjet when measured.

As discussed at the outset of this chapter, knowing exactly where you are in treatment is paramount to guaranteeing success. Every time the patient comes into the clinic for a review, the following sequence of measurements should be made: overjet, overbite, centreline, reverse overjet, molar relationship and canine relationship. Considering these, as well as how well the patient has adapted to the appliance will allow the clinician to monitor progress. Using a correctly designed and constructed Twin Block appliance in an appropriate case, with a cooperative patient, the overjet should be reducing by 1–2 mm every 6 weeks with the overbite, in deep bite case, showing a similar reduction of 1–2 mm every visit. As the overjet reduces the reverse overjet (overjet measurement with the patient maximally protruded) should be increasing by the same amount. The canine and molar relationship should also be showing concomitant changes in the appropriate direction.

The most important measurement, when assessing progress, is the reverse overjet because the overjet measurement can be misleading [11] (Fig. 4.5). Patients will develop a

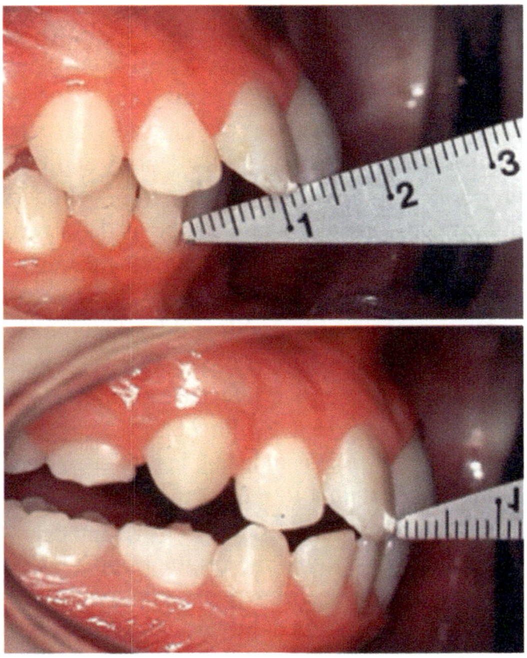

Fig. 4.5 Measurement of the overjet and overjet at maximum posture to ascertain progress during functional appliance treatment

tendency to posture the mandible forward giving a false impression of progress. The reverse overjet measurement however, with the patients protruding their mandible maximally, cannot be faked. Ideally, if the patient is being successfully encouraged into retruded contact then the difference in the measurement between overjet and reverse overjet will remain constant throughout treatment. Both of these measurements should be accurately recorded at every visit.

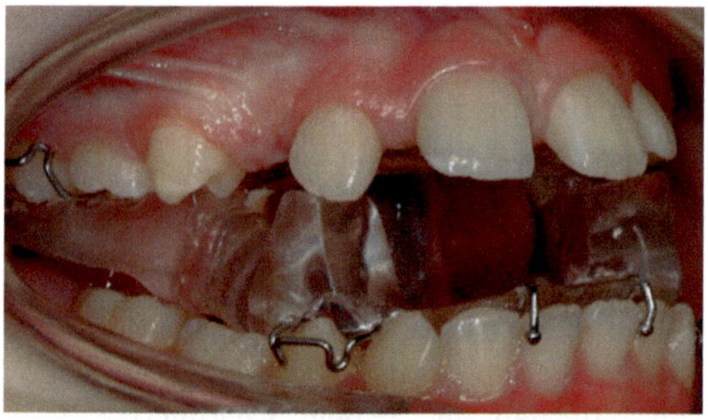

Fig. 4.6 Reactivation of a Twin Block using pre-cut blocks of acrylic attached to the mesial of the upper block

4.7 Twin Block Reactivation

Due to the positive Class II correction of the appliance following fitting, Twin Blocks can become less effective after the first 3 or 4 months of functional appliance treatment. If a satisfactory bite registration is taken at the first visit, they should not be able to posture much further forward on the appliance fit visit. Usually on the third or fourth visit however, the patient will be able to posture significantly further forward opening a gap between the two blocks. The appliance should at this point be reactivated using acrylic to the upper block. This can either be done free hand, by adding cold-cure acrylic to the inclined plane of the upper block, or by adding a pre-formed block of acrylic made from cylinders of heat-cured acrylic. These can be made in various sizes between 3 and 5 mm and attached to the Twin Block with cold cure acrylic (Fig. 4.6). Activation in this manner should be done on the inclined plane of the upper block. This is because when there is a deep overbite and increased curve of Spee often associated with Class II malocclusions, as the overjet is reduced, lateral open bites result. In an attempt to reduce these, the Adams clasps can be removed from the lower molars and the occlusal surface of the original upper block trimmed to allow differential eruption of the lower first and second molars. It is therefore important that the lower block does not extend distally beyond the lower second premolar to cover the surface of the lower first molar as this will prevent its eruption.

The Twin Block occasionally requires activation a second time in treatment, particularly if the original overjet is over 15 mm. In most cases, the endpoint of the initial phase of Twin Block is with the patient in and edge-to-edge bite with a 0 mm overjet, and a 0 mm overbite. The patient may also have lateral open bites in the buccal segments if despite differential trimming of the upper block there is still an increased curve of Spee. This is rarely if ever a significant challenge to close these down during the subsequent fixed appliance treatment.

4.8 Transition to Fixed Appliances

In the vast majority of cases, it is desirable to undertake a course of fixed appliances following successful treatment with a Twin Block. This will be to level and align the arches and detail the occlusion consolidating the Class I buccal segment and incisor relationships. There are numerous strategies that can be employed but a useful way to transition to the straight wire appliance is to use an upper removable appliance with an inclined anterior bite plane to maintain the postured position of the mandible [12, 13]. This can be held in place using Plint or flyover clasps engaging with the headgear tubes on bands placed on the upper first molars for retention and ball-ended clasps engaging with the buccal segment or anterior dentition (Fig. 4.7). The bite plane should be steep and deep ensuring the patient occludes in front of it as opposed to

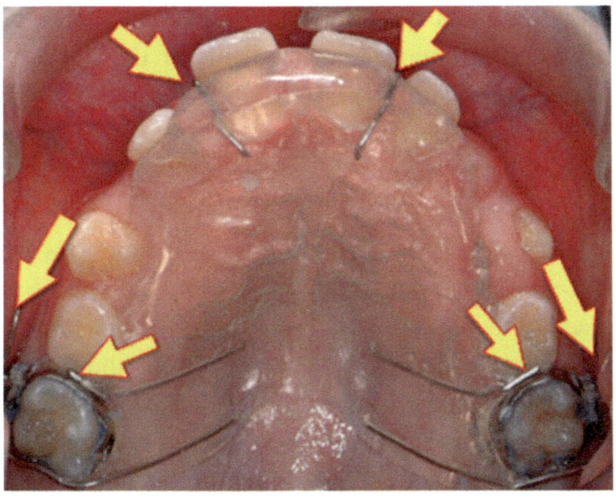

Fig. 4.7 An upper removable appliance with an inclined bite plane with flyover cribs and ball-ended clasps highlighted for retention used during the transition from functional to fixed appliances to maintain the mandibular position

behind it. The patient is asked to wear the inclined plane full time initially, apart from eating, swimming and during contact sport. This steep and deep clip bite plane serves to remind the patient to close in the position achieved during the 9-month Twin Block therapy, but at the same time it allows placement of upper and lower fixed appliances, and with careful trimming of the palatal interproximal acrylic some premolar derotation and space closure in the buccal segments can be undertaken. The inclined bite plane is continued during the initial aligning phase of treatment until the placement of the working archwires. If using a 0.022 × 0.028 in. bracket slot these are usually 0.019 × 0025 in. stainless steel arch wires. This is when Class II elastics can be used. The Class II elastics will then continue to help maintain any sagittal correction achieved, assisting space closure in the upper and lower arches and maintain the overjet and overbite correction achieved by contributing to lateral open bite closure (Fig. 4.8).

Alternative strategies include part-time wear of the appliance at night for a period of time before moving into fixed appliances. While this has the benefit of maintaining the Class II correction achieved, it will inevitably lead to unnecessary extension of overall treatment time while allowing only limited occlusal settling.

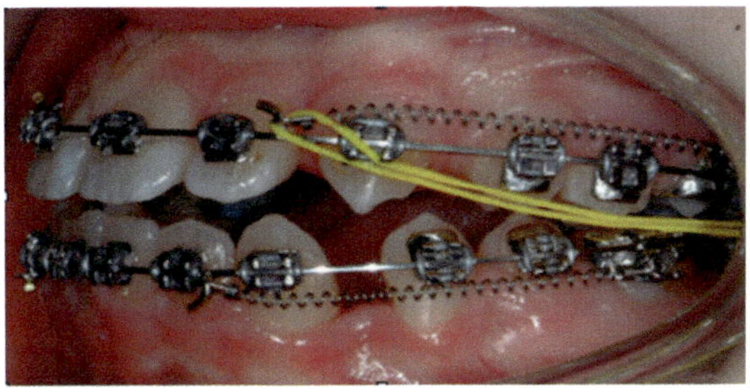

Fig. 4.8 Use of Class II intermaxillary traction during fixed appliances following initial treatment with a functional appliance once into rectangular steel wires

4.9 Finishing Twin Block Cases

As in all comprehensive orthodontic treatment, the aim is to finish to a high standard, to optimise the aesthetic and functional result. This will usually involve dropping down from the 0.019 × 0.025-in. stainless steel working archwires into light wires such as 0.016-in. Australian regular stainless steel wire that allow occlusal settling. Finishing bends can be placed in these wires to correct any slight inaccuracies in bracket position, to make any adjustments to the tip or in-out of teeth, thus correcting both the contact points and the marginal ridge positions. Two or three finishing visits in 0.016-in. stainless steel wires are usually sufficient to allow full correction of the malocclusion. The average treatment time would be about 9 months in Twin Blocks followed by 12–15 months in fixed appliances. This is comparable to overall treatment times found with fixed Class II correctors such as the Herbst or Forsus appliances [14, 15].

4.10 Evidence for Twin Block Treatment Effects

How functional appliances work and whether they affect meaningful skeletal change has been one of the core questions at the heart of orthodontics. Historically animal experiments in rats and primates had shown by placing hyper-propulsive appliances in otherwise normal dentitions, skeletal change and remodelling was found in the condyle and at the glenoid fossa [16–18]. This led many to believe functional appliances could actually increase the growth of the mandible. There is however now a body of high-quality evidence from several large RCTs that has questioned this [19–21]. It appears, as with other functional appliances, that the short-term effects of the Twin Block appliance are mostly dentoalveolar, effecting Class II correction by retroclination of the maxillary incisors and distal tipping of the buccal dentition and proclination of the mandibular incisors [4, 22–26]. There does appear to be a small but significant effect on the position and growth of the mandible most of which is directed vertically. Use of high-pull headgear has been advocated in an attempt to control this vertical growth and optimise the antero-posterior change but this requires even greater compliance from the patient in what is already very demanding treatment [27, 28]. Therefore, the risks tend to outweigh the benefits and headgear is not routinely used except in high-angle cases with a hyperdivergent growth pattern.

The 'extra growth' seen during the functional phase of treatment seems to disappear in the post-functional period with less growth of the mandible in patients treated with Twin Blocks during that period [29]. Therefore, in the long term, it appears the Twin Block as with all functional appliances does not affect the underlying size or shape of the mandible. What appears to happen is that by using a functional appliance such as a Twin Block, the occlusion is changed from Class II to Class I utilising the underlying cephalocaudal growth pattern whereby on average the mandible grows more than the maxilla during the adolescent growth spurt. Without the use of a functional appliance, the occlusion maintains the Class II relationship despite this growth [30]. Therefore, it appears that Kingsley's original concept of 'jumping the bite' was indeed correct.

4.11 Twin Blocks: A Patient-Centred Approach

The authors firmly believe that the most important factor when providing Twin Block appliance therapy is a positive attitude. This means that the clinicians and the nurses should be very careful with the language used in front of the patients and the parents when initially fitting the Twin Block appliance. Our advice is to keep the parents out of the surgery when the Twin Block is initially being fitted. The patient should be instructed to keep their teeth together and to wear the appliance '24 h a day.' It should be emphasised, the outcome of their treatment is totally within their control and if they wear the appliance as instructed, in a short period of time, they will see a dramatic changes to the position of the teeth and the jaws. Patients who have an internal locus of control whereby they feel treatment is being done for them and not just to them tend to do very well with Twin Block treatment.

A demonstration should be given to the patient of how they can in fact speak with their teeth together as a small number of patients are really reluctant to start talking with the appliance in place. Our advice is to start immediately with full-time wear, as it can be confusing to ask the patients to wear it a couple of hours this week, and then increasing the number of hours in subsequent weeks. It is also easy for patients to find excuses not to wear the appliances. With full-time wear, there can be no such excuses. Once the patient is fully familiar with fitting the appliance, how they are to occlude forward into it, the parents can now be invited into the surgery. We then leave it to the child to explain to the parents how the appliances work. This again gives the patient control and responsibility for the success of their own treatment, enhancing further an internal locus of control. This patient-centred approach has been found to be successful even in the most challenging cases.

4.12 Summary

The Twin Block is an extremely effective appliance for Class II correction in growing patients. While in the short term most of the effects are dentoalveolar, the Twin Block appliance does seem to have an effect on the position and possibly growth of the mandible. However, in the long term this disappears. The effectiveness of the appliance is dictated by the height and inclination of the blocks and like all removable appliances its efficiency is also dictated by good compliance. By developing a patient-centred approach this can be optimised. Accordingly, we recommend full-time wear from the outset. With a well-designed and constructed appliance and with good compliance, the Twin Block appliance can be used even in the most severe Class II malocclusions.

References

1. Schmuth GPF. Milestones in the development and practical application of functional appliances. Am J Orthod. 1983;84:48–53.
2. Fränkel R. The treatment of class II, Divison 1 malocclusion with functional correctors. Am J Orthod. 1969;55:265–75.
3. Clark WJ. The twin block technique. A functional orthopedic appliance system. Am J Orthod Dentofacial Orthop. 1988;93:1–18.
4. Lund DI, Sandler PJ. The effects of twin blocks: a prospective controlled study. Am J Orthod Dentofacial Orthop. 1998;113:104–10.
5. Dyer FM, McKeown HF, Sandler PJ. The modified twin block appliance in the treatment of class II division 2 malocclusions. J Orthod. 2001 Dec;28(4):271–80.
6. Gill SD, Lee RT. Prospective clinical trial comparing the effects of conventional twin-block and mini-block appliances: part 1. Hard tissue changes. Am J Orthod Dentofacial Orthop. 2005;127:465–72.
7. Clark W. Design and managements of twin blocks: reflections after 30 years of clinical use. J Orthod. 2010;37:209–16.
8. Yaqoob O, DiBiase AT, Fleming PS, Cobourne MT. Use of the clark twin block functional appliance with and without an upper labial bow: a randomized controlled trial. Angle Orthod. 2012;82:363–9.
9. Parekh J, Counihan K, Fleming PS, Pandis N, Sharma PK. Effectiveness of part-time vs full-time wear protocols of Twin-block appliance on dental and skeletal changes: A randomized controlled trial. Am J Orthod Dentofacial Orthop. 2019;155:165–72.
10. Frilund E, Sonesson M, Magnusson A. Patient compliance with twin block appliance during treatment of class II malocclusion: a randomized contolled trial on two check-up prescriptions. Eur J Orthod. 2022;45:142–9. https://doi.org/10.1093/ejo/cjac046.
11. Petit HP, Chateau M. The K test and the condylar test. J Clin Orthod. 1984;18:726–32.
12. Fleming P, Scott P, DiBiase A. How to…manage the transition from functional to fixed appliances. J Orthod. 2007;34:252–9.
13. Sandler PJ, DiBiase DD. The inclined bite plane—a useful clinical tool. Am J Orthod Dentofacial Orthop. 1996;110:339–50.
14. O'Brien K, Wright J, Conboy F, et al. Effectiveness of treatment for Class II malocclusion with the Herbst or Twin-block appliances: a randomised, controlled trial. Am J Orthod Dentofacial Orthop. 2003;124:128–37.
15. Giuntini V, Vangelisti A. Masucci et al treatment effects produced by the twin-block appliance vs the Forsus fatigue resistant device in growing class II patients. Angle Orthod. 2015;85:784–9.
16. Charlier JP, Petrovic A, Herrmann-Stutzmann J. Effects of mandibular hyperpropulsion on the prechondroblastic zone of young rat condyle. Am J Orthod. 1969;55:71–4.
17. McNamara JA Jr, Bryan FA. Long-term mandibular adaptations to protrusive function: an experimental study in Macaca mulatta. Am J Orthod Dentofacial Orthop. 1987;92:98–108.
18. Voudouris JC, Woodside DG, Altuna G, Kuftinec MM, Angelopouus G, Borque PJ. Condyle fossa modifications and muscle interactions during Herbst treatment. Part 2. Results and conclusions. Am J Orthod Dentofacial Orthop. 2003;124:13–29.
19. Tulloch JF, Proffitt WR, Phillips C. Outcomes in a 2-phase randomized clinical trial of early class II treatment. Am J Orthod Dentofacial Orthop. 2004;125:657–67.
20. Dolce C, MCGorray SP, Brazeau L, et al. Timing of class II treatment: skeletal changes comparing 1-phase and 2-phase treatment. Am J Orthod Dentofacial Orthop. 2007;132:481–9.
21. O'Brien K, Wright J, Conboy F, et al. Early treatment for class II division 1 malocclusion with twin-block appliance: a multi-center, randomized, controlled trial. Am J Orthod Dentofacial Orthop. 2009;135:573–9.
22. DeVincenzo JP. Changes in mandibular length before, during and after successful orthopedic correction of class II malocclusions using a functional appliance. Am J Orthod Dentofacial Orthop. 1991;99:241–57.
23. Mills CM, McCulloch KJ. Treatment effects of the twin block appliance: a cephalometric study. Am J Orthod Dentofacial Orthop. 1998;114:15–24.
24. O'Brien K, Wright J, Conboy F, et al. Effectiveness of early orthodontic treatment with the twin-block appliance: a multicentre, randomised, controlled trial. Part 1. Dental and skeletal effects. Am J Orthod Dentofacial Orthop. 2003;124:234–43.
25. Lee RT, Barnes E, Dibiase A, Govender R, Qureshi U. An extended period of functional appliance therapy: a controlled clinical trial comparing the twin block and dynamax appliances. Eur J Orthod. 2014;36:512–21.
26. Ehsani S, Nebbe B, Normando D, Lagravere MO, Flores-Mir C. Short-term treatment effects produced by the twin-block appliance: a systematic review and meta-analysis. Euro J Orthod. 2015;37:170–6.
27. Teuscher U. A growth related concept for skeletal class II treatment. Am J Orthod. 1978;74:258–75.

28. Parkin NA, McKeown HF, Sandler PJ. Comparison of 2 modifications of the twin-block appliance in matched class II samples. Am J Orthod Dentofacial Orthop. 2001 Jun;119(6):572–7.
29. DiBiase AT, Lucchesi L, Qureshi U, Lee RT. Post-treatment cephalometric changes in adolescent patients with class II malocclusion treated using 2 different functional appliance systems for an extended time period: a randomized clinical trial. Eur J Orthod. 2020;42:135–43.
30. You ZH, Fishman LS, Rosenblum RE, Subtelny JD. Dentoalveolar changes related to mandibular forward growth in untreated class II persons. Am J Orthod Dentofacial Orthop. 2001;120:598–607.

Fixed Functional Appliances in the Management of Class II Malocclusion

5

Mithran S. Goonewardene

5.1 Introduction

Clinicians across all health disciplines are often challenged with compliance issues with any proposed therapy, including patients with serious health problems [1]. Compliance with removable orthodontic appliances has been shown to be sub-optimal with many patients exaggerating the period of reported wear. Moreover, predicting compliance in the orthodontic patient has been shown to be difficult [2, 3].

Although the overall prevalence of class II malocclusion is reported between 15 and 20% of the population [4–7], approximately 30–40% of the patient's presenting for treatment in clinical practice are class II [8]. As with any treatment approach, compliance with orthodontic appliances is essential for success. With class II malocclusion patients often face the prospect of wearing removable appliances and/or adjuncts such as headgears and elastics for which excellent compliance is necessary.

Many clinicians are challenged with predicting the compliance in a specific patient prior to initiating a course of treatment [9]. Therefore with the perception of progressively reducing compliance in the patient population, there has been a trend to select appliances that do not rely as much on patient compliance.

In choosing the type of appliance (removable or fixed) the clinician has to consider the relative efficacy of these appliances from a dentofacial morphological perspective and patient-centred outcomes. However sound recommendations have not been reported due to the lack of robust studies [10]. Moreover, the cost of fixed class II correctors and the associated fixed appliance components may be prohibitive in some environments when compared to the laboratory costs of a removable appliance [11, 12].

It is critical for the clinician to recognise the numerous skeletal and dental characteristics of a specific malocclusion and clearly establish treatment goals that satisfy the individual patient's needs. Although clinicians often feel the necessity to establish efficient systems in their offices and can be tempted to select a consistent universal strategy for all class II patients, this may not satisfy the individual patient-centred goals. A "one size fits all" approach that simply fits the teeth together without considering issues such as lip support, incisor inclinations and chin position may not satisfy the patient-centred goals, then it has been said that "everything works" and "nothing really matters" when it comes to choice of strategy [13].

Management of class II discrepancies can be divided into three broad categories: Growth

M. S. Goonewardene (✉)
Discipline Lead and Graduate Program Convener in Orthodontics, UWA Dental School, The University of Western Australia (M512), Perth, Australia
e-mail: mithran.goonewardene@uwa.edu.au

M. T. Cobourne (ed.), *Orthodontic Management of Class II Malocclusion*,
https://doi.org/10.1007/978-3-031-57530-3_5

modification, orthodontic camouflage or combined surgery and orthodontics. In growth modification, facial and dentoalveolar growth and maturation are attempted to be utilised during sagittal correction; with orthodontic camouflage, compensatory tooth movements are effected by appliances that reposition the teeth in the best "compromised position" within existing skeletal envelope. The distinction between these categories is not so clear as components of dental compensation generally accompany growth modification strategies. In significant skeletal discrepancies, growth modification and/or orthodontic camouflage may not be able to achieve a desired outcome without significant compromise to aesthetics, health of the supporting soft and hard tissues of the alveolus or significant instability. In these circumstances, combined surgery and orthodontics may be considered carefully with its associated risks.

Clinicians have long held the belief that fixed and removable class II appliances have the capacity to stimulate jaw growth beyond the genetically determined plan. Theoretically, the mandible may express its innate capacity to grow at an earlier stage than originally patterned [14]. A favourable magnitude and direction of growth may effect the possibility for significant dentoalveolar compensation; however, the long-term alteration in the skeletal pattern has not been demonstrated in the literature [15].

The timing of initiating treatment for growing class II patients may vary between the choice of removable or fixed appliances. Removable appliances are generally inserted in the late mixed dentition with the expectation that the overjet will be corrected and the occlusion stabilised by the time that the child is in the early permanent dentition and ready to proceed with fixed appliances. Fixed appliances often rely on the presence of fully erupted permanent teeth for accurate and comfortable placement. Timing for both strategies focuses on reported favourable patterns of differential growth when the mandible outgrows the maxilla However, the overall changes are often minimal due to anterior and downward dentoalveolar compensatory mechanisms in the maxillary dentition [16, 17].

The treatment effects of the various reported appliances appear to be related to their ability to limit the compensatory movements of the maxillary dentition to follow the growing mandible [18, 19]. It is clear from high-quality reports that regardless of treatment timing, fixed or removable functional appliances do not provide any additional long-term growth [20].

5.2 Historical Perspectives in Fixed Class II Correctors

The concept of "bite jumping" to address class II malocclusion was reported by Kingsley in the 1860s [21] and his textbook "A Treatise of Oral Deformities as a Branch of Mechanical Surgery" was published in New York and Germany. Kingsley's application of a fixed bite plane influenced several Europeans including Pierre Robin, who introduced the monobloc appliance, specifically to posture the mandible forward and address issues related to the Pierre Robin syndrome (Fig. 5.1). Andresen independently developed an analogous appliance, the "activator" after an experience with his daughter's treatment. His daughter's fixed appliances were removed for the summer vacation and he placed a removable "Hawley" type appliance with a lingual flange to force the mandible forward 3–4 mm. After the summer, Andresen was surprised to see the class II relationship resolved and stable. These appliances were the forerunners to many of the contemporary functional appliances.

Emile Herbst introduced a fixed bite jumping appliance called the "Scharnier" (English translation-hinge) at the International Dental Congress in Berlin in 1909 (Fig. 5.2). He later

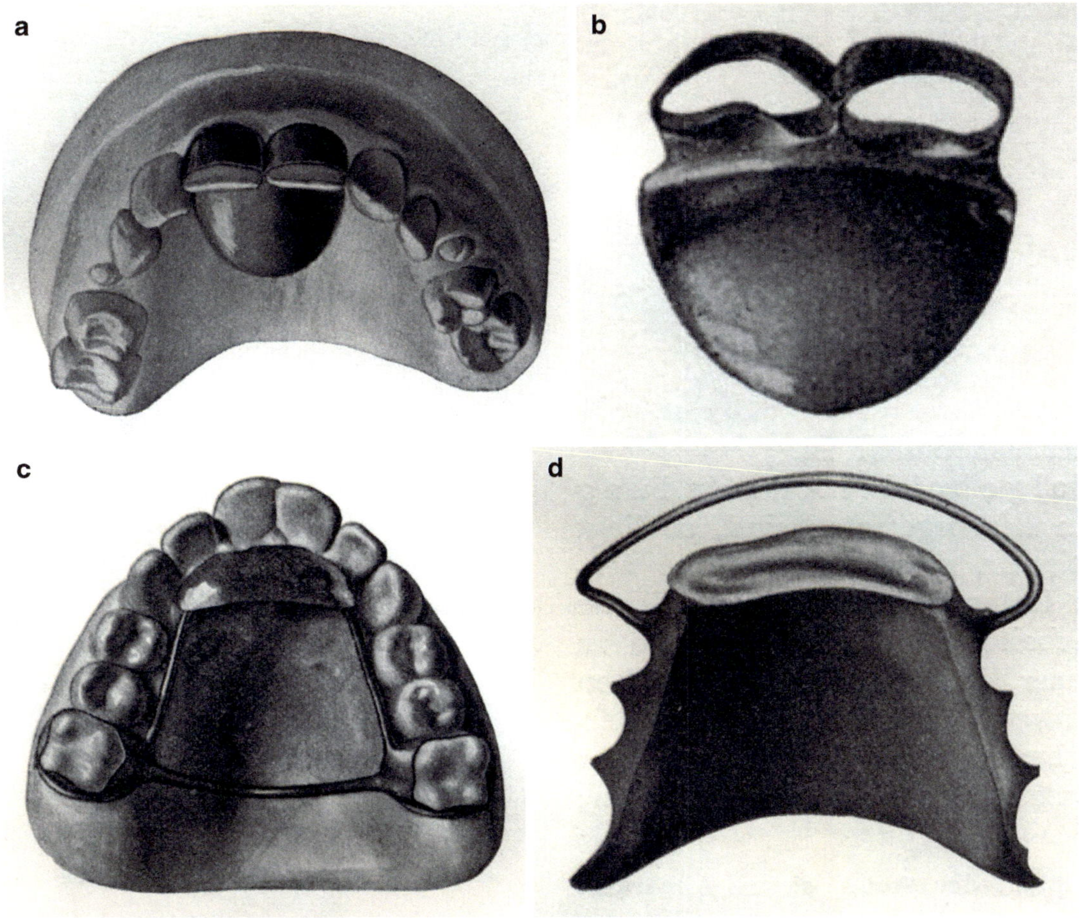

Fig. 5.1 Fixed inclined plane attached with gold clasps to the upper incisors (**a**, **b**). A modification of a fixed inclined plane attached to the molars (**c**) and a removable inclined bite plane (**d**) (From Herbst E. Atlas and Grundriss der Zahnärztlichen Orthopädie. J.F.Lehmann, Munich. 1910)

published a text in orthodontics in 1910 that included the "Scharnier" and a number of variants of bite jumping appliances that resemble many of the current fixed functional appliances [22] (Fig. 5.3).

In more than 30 years numerous designs of fixed functional appliances have been reported and a number of conclusions have been drawn. Although there are minor differences in the dental effects of these appliances, these differences have not been shown to be clinically significant in the long term. These effects include:

1. Distal movement of the upper dentoalveolus and proclination of the lower dentoalveolus, and this cannot be avoided.
2. Anterior positioning of the mandible with significant individual variation in the pattern and magnitude of change. The length of the mandible increased consistent with the normal variation in mandibular growth.
3. An increase in lower face height both anteriorly and posteriorly.
4. Clinically insignificant but mild restriction of maxillary growth.

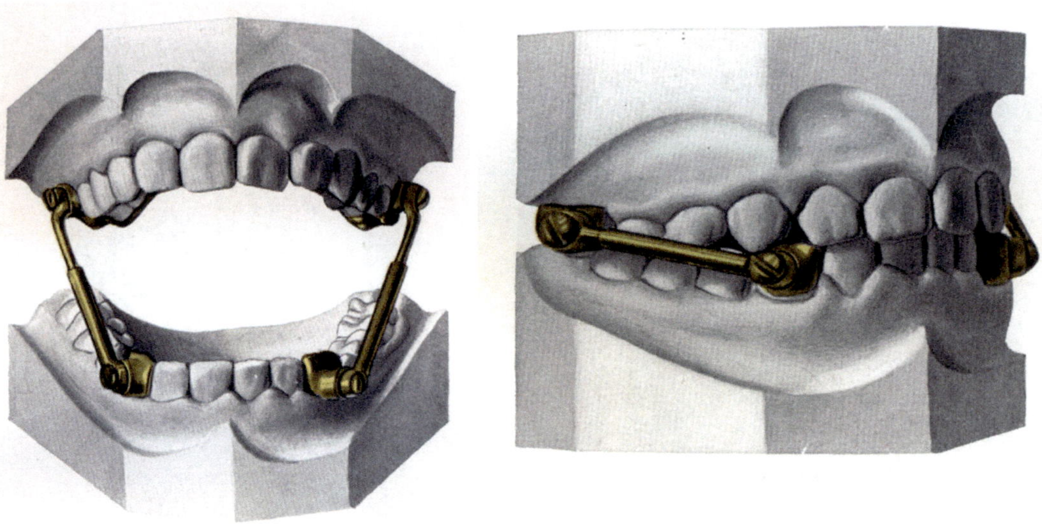

Fig. 5.2 Herbst's original appliance constructed in gold alloy, attached to crowns on the upper molars and lower premolars. (From Herbst E. Atlas and Grundriss der Zahnärztlichen Orthopädie. J.F.Lehmann, Munich. 1910)

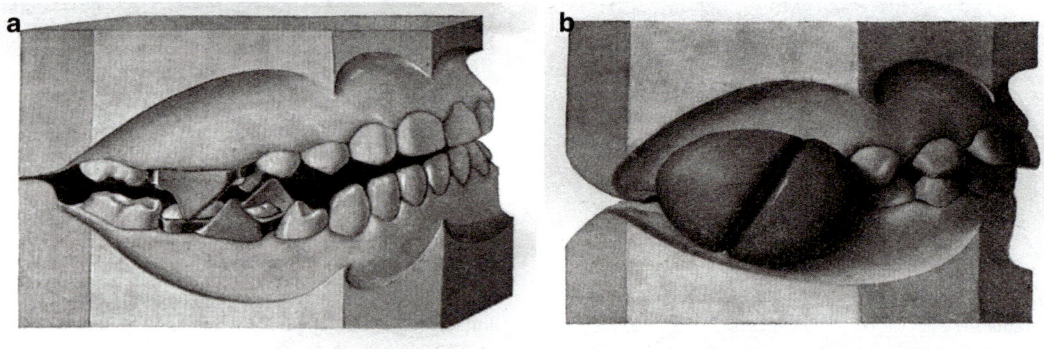

Fig. 5.3 A number of early variants of fixed mandibular protruding devices have been described by Herbst. An inclined plane attached to molar teeth with gold attachments (**a**). An inclined plane, rubber blocks attached to 3 gold rings on both the upper and lower arches (**b**). (From Herbst E. Atlas and Grundriss der Zahnärztlichen Orthopädie. J.F.Lehmann, Munich. 1910)

5.3 The Saif Spring

The use of multibracket appliances and class II elastic traction has been the mainstay for many clinicians since introduced by Dr. H Baker in Boston in the early 1900s [23]. Compliance has been and continues to be a challenge for both historical and current clinicians.

The Saif Spring was introduced in the 1960s by Armstrong [24]. A stainless steel spring of various lengths was attached to the banded appliances in a class II elastic configuration to overcome poor compliance (Fig. 5.4). The spring applied 200–400 g of force but its limited capacity to stretch and adapt to a range of mandibular excursions resulted in significant appliance breakage, although it had been reported to be very effective if the spring remained intact. In addition to the frequent breakages, the bulk of the spring posed an oral hygiene challenge so its popularity and modifications to its design rapidly waned.

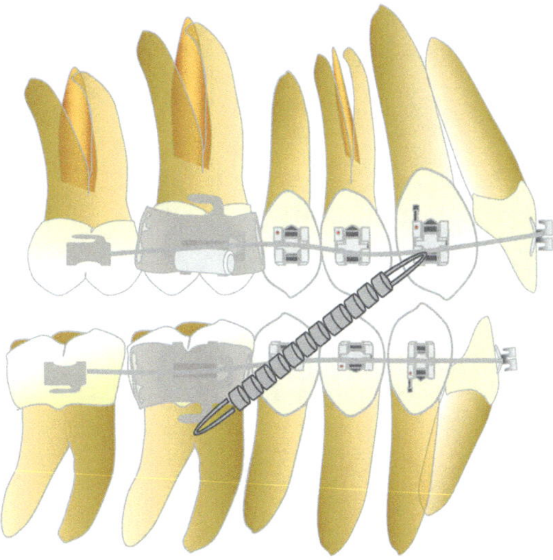

Fig. 5.4 A number of fixed adjuncts to address the class II malocclusion have been developed. The Saif Spring is attached to the fixed appliances similar to class II elastics

5.4 Contemporary Application of the Herbst Appliance

The contemporary Herbst appliance and its variants have only deviated minimally from the initial design described in the early 1900s [25]. The mandible is usually postured forward to an edge-to-edge relationship, or some clinicians routinely advance the mandible forward in a progressive manner. Progressive mandibular advancement is recommended for patients with a large overjet with some investigators suggesting that there is an enhanced growth effect [26]. This finding in the rat model has not been replicated in humans. Except for the replacement of stainless steel alloys for the original gold alloy, a passive right and left telescopic male and female arm system is still utilised (Figs. 5.5 and 5.6). Stainless steel crowns are trimmed and fitted to the upper first molars and lower premolars. Orthodontic bands are also fitted to the upper first premolars and lower first molars and pick-up impressions taken and cast in plaster (Fig. 5.7). An edge-to-edge bite registration is usually recorded. The casts are mounted on an articulator and the arms soldered or laser welded to crowns or thickened bands on the upper first molar to the lower first premolars.

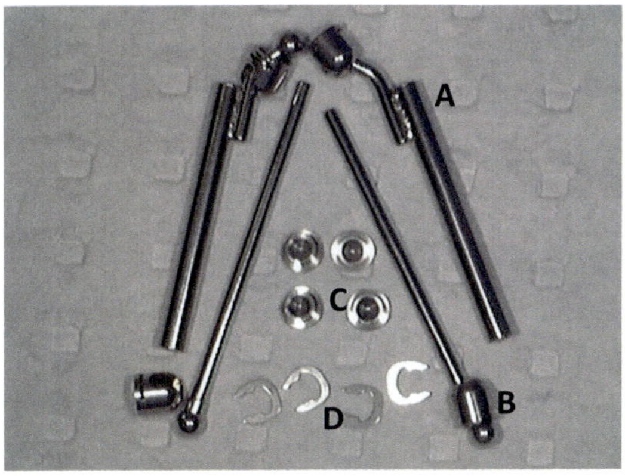

Fig. 5.5 The Herbst IV kit comprises several components. The female tube (**a**) and the male rod (**b**) are joined to a rod with a ball joint that has a cover to engage lugs that are welded to the crowns/bands (**c**). "C" clips (**d**) secure the covers to the lugs

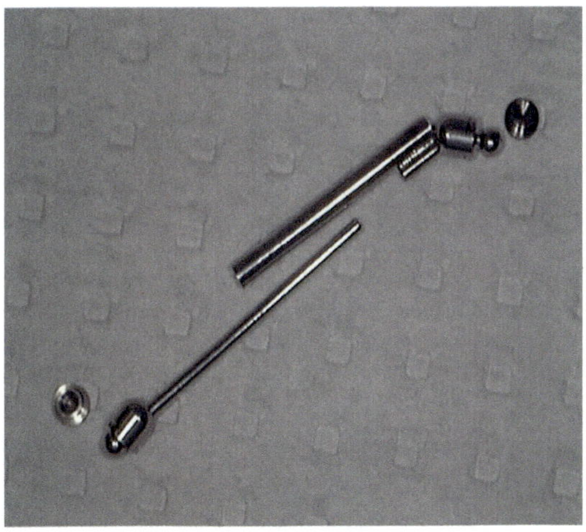

Fig. 5.6 The male and female piston configuration with the lugs that are welded to the stainless steel crowns. The ball and socket arrangement facilitates lateral movements with minimal torquing effects on the welded attachments

Fixed lingual and palatal arches are soldered to unify the maxillary and mandibular dentition with additional attachments on the lower first molars and upper first premolars (Fig. 5.8). In the contemporary Herbst IV appliance, "C" clips are used to secure the ball into the socket through a slit in the covering head (Fig. 5.9).

Fixed class II correctors such as the Herbst appliance are usually inserted during the period of maximal facial growth (Fig. 5.10). The short-

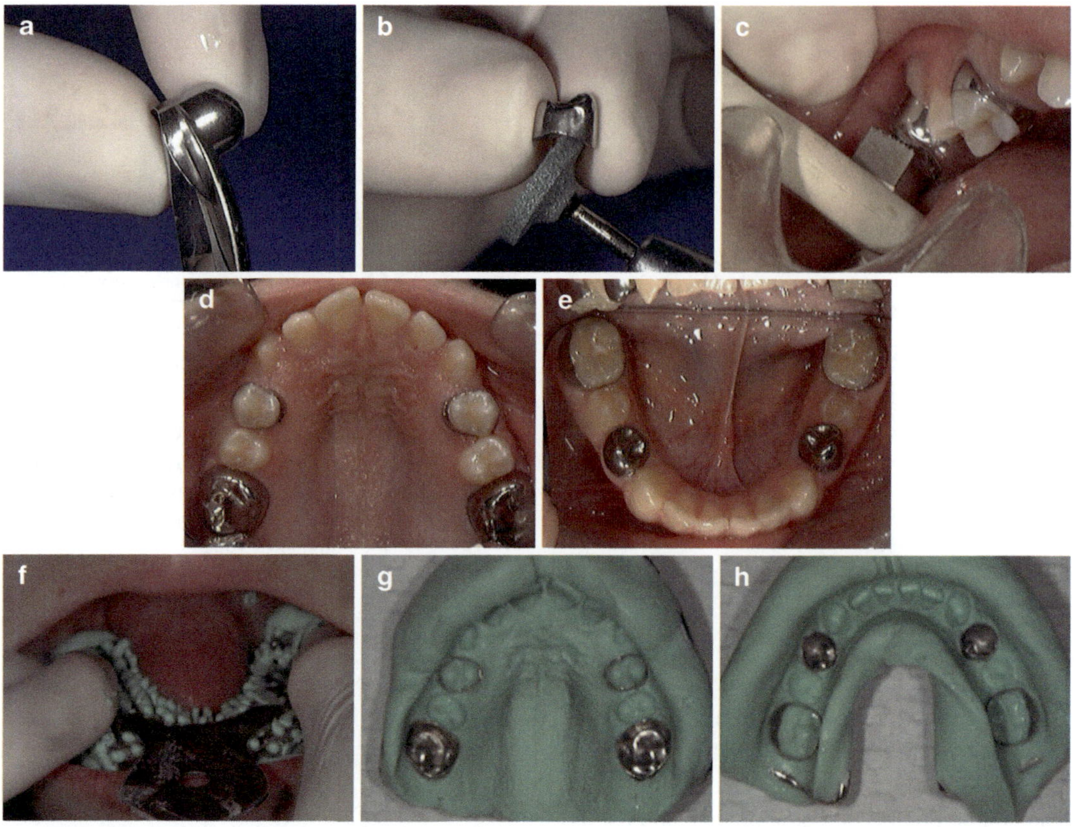

Fig. 5.7 Preparation of the crowns and bands for the Herbst appliance. Crowns are firstly trimmed to the clinical crown height with crown scissors (**a**) and the interdental col. region contoured to avoid gingival impingement (**b**). Crowns are placed on the upper molars and lower premolars and bands placed on the upper premolars and lower molars (**c–e**). Impressions are taken and the crowns/bands placed in the impression for pour up (**f–h**)

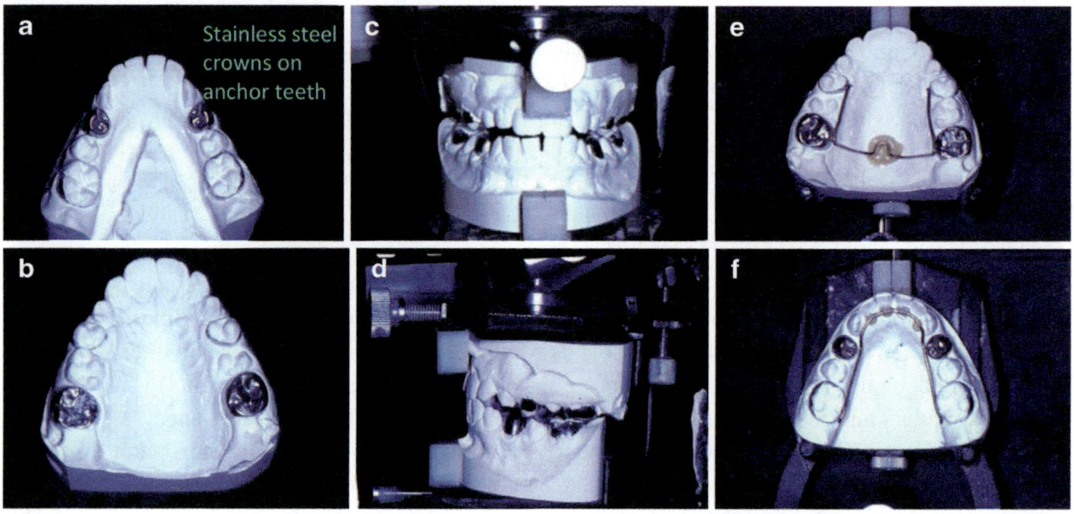

Fig. 5.8 Fabrication of the Herbst IV Appliance. Stone models are cast with the crown/bands in place (**a**, **b**) and the models mounted on a plaster-less articulator using a construction bite (**c**, **d**). 1–1.25 mm stainless steel wire is formed and approximated to oppose the crowns/bands (**e**, **f**). After covering the wire with heat-resistant gel (**g**, **h**), the wires are soldered to the bands/crowns (**i**, **j**) and the pistons attached to the lugs in the articulated models (**k**, **l**)

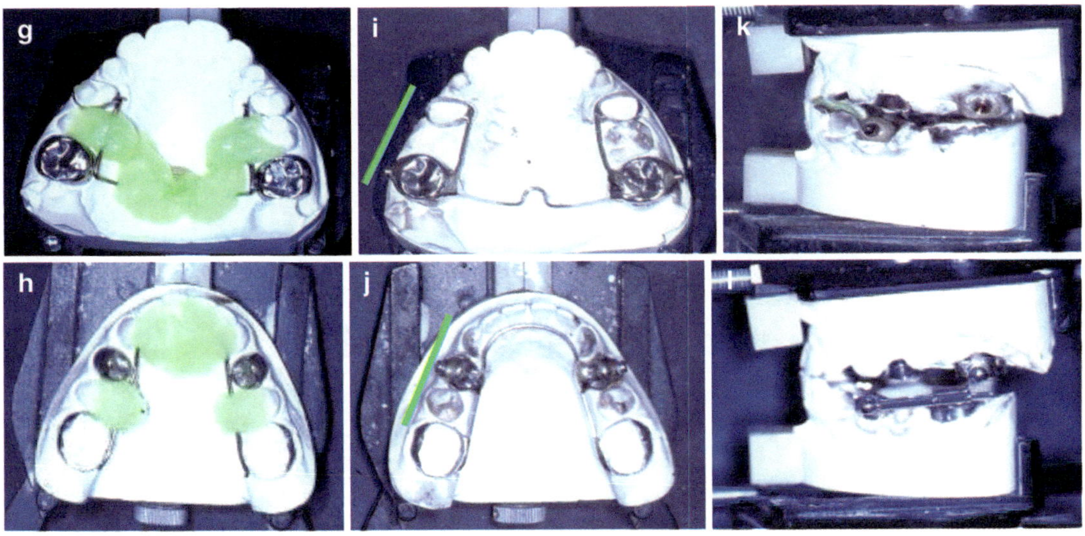

Fig. 5.8 (continued)

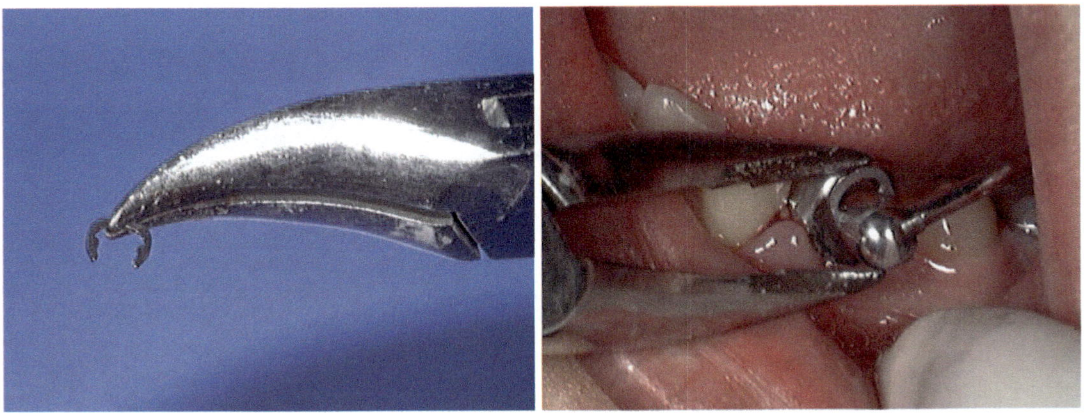

Fig. 5.9 "C" Clips are used to engage the undercuts on the lugs and secure the caps to the crowns to the Herbst IV appliance. The ball joint on the rods facilitates lateral movements to minimise the likelihood of torquing the attachments that can lead to appliance breakage

term effects of the Herbst include a combination of enhancement of the cephalocaudal gradient of maxillo-mandibular growth and dental compensation. Theoretically, effecting maximal skeletal changes reduces the magnitude of dental compensation. The necessity to select individuals who are growing has been brought into question with satisfactory clinical changes following Herbst appliance treatment in adults with mild to moderate skeletal class II relationships [27]. Although the treatment times were extended when compared to growing children, the results compared favourably with patients treated with orthognathic surgery [28]. The long-term reports of patients treated with the Herbst appliance reveal outcomes similar to almost all other functional appliances, with the only significant treatment effects represented by dentoalveolar compensation, reported to remain over 30 years of observation. When the effects of normal

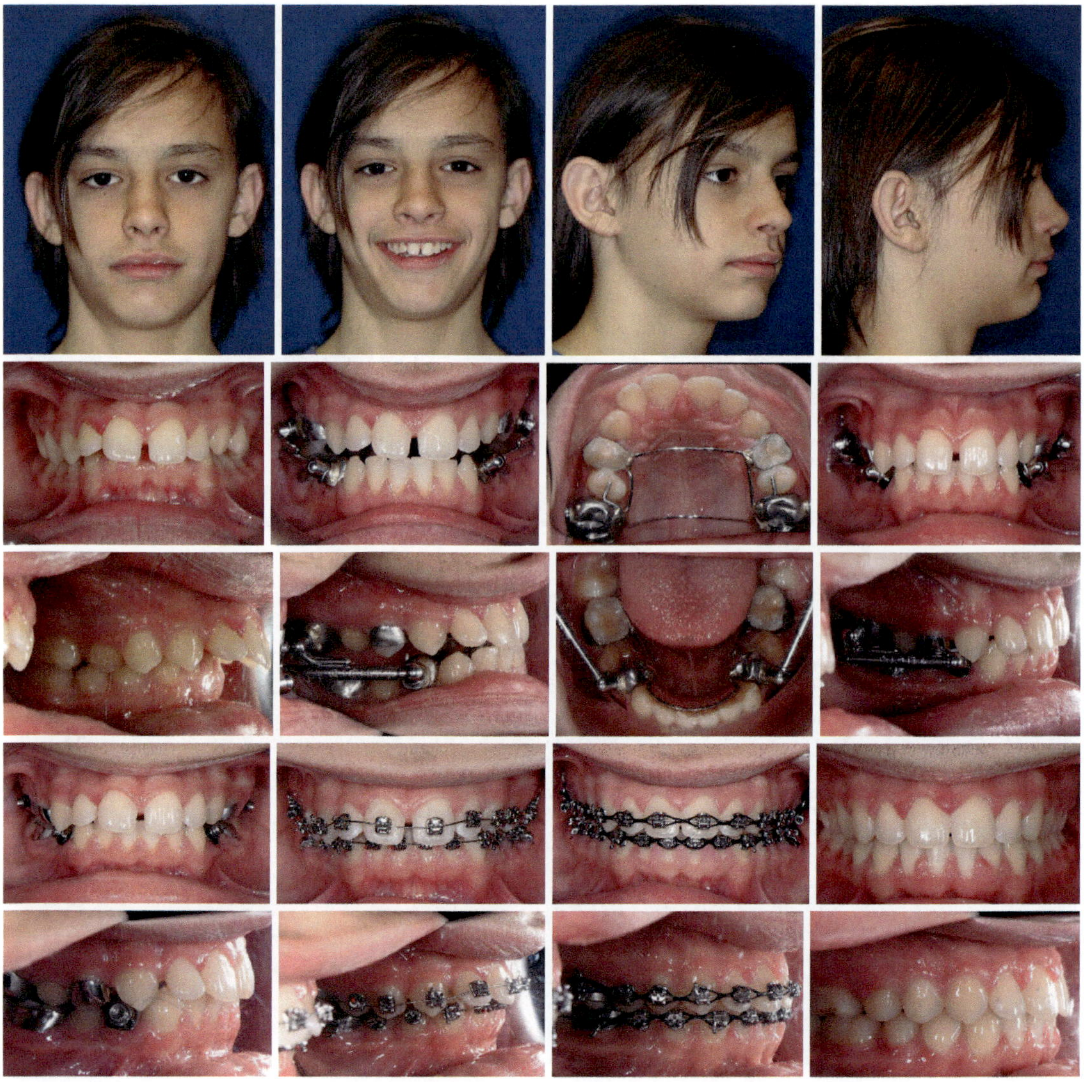

Fig. 5.10 A 13-year-old male presented with a class II division 1 malocclusion with increased overjet and mild upper arch irregularity. The goals of treatment included addressing the class II relationship by a combination of upper molar distalisation and mesial movement of the lower arch with any complimentary growth of the mandible. Upper and lower components of the Herbst appliance with stainless steel crowns on the upper molars and lower first premolars were placed with associated palatal and lingual arches. After 8–9 months, the antero-posterior correction was achieved and the Herbst appliance removed. Full fixed edgewise appliances were placed with archwires progressing from round to rectangular nickel titanium through to 19 × 25-in. titanium molybdenum alloy (TMA) to finalise tooth positions. The upper panels show the pre-treatment facial appearance with subsequent panels organised in vertical pairs from left to right showing treatment progression

growth are taken into account, the long-term skeletal effects are of minimal clinical significance [29, 30].

Managing patients with poor oral hygiene is a challenge for all clinicians, particularly when class II correction is desired. Like the twin-block appliance, the Herbst appliance may be placed to address the class II relationship without the significantly increased decalcification risk associated with multi-bracketed appliances. Moreover, the Herbst appliance requires minimal compliance and there is an immediate improvement in profile at the time of insertion. The clinician may be able to make significant progress whilst the patient is growing and have the time to consolidate oral hygiene measures before detailing the occlusion with multi-bracketed appliances. The reported treatment time of approximately 9 months followed by fixed appliances is significantly shorter than two-stage treatment with either removable appliances or comprehensive fixed appliances alone [30].

Incorporating the Herbst appliance into clinical practice necessitates an experienced clinical and laboratory team to firstly fit the crowns and bands and construct the appliance, as the precise orientation of the components is essential (Fig. 5.8). Moreover, the management of complications such as soft tissue irritation, distortion or fracture of components and debonding of attachments requires experience in troubleshooting these issues [31, 32]. These complications have undoubtedly contributed to some reluctance in utilising this appliance.

The historical Herbst design has been modified significantly. This may include more robust orthodontic bands, stainless steel crowns, cast frameworks and acrylic splint-type appliances. Moreover, more compact designs, such as the cantilever Herbst and the mini Herbst appliance have also been reported [33, 34] (Fig. 5.11).

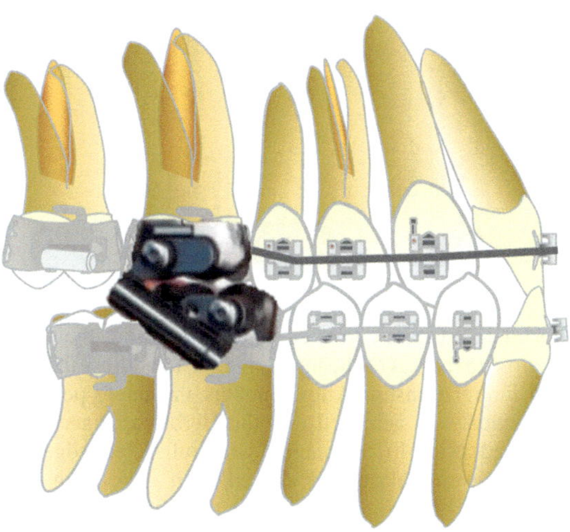

Fig. 5.11 A mini Herbst design that may be simultaneously inserted with multi-bracketed appliances

5.5 Application in Class II Subdivision Malocclusions

The morphology of class II subdivision malocclusions is complex and variable with both maxillary and/or mandibular dental and skeletal asymmetries [35]. However, it appears that a component of skeletal and dentoalveolar mandibular asymmetry, with a midline deviation, is most frequently encountered [36, 37].

The treatment options of class II subdivision malocclusions include:

- Asymmetrical extractions and fixed appliances, as changing the molar relationship was considered to be more challenging and less stable [38, 39].
- Asymmetrical elastic traction, with or without extra-oral traction. This option requires excellent cooperation.
- A fixed class II corrector that reduces the need for excellent compliance.
- Orthognathic surgery to address the asymmetry but patients are less likely to choose a surgical plan because of the associated risks and financial impost [40].

The choice of strategy may be further complicated by the presence of significant upper and lower crowding when extractions may be a necessary consideration.

In the presence of a class II subdivision type malocclusion with minimal arch length discrepancy, a fixed class II corrector such as the Herbst type appliance provides a robust and predictable mechanism by which dentoalveolar compensations may be achieved with associated growth changes (Fig. 5.12). The mandible is advanced to an over-corrected position with the midline deviated to the opposite side; however, a degree of incomplete correction of the midline deviation has been reported as well as routine proclination of the mandibular dentition [40].

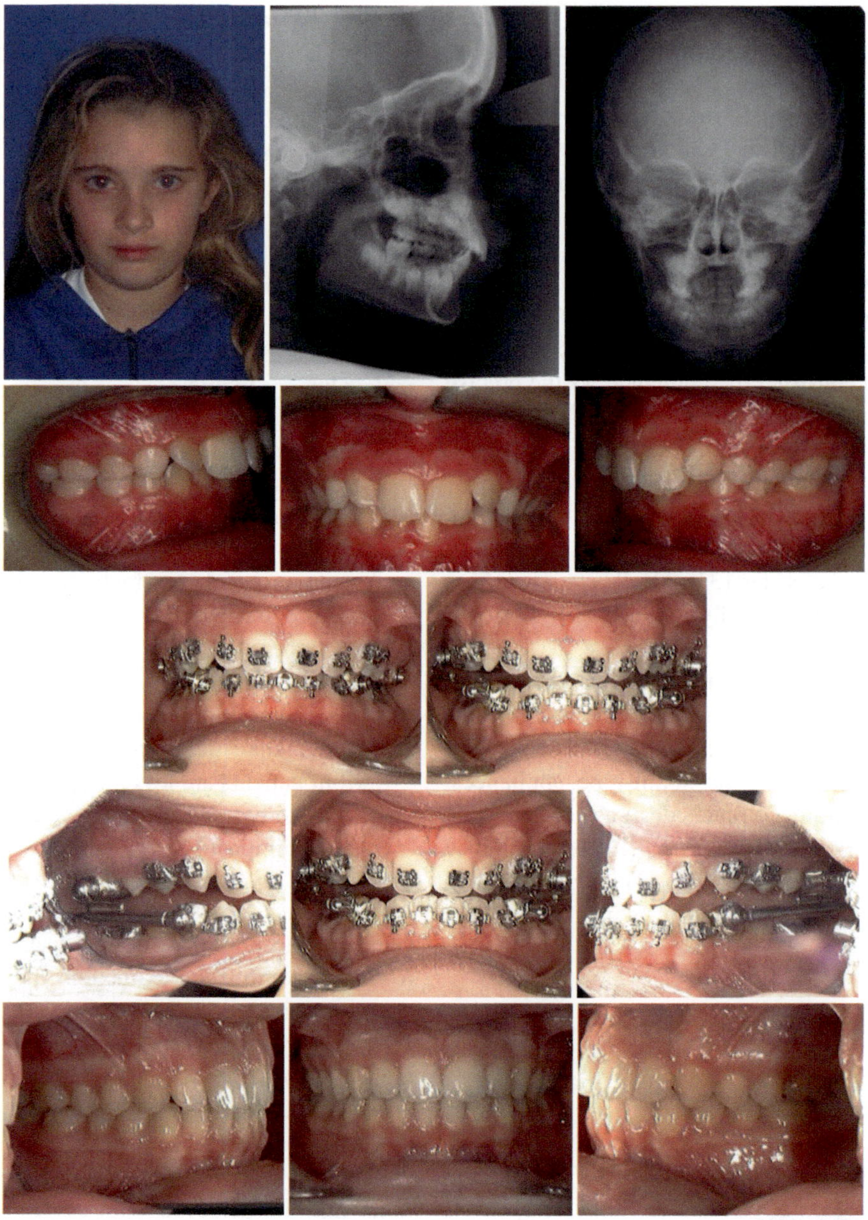

Fig. 5.12 A 9-year-old female initially presented with a class II division 2 subdivision right malocclusion related to mandibular asymmetry. The patient was left for review until the permanent teeth had emerged and permanent teeth accessible for fixed appliances. The goals of treatment included addressing the class II relationship by a combination of upper molar distalisation and mesial movement of the lower arch differentially. Full fixed edgewise appliances were placed simultaneously with the Herbst appliance with archwires progressing from round to rectangular nickel titanium through to 19 × 25-in. titanium molybdenum alloy (TMA). The Herbst appliance was constructed with stainless steel crowns on the upper and lower molars were placed with a maxillary and lower lingual arches. The functional bite registration was positioned in an over-corrected position, relating the lower midline to the left of the upper midline to address the subdivision relationship. After 9 months, the antero-posterior correction was achieved and the Herbst appliance was removed prior to continuing with full fixed edgewise appliances and elastics as needed, with 19 × 25-in. titanium molybdenum alloy (TMA) to finalise tooth positions. The upper panels show the pre-treatment facial appearance with mild asymmetry with chin deviated to the right and lateral and PA cephalogram. With subsequent panels organised in rows from left to right showing treatment progression

5.6 The Cantilever Bite Jumper Herbst Appliance

The Cantilever Bite Jumper (CBJ; Ormco Corporation, Orange, Calif) is one of the modifications to the original Herbst appliance design [41]. The CBJ Herbst does not attach to the lower premolar but attaches to a cantilever arm extended from a crown on the lower first molar (Fig. 5.13). This enables clinicians to extend the application of this appliance to the mixed dentition. Moreover, the appliance may be used when the first premolar is either partially erupted or difficult to secure a band or crown, particularly if the arches are significantly irregular (Fig. 5.14). This appliance is available in prefabricated components of various

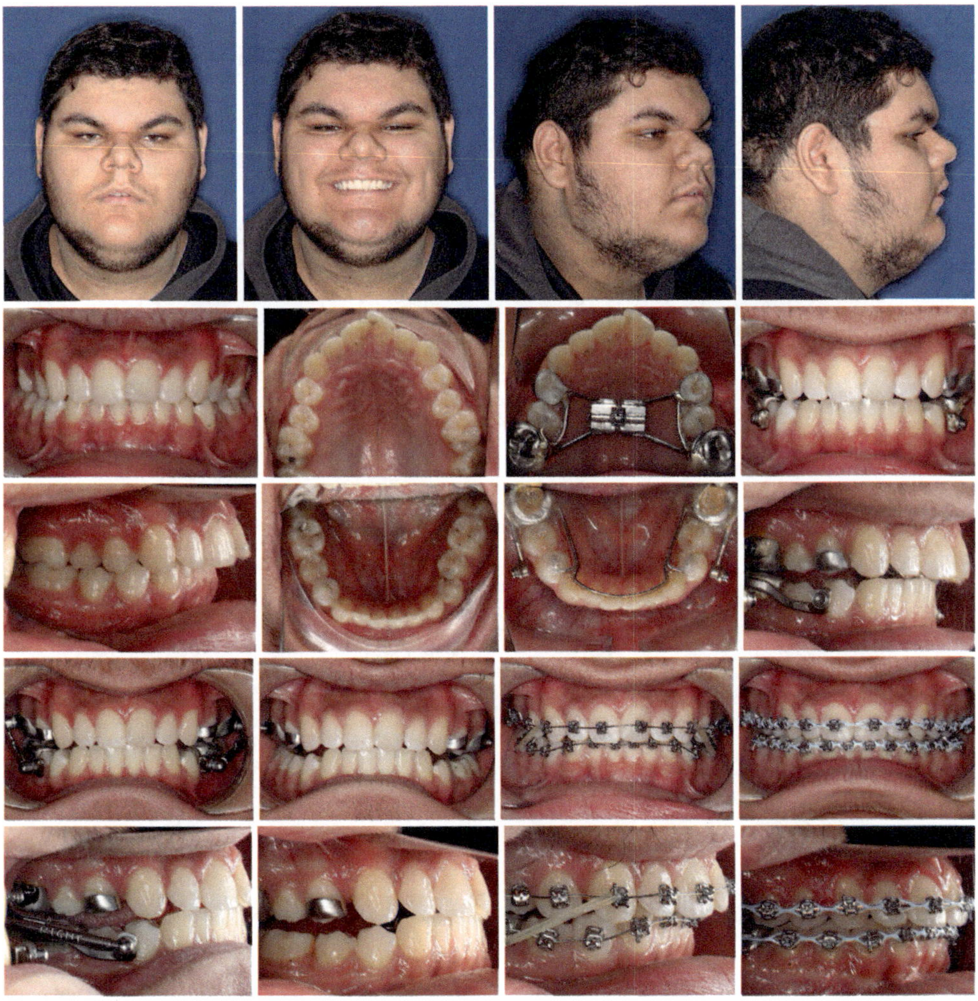

Fig. 5.13 A 15-year-old male presented with a class II division 1 malocclusion with increased overjet, a narrow maxilla and upper arch crowding. The goals of treatment included expanding the maxilla, addressing the class II relationship by a combination of upper molar distalisation and mesial movement of the lower arch with any complimentary growth of the mandible. Upper and lower components of the cantilever (CBJ) Herbst appliance with stainless steel crowns on the upper and lower molars were placed with a maxillary expansion component and a lower lingual arch. The CBJ Herbst appliance was chosen because of difficulty fitting crowns to the irregular lower first premolars The maxillary arch was firstly expanded before the pistons were placed. After 12 months, the antero-posterior correction was achieved and the CBJ Herbst appliance removed. Full fixed edgewise appliances were placed with archwires progressing from round to rectangular nickel titanium through to 19 × 25-in. titanium molybdenum alloy (TMA) to finalise tooth positions. The upper panels show the pre-treatment facial appearance with subsequent panels organised in vertical pairs from left to right showing treatment progression

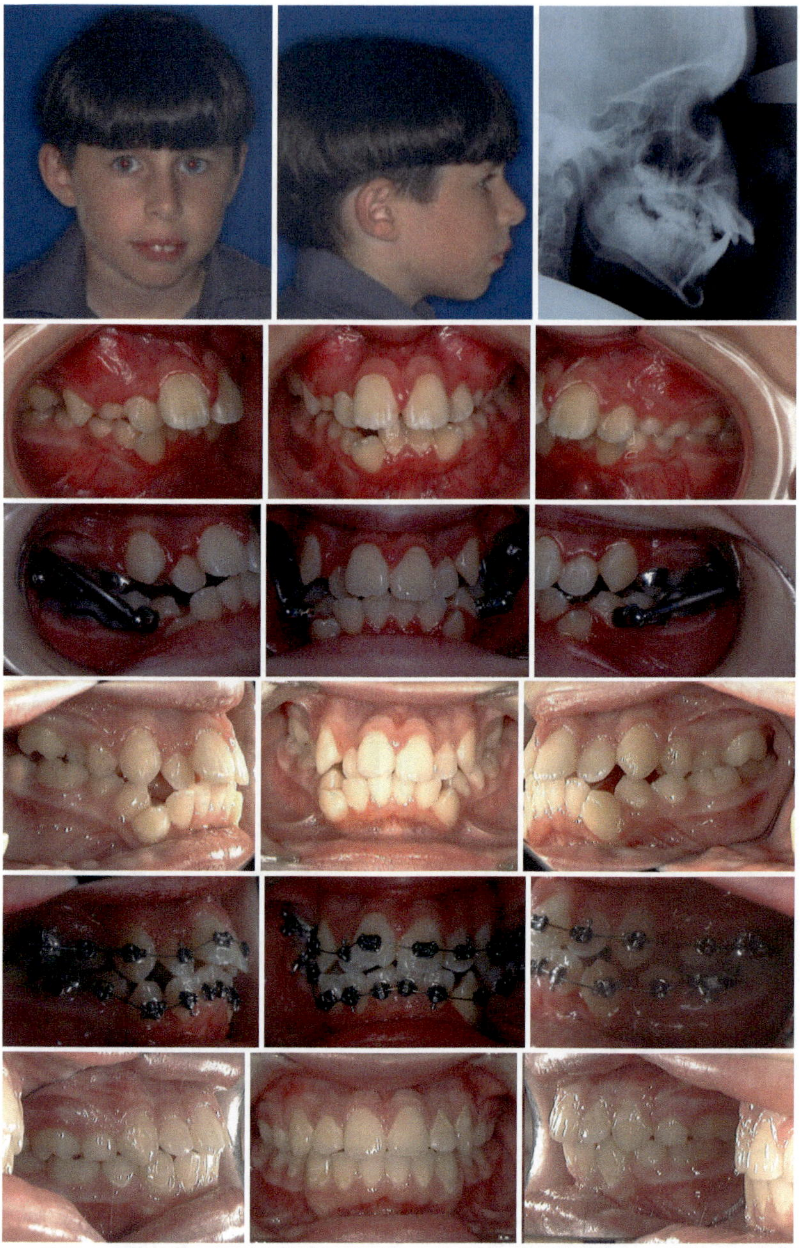

Fig. 5.14 A 13-year-old male presented with a class II division 1 malocclusion with increased overjet and significant upper and lower arch crowding. There was significant concern with compliance so a fixed class II corrector was chosen for treatment. The goals of treatment included addressing the class II relationship by a combination of upper molar distalisation and mesial movement of the lower arch with any complimentary growth of the mandible. Extraction of teeth and fixed edgewise appliance treatment would then be considered, dependent on levels of compliance. Upper and lower components of the cantilever (CBJ) Herbst appliance with stainless steel crowns on the upper and lower molars were placed with a maxillary and lower lingual arches. The CBJ Herbst appliance was chosen because of difficulty fitting crowns to the irregular lower first premolars The maxillary After 9 months, the antero-posterior correction was achieved and the CBJ Herbst appliance removed. Upper and lower premolar extractions were performed prior to full fixed edgewise appliances with archwires progressing from round to rectangular nickel titanium through to 19 × 25-in. stainless steel appliances to close spaces followed by titanium molybdenum alloy (TMA) to finalise tooth positions. The upper panels show the pretreatment facial appearance and cephalogram with subsequent panels organised in rows from left to right showing treatment progression. Please note the decalcification in the final photographs related to compromised oral hygiene

sizes and the placement of the anterior attachment gingivally enables a longer rod to be incorporated that minimises displacement of the rod from the tube during function [42, 43]. Unfortunately, the disadvantage of the longer extension arm and the more vertically directed force results in a tendency for the mandibular molar to tip mesially [44].

5.7 The Mandibular Protraction Appliance

The mandibular protraction device is a simple rigid device introduced in 1995 by Filho and colleagues, which may be constructed chairside by preparing two interlocking rods from 0.032 in. stainless steel with a compressed coil separating the two rods [45, 46]. This rigid device is attached to full arch bonded and banded appliances to posture the mandible forward, analogous to the Herbst appliance mechanism. Typically the lower premolars are not initially included in the set-up (Fig. 5.15). The fabrication cost is minimal rather than purchasing one of the numerous commercially available class II correctors. However, the appliance's rigidity contributes to an increased rate of breakage and inconvenience to the clinician.

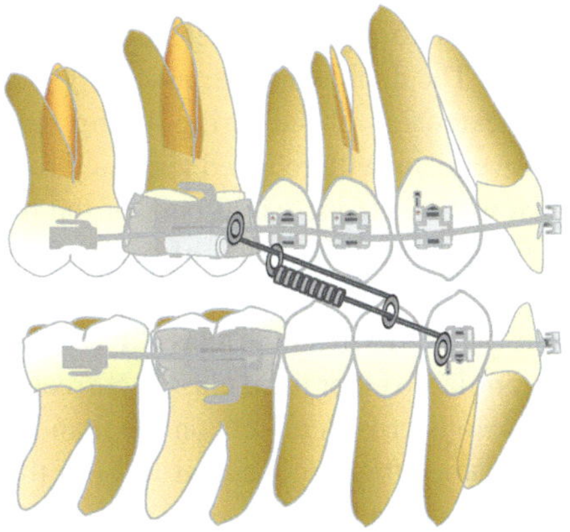

Fig. 5.15 The mandibular protraction device is a simple rigid device that may be constructed from 0.032-in. stainless steel with a compressed coil separating the two rods. This rigid device is attached to full arch bonded and banded appliances to posture the mandible forward

5.8 Jasper Jumper

The Herbst appliance's rigidity resulted in numerous attempts to improve the range of lateral movements that tended to contribute to appliance breakage. The screw holes in the rods were enlarged to afford greater flexibility but breakages remain a constant challenge. The Jasper Jumper was developed to overcome the rigidity experienced with the Herbst pistons [47]. The Jasper Jumper is an open coil spring of 5 different sizes, embedded in a soft synthetic polymer jacket, soldered to eyelets at each end. The spring was initially directly attached to the fixed appliance components. Unlike the Saif spring and class II elastics, this delivered a compressive force analogous to the Herbst appliance, however without the rigidity (Fig. 5.16). Theoretically, this force would not extrude the maxillary anterior teeth and steepen the occlusal plane as the vertical forces are closer to the centre of resistance of the dental units. The original configuration was fraught with numerous breakage complications that often detached numerous fixed appliance components and its popularity with clinicians slowly waned.

The Jasper jumper design has been modified to place an "outrigger" type wire for the spring to be attached to the mandibular component. When this outrigger component is combined with attachment distal to the maxillary archwire, this

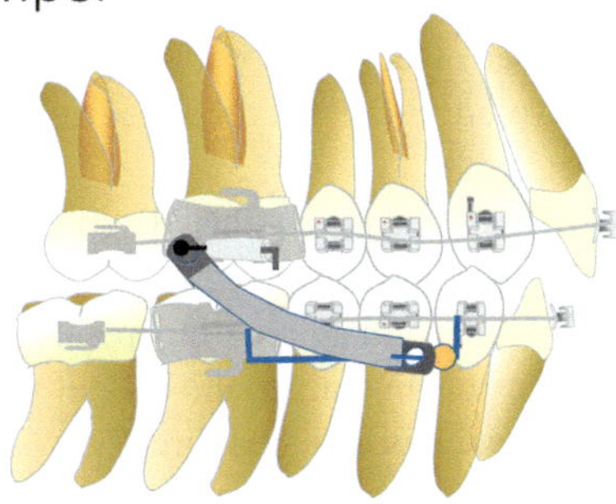

Fig. 5.16 The Jasper Jumper is an open coil spring of 5 different sizes, embedded in a soft synthetic polymer jacket, soldered to eyelets at each end. It is attached to the upper molar and may be modified to attach to an "Outrigger" segment in the lower arch to decrease direct forces to the lower appliances and assist to reduce breakages

dissociated any breakages from the main archwire and brackets. The clinical effects of the Jasper jumper appear to be similar to most other fixed class II correctors, but superior to removable functional appliances [48–50]. A combination of normal horizontal mandibular growth, mild maxillary distalisation and anterior movement of the lower dentition is reported. But the overwhelming issue relates to appliance breakage and denaturation of the polymer coating surrounding the spring. The Adjustable Bite Corrector and The Bite Fixer (Ormco Pty Ltd) are variations of the Jasper Jumper design and concept that have similar issues to the Jasper Jumper.

5.9 The Eureka Spring and Twin Force

The Eureka Spring was the first interarch compressive spring that enabled a male and female component to establish a protrusive position [51]. The differences between the Eureka spring and the Herbst appliance lie in a spring that compresses when the male and female components engage. This flexible engagement reduced the stresses on the appliances and encouraged clinicians who had disappointing experiences with the Jasper Jumper breakages. The appliance is attached directly to the fixed multibracket appliances so independent intra-arch tooth movements could be effected as the class II correction occurred. This appliance was the forerunner to a number of contemporary class II correctors that delivered more predictable results with fewer breakages.

The Twin Force class II corrector progressed from the Eureka spring to comprise two plunger assemblies that are independently the same dimension, but larger and bulkier when combined. The device is attached directly to the archwire by two locking components (Fig. 5.17). The distal attachment does not attach to the band or bracket but attaches to a distal extension of the upper archwire. The double plunger assembly facilitates greater extension of the spring during functional jaw movements with reduced tendency for breakage. However, the increased bulk of the plungers does increase the likelihood of occlusal interference and discomfort for the patient. The clinical effects of the Twin Force class II corrector are again similar to other fixed class II correctors with simultaneous growth effects on the mandible and compensatory tooth movement in both the mandible and maxilla [52–54].

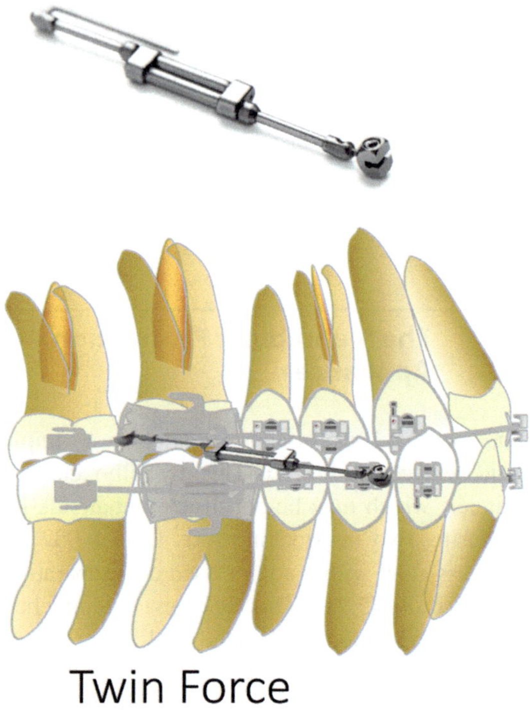

Fig. 5.17 Twin Force device comprises two plunger assemblies that are independently the same dimension as the Eureka spring with an active compressive spring component but essentially effecting the same mandibular protrusion effect. The device is attached directly to the archwire by two locking components. The distal attachment does not attach to the band or bracket but attaches to a distal extension of the upper archwire

5.10 Forsus™ Fatigue Resistant Module

The Forsus™ (Fatigue Resistant) module is one of the many commercially available class II corrector devices. Its effects are analogous to other types of functional appliances in growing children. The treatment effects combine minor skeletal effects, related to the magnitude and direction of growth and the typical dentoalveolar compensation of upper arch retraction and mesial movement of the lower arch [55]. Clinicians are able to simultaneously combine alignment, levelling and arch coordination with fixed appliances and simultaneous antero-posterior correction with the Forsus™ module, with the potential of reducing treatment time and the associated patient compliance issues. Unlike rigid Herbst-type appliances, the Forsus™ module comprises right and left springs that are inserted into the headgear tube of the upper molar and a male rod that inserts into a nickel-titanium spring (Fig. 5.18). It has been suggested that the forward positioning effected by the Herbst appliance potentially places large continuous loads on the temporomandibular joint, and may compromise joint integrity more than the flexible spring from the Forsus™ [56, 57].

The combination of fixed appliances and Forsus™ module has been reported to effect significant changes in upper and lower incisor position and steepening of the occlusal plane [58, 59]. Technical modifications have been recommended to reduce these side-effects and studies reporting effects are often complicated by these individual approaches. Significant retraction and uprighting of upper incisor position has been reported and it has been suggested to prepare the upper wire to effect palatal root movement or place high torque upper incisor brackets. On the lower wire, labial root movement in the lower incisors either by archwire bending or varying the third-order prescription of the lower incisor brackets have all been suggested as mechanisms to control this perceived anchorage loss (Figs. 5.19 and 5.20). Positioning of the male component of the module against the first premolar instead of the canine will reduce the rotational moment on the lower occlusal plane (Fig. 5.21). Placement of temporary anchors in the lower arch has also been reported to reduce the loss of lower incisor control [60].

There is insufficient evidence to draw any sound conclusion because of the absence of carefully considered studies. The Forsus™ module can be used to manage class II division 1 and attached to the lower canine (Fig. 5.22) and may have simultaneous expansion and attachment to the lower first premolars (Fig. 5.23). Class II division 2 type malocclusions may have the forsus module attached after multi-bracketed appliances have converted division 2 into division 1 (Fig. 5.24). Simultaneous maxillary expansion may also be performed in conjunction with the fixed multi-bracketed appliances to "telescope" the components of the treatment with the potential to shorten overall treatment time (Fig. 5.24). The Forsus™ module can also be utilised for the correction of significantly crowded class II problems combined with fixed appliances and premolar extractions (Figs. 5.25 and 5.26).

As with the Herbst appliance, the Forsus™ module may be utilised to address class II subdivision-type malocclusion (Fig. 5.27). The distance from the upper first molar to the canine on the class II side is decreased therefore symmetrical modules will effect a greater protruding force on the class II side. However, it is recommended to over-advance the mandible to an over-corrected position with the midline deviated to the opposite side, using a shim on the male component. Similar to the findings with the Herbst appliance, a degree of incomplete correction of the midline deviation has been reported and routine proclination of the mandibular dentition [40].

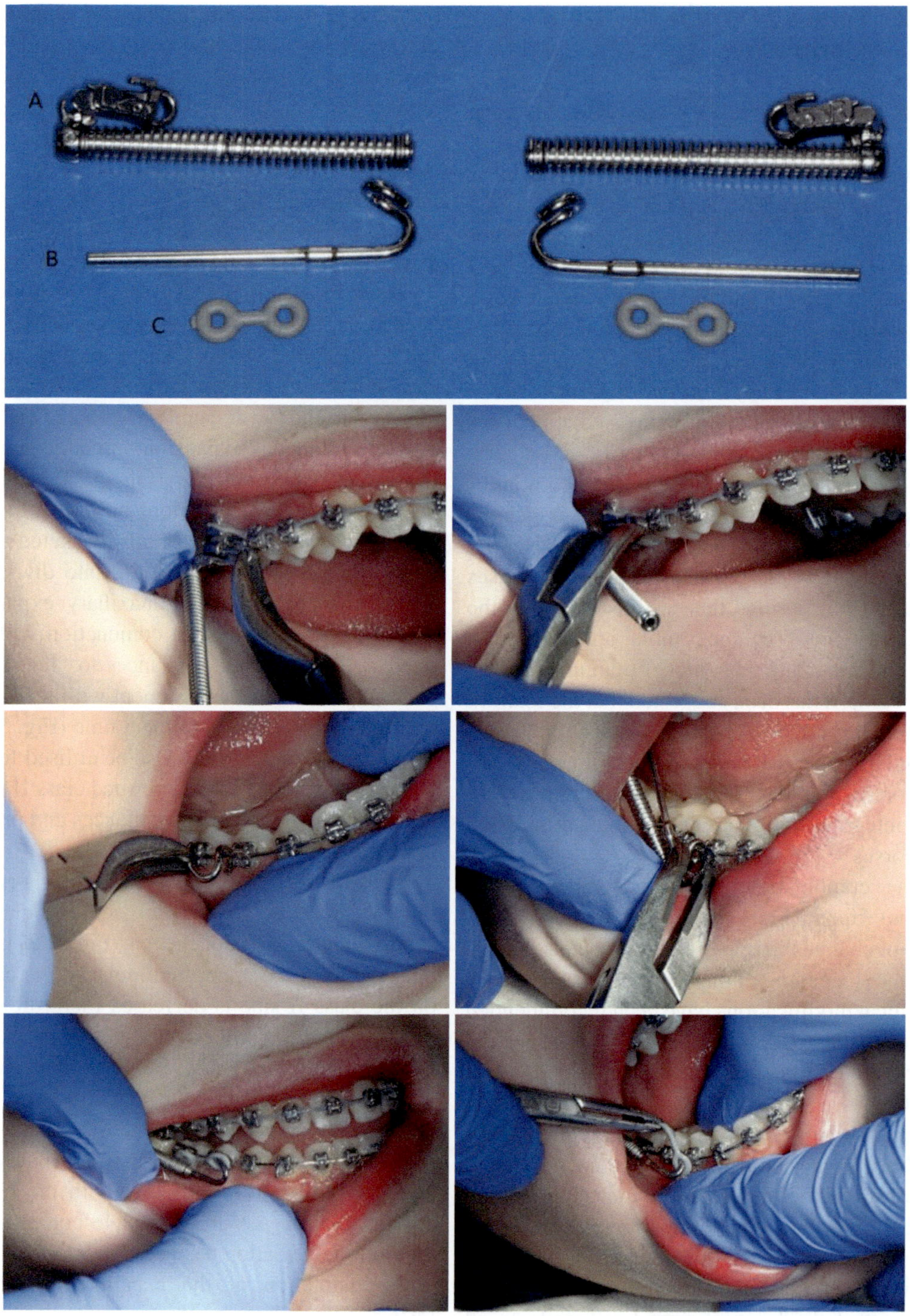

Fig. 5.18 The Forsus™ module comprises right and left springs (**a**) inserted into the headgear tubes of the upper molars and male rods (**b**) that are inserted into the springs. The springs have a male component that clips onto the headgear tube using a utility plier and a male component that is crimped onto the archwire either between premolars or premolar and canine. The dumbbell elastic (**c**) is attached from the anterior of the male component back to the first molar tube to minimise breakages of the premolar/canine brackets and prevent space from opening in the lower arch secondary to the mesial force on the anterior dentition

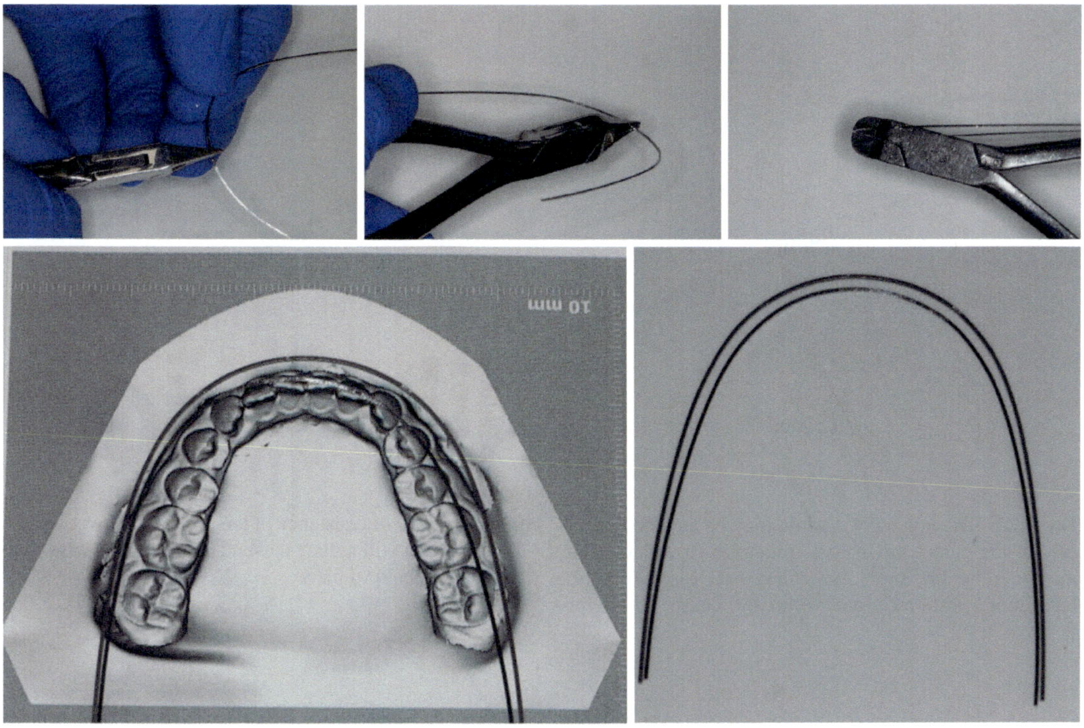

Fig. 5.19 Archwires are prepared specifically to support the Forsus™ module. Approximately 10–15 ° of lingual root torque is added to the upper incisors and approximately 10 ° of labial root torque to the lower incisors to reduce the significant uprighting and proclination of the upper and lower incisors respectively, secondary to the antero-posterior forces generated with this appliance

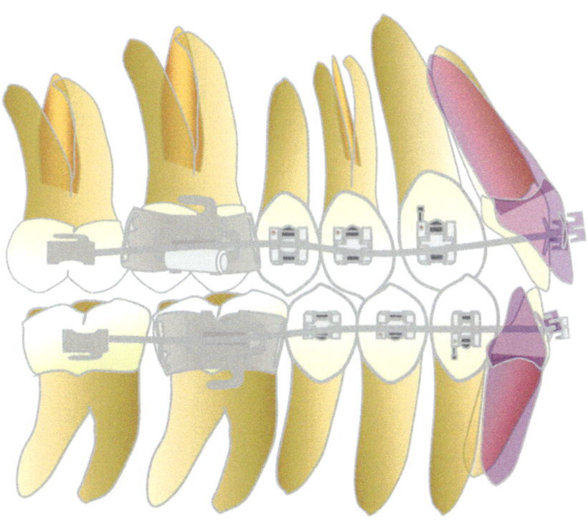

Fig. 5.20 The effects of twist in the wire to twist the upper and lower incisors to resist the relative displacement effected by the Forsus™ module

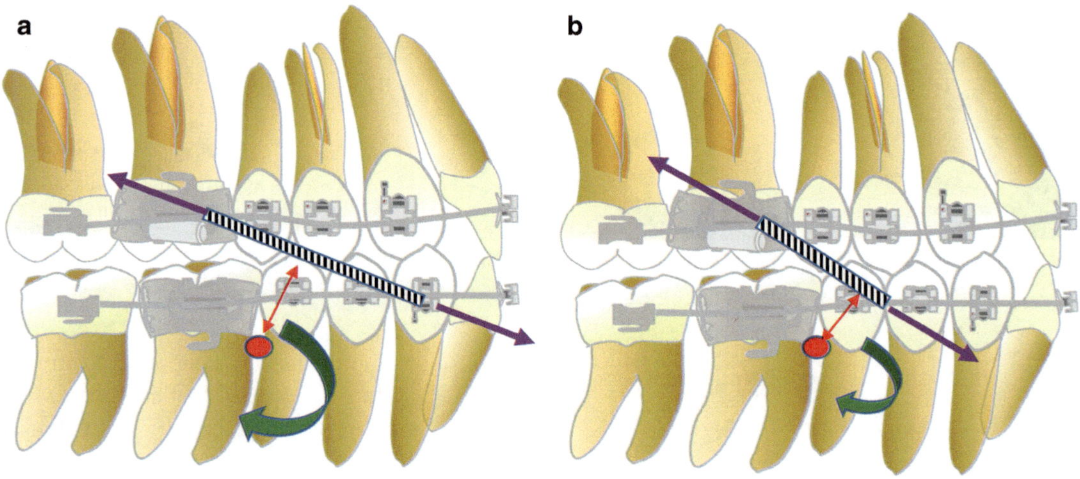

Fig. 5.21 The Forsus™ module may be attached anteriorly to the canine (**a**) or first premolar (**b**). Placing the module to the first premolars changes the direction of the force more posteriorly and vertically relative to a hypothetical centre of resistance of the upper and lower arches. This in effect will reduce the tendency for clockwise rotation of the occlusal plane

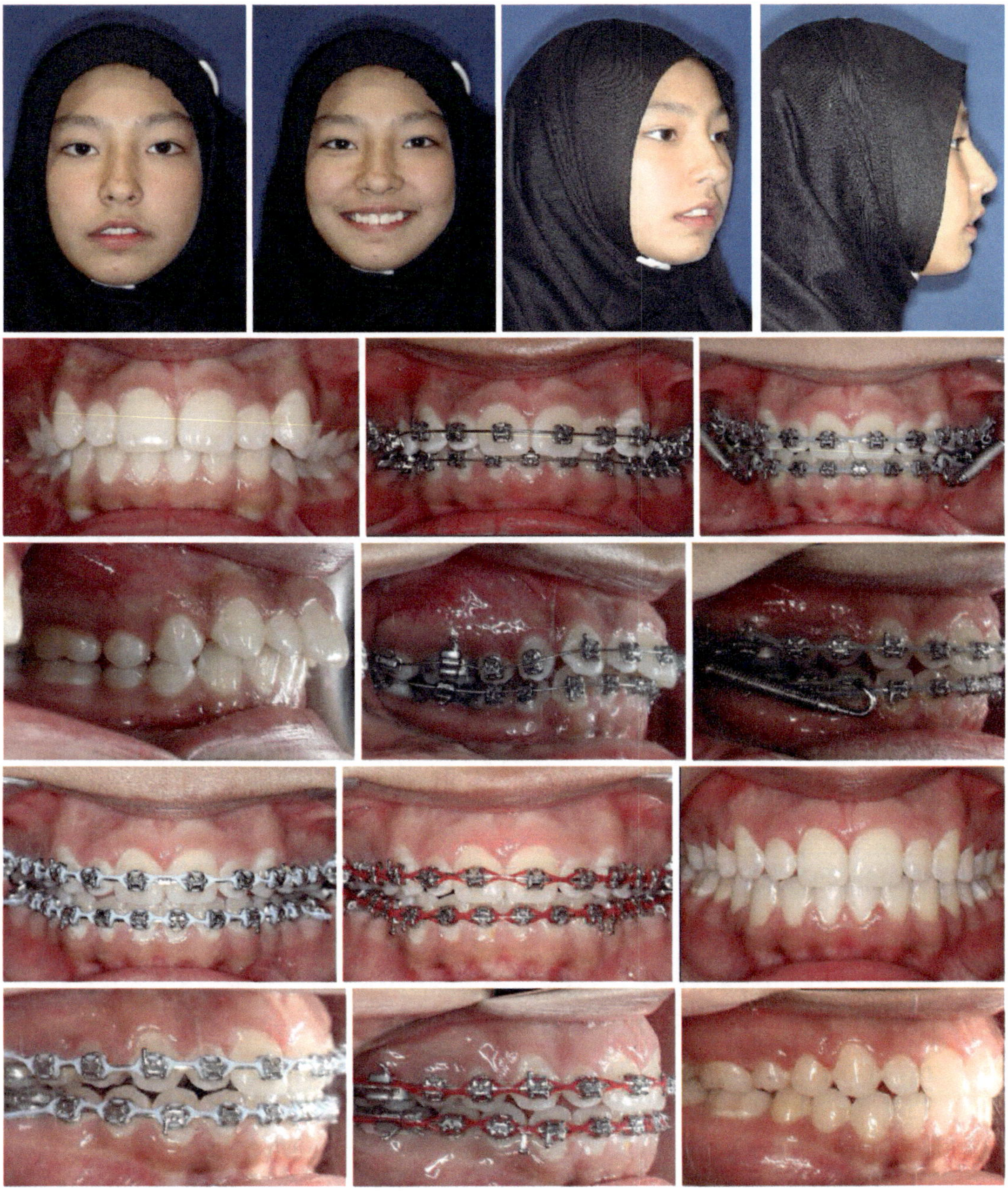

Fig. 5.22 A 12-year-old female presented with a class II division 1 malocclusion with increased overjet and upper irregularity. The goals of treatment included addressing the class II relationship by a combination of upper molar distalisation and mesial movement of the lower arch with any complimentary growth of the mandible. Upper and lower fixed edgewise appliances were placed with archwires progressing from round to rectangular nickel-titanium archwires through to 19 × 25-in. TMA upper and 19 × 25-in. stainless steel lower. The upper arches were prepared with third-order adjustments to effect palatal root movement in the upper incisors and mild labial root movement in the lower incisors. A Forsus™ module was placed to the lower canines. A stainless steel wire is necessary in the lower arch to prevent fracture from the male arm of the module. After 6 months, antero-posterior correction was achieved and the Forsus™ module removed, anterior seating elastics were worn at night and new 19 × 25-in. TMA archwires used to detail the occlusion. The upper panels show the pre-treatment facial appearance with subsequent panels organised in vertical pairs from left to right showing treatment progression

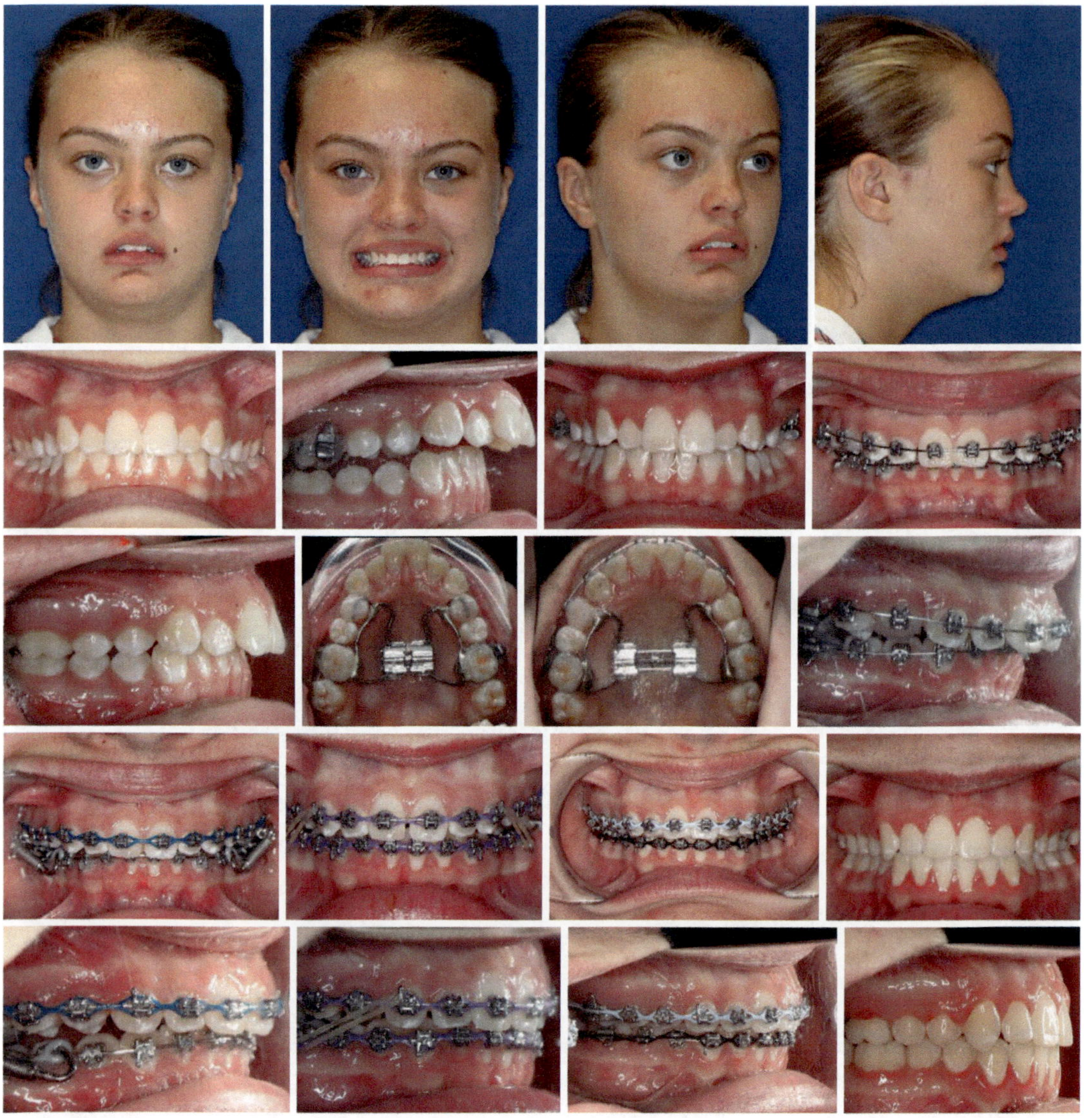

Fig. 5.23 A 13—year-old female presented with a class II division 1 malocclusion with increased overjet, a narrow maxilla and upper irregularity. The goals of treatment included expansion of the narrow maxilla, and addressing the class II relationship by a combination of upper molar distalisation and mesial movement of the lower arch with any complimentary growth of the mandible. A fixed maxillary expansion appliance was placed and activated for 10 weeks to achieve a slightly over-expanded transverse dimension. Upper and lower fixed edgewise appliances were placed during the 4–5 months or retention of the expander, with archwires progressing from round to rectangular nickel-titanium archwires through to 19 × 25-in. TMA upper and 19 × 25-in. stainless steel lower. The upper arches were prepared with third order adjustments to effect palatal root movement in the upper incisors and mild labial root movement in the lower incisors. A Forsus™ module was placed to the lower premolars in this instance to minimise the rotation of the occlusal plane. A stainless steel wire is necessary in the lower arch to prevent fracture from the male arm of the module. After 6 months, antero-posterior correction was achieved and the Forsus™ module removed, anterior seating elastics were worn at night and new 19 × 25-in. TMA archwires used to detail the occlusion. The upper panels show the pre-treatment facial appearance with subsequent panels organised in vertical pairs from left to right showing treatment progression

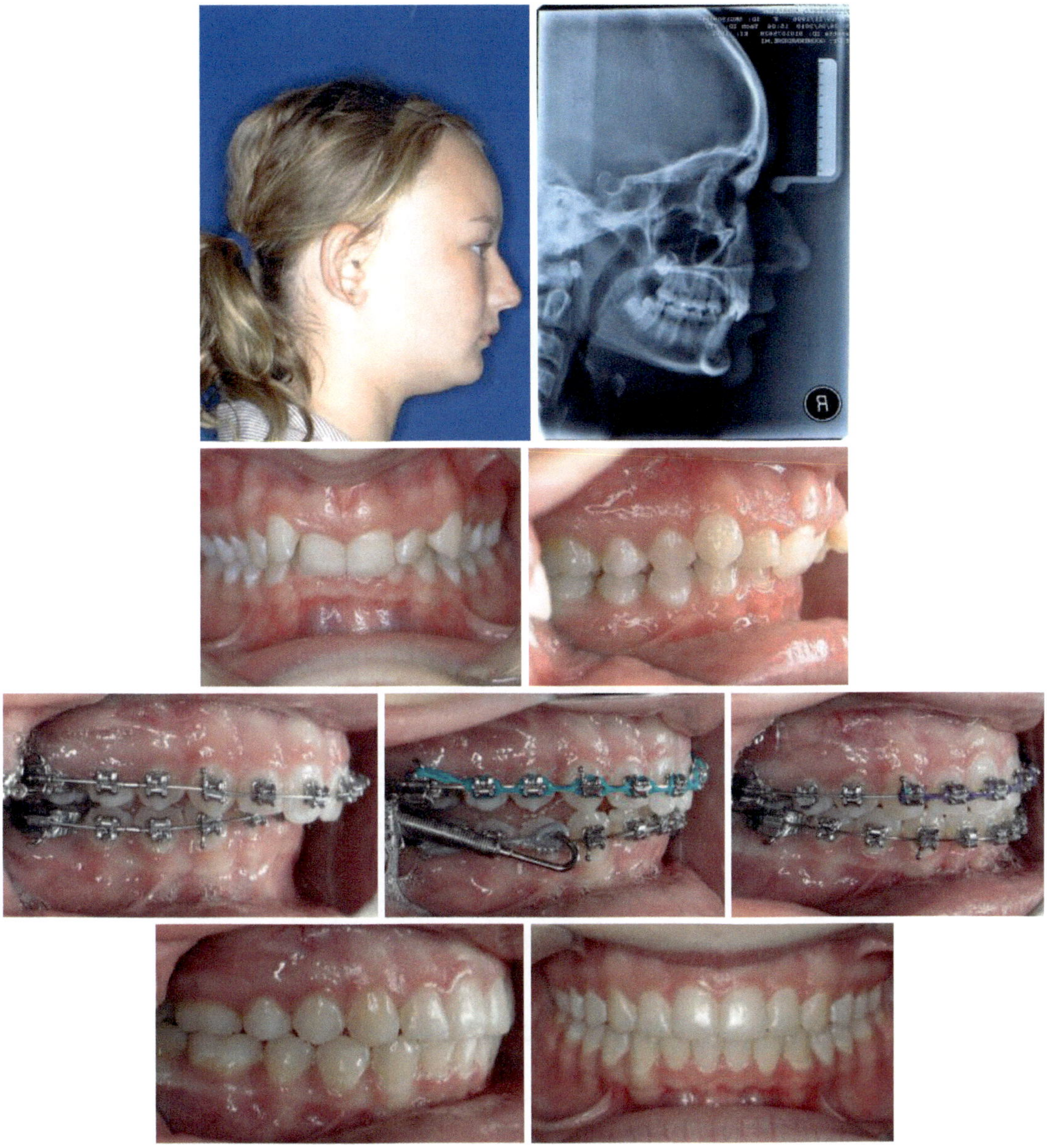

Fig. 5.24 A 12-year-old female presented with a class II division 2 type malocclusion with increased overbite, mandibular retrognathism and upper irregularity. This case demonstrates the side effect of excessive lower incisor proclination when labial root torque or large dimension lower rectangular wires are not added to the lower archwire. The goals of treatment included proclining the upper incisors to a class II division 1 relationship prior to addressing the class II relationship by a combination of upper molar distalisation and mesial movement of the lower arch with any complimentary growth of the mandible. Upper and lower fixed edgewise appliances were placed with archwires progressing from round to rectangular nickel-titanium archwires through to 19 × 25-in. TMA upper and 19 × 25-in. stainless steel lower. A Forsus™ module was placed to the lower canine. A stainless steel wire is necessary in the lower arch to prevent fracture from the male arm of the module. After 9 months, antero-posterior correction was achieved and the Forsus™ module removed, anterior seating elastics were worn at night and new 19 × 25-in. TMA archwires used to detail the occlusion. The upper panels show the pre-treatment facial profile appearance and lateral cephalogram as well as the pr-treatment dental relationships. The treatment progression with fixed appliances appears most satisfactory but the lower panels reveal excessive lower incisor proclination in the lateral cephalogram and cranial base superimposition

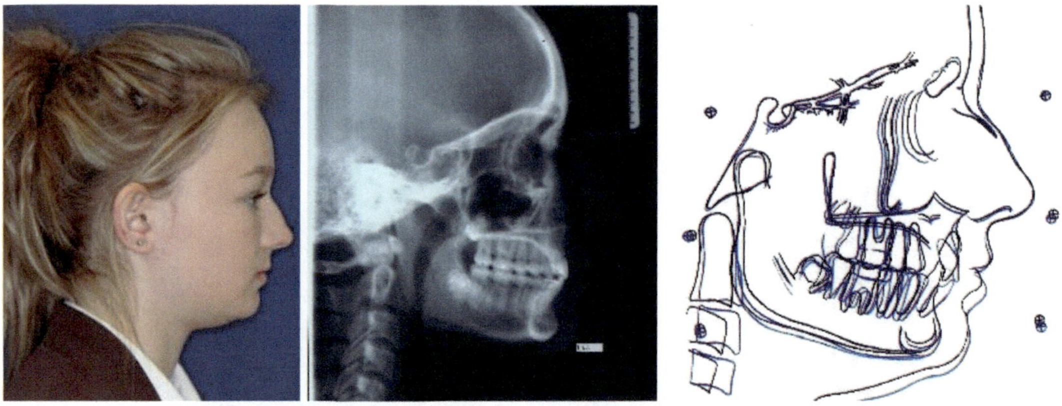

Fig. 5.24 (continued)

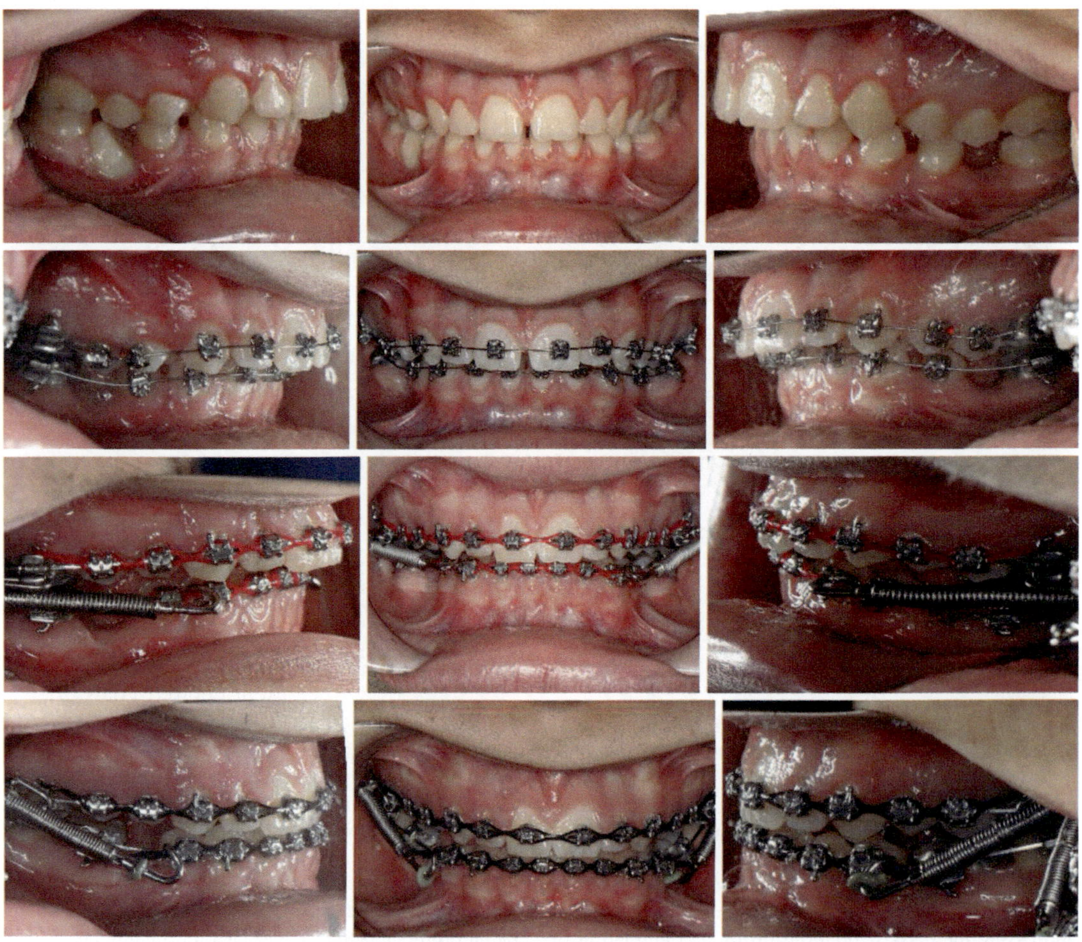

Fig. 5.25 The Forsus™ module may be used as anchorage to maintain the lower incisor position during space closure after extraction in the lower arch. A 14-year old male patient presented with missing lower second premolars. A Forsus™ module was placed to simultaneously keep the lower incisors forward whilst the lower posterior teeth were protracted

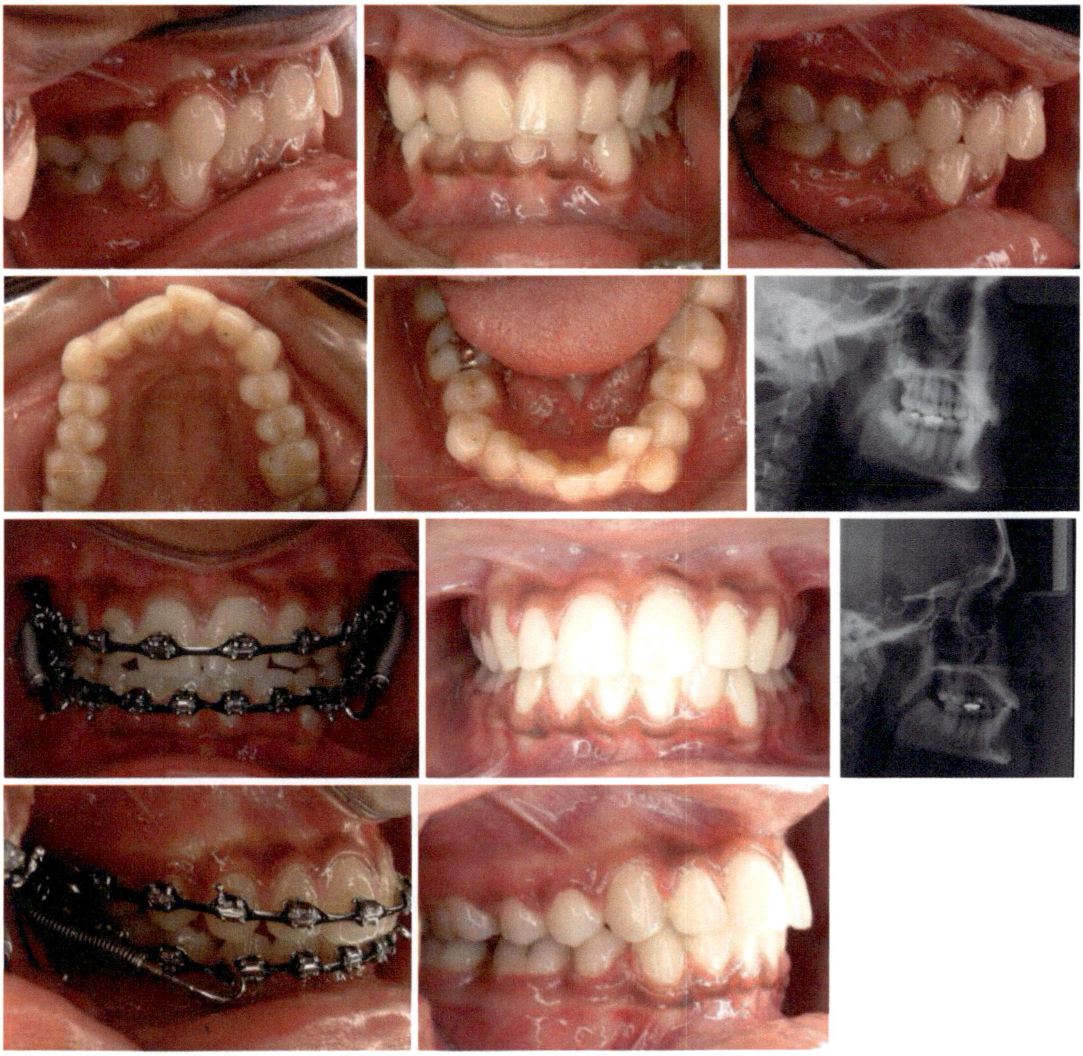

Fig. 5.26 The Forsus™ module may be used as anchorage to maintain the lower incisor position during space closure after extraction in the lower arch. A 13-year-old female patient presented with significant lower crowding and a thin gingival phenotype. Moreover, the lips were relatively flat. Extraction of lower first premolars was considered and a Forsus™ module was placed to simultaneously keep the lower incisors forward whilst the reciprocal effect on the upper arch distalised the upper molar. The upper panels exhibit the pre-treatment intraoral photographs and lateral cephalogram. The lower panels demonstrate the Forsus™ module in use to maintain lower incisor position and the post-treatment lateral cephalogram exhibits maintenance of upper and lower incisor positions

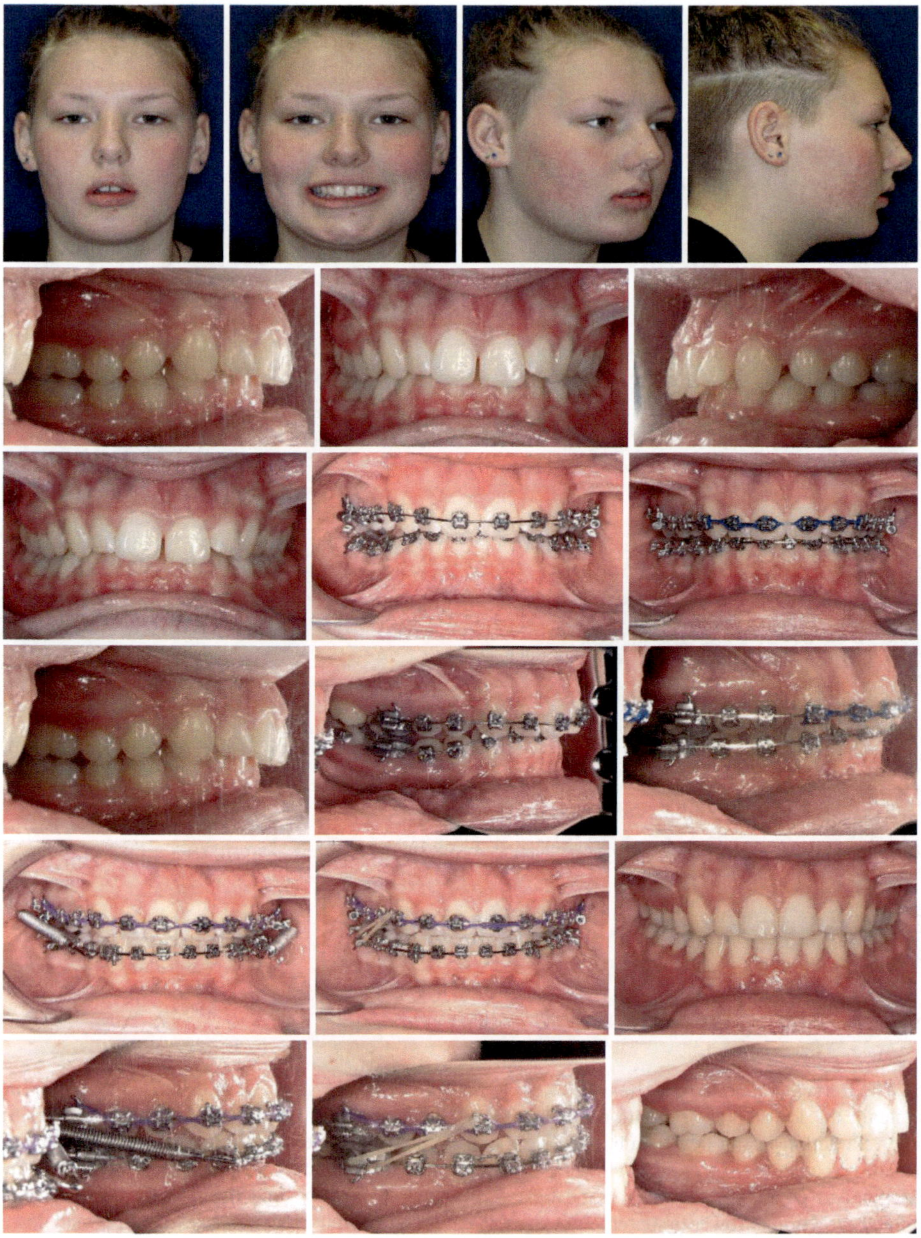

Fig. 5.27 A 13-year-old female presented with a class II division 1 subdivision right malocclusion with increased overjet and upper irregularity. The goals of treatment included addressing the class II relationship by a combination of asymmetrical upper molar distalisation and mesial movement of the lower arch with any complimentary growth of the mandible. Upper and lower fixed edgewise appliances were placed with archwires progressing from round to rectangular nickel-titanium archwires through to 19 × 25-in. TMA upper and 19 × 25-in. stainless steel lower. The upper arches were prepared with third-order adjustments to effect palatal root movement in the upper incisors and mild labial root movement in the lower incisors. A Forsus™ module was placed to the lower canines. The asymmetrical molar relationship on the right results in greater compression of the spring on the right side facilitating asymmetrical dental changes. A stainless steel wire is necessary in the lower arch to prevent fracture from the male arm of the module. After 9 months, antero-posterior correction was achieved and the Forsus™ module removed, anterior seating elastics were worn at night and new 19 × 25-in. TMA archwires were used to detail the occlusion. The upper panels show the pre-treatment facial appearance and the asymmetrical buccal segment relationships with subsequent panels organised in vertical pairs from left to right showing treatment progression

5.11 Modified Crossbow Appliance

The crossbow appliance comprises a lingual and buccal metallic framework that has protrusive compressive springs attached to the framework [61]. The maxillary component usually comprises a fixed maxillary expansion device.

The skeletal effects were minimal with reduction of maxillary protrusion without mandibular advancement and an increase of the vertical dimension. The dental effects contributing to overjet reduction included an increase in mandibular incisor protrusion without maxillary incisor movement. The maxillary molars were distalised whereas the mandibular molars were mesialised. These changes although statistically significant were not found to be clinically significant as the changes again followed the general effect of most fixed class II correctors.

The crossbow may be used as a first stage of class II treatment followed by a second stage of fixed multibracket appliances. This may even extend to patients who require extraction (Fig. 5.28).

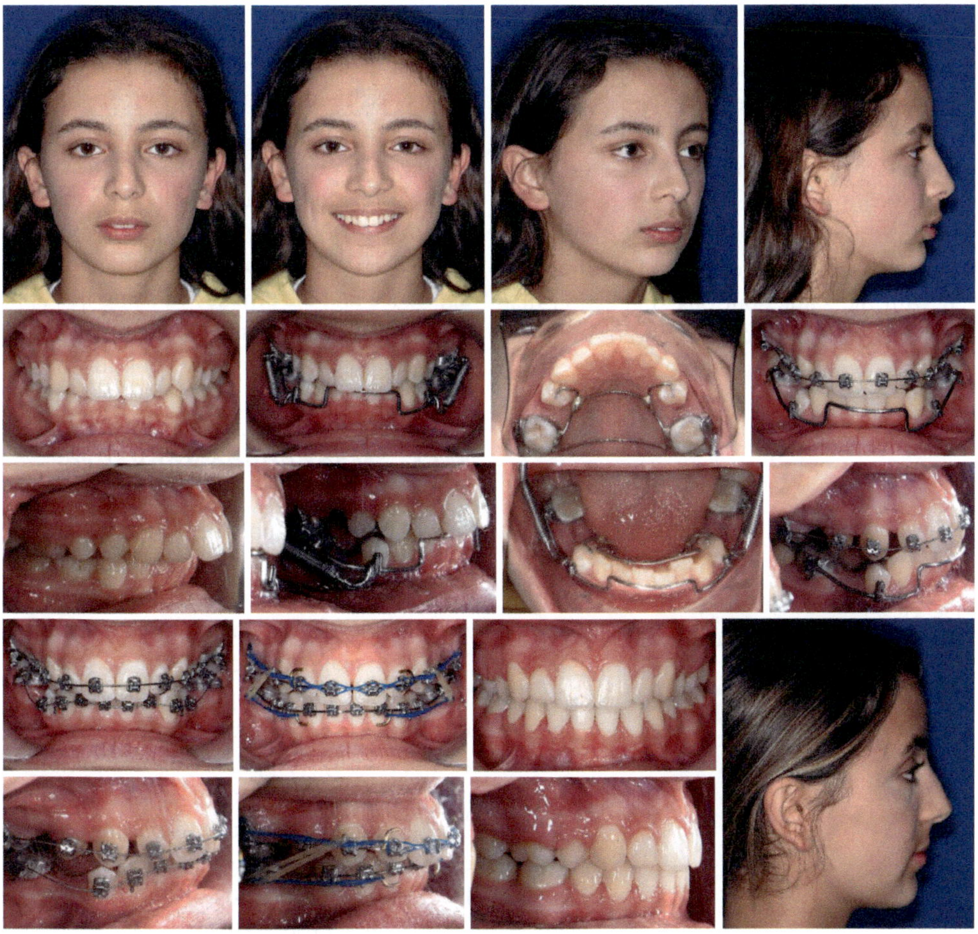

Fig. 5.28 A 13-year-old female presented with a class II division 1 malocclusion with increased overjet, mild upper crowding and hypodontia with absence of the lower second premolars. The goals of treatment included addressing the class II relationship by a combination of upper molar distalisation and mesial movement of the lower arch with any complimentary growth of the mandible. Extraction of the upper second premolars and the lower second deciduous molars was performed. A crossbow appliance that comprised of an upper palatal and lower lingual framework and Forsus™ module was inserted for initial class II correction for 8 months. Full fixed edgewise appliances were then placed in tandem with the crossbow appliance. After progression to rectangular nickel-titanium archwires, the framework was removed and routine space closure was performed on 19 × 25 stainless steel archwires, sliding mechanics and support with class II elastics. The upper panels show the pre-treatment facial appearance with subsequent panels organised in vertical pairs from left to right showing treatment progression

5.12 Mandibular Repositioning Appliance (MARA)

The MARA appliance is a relatively new appliance but has a minimalistic impact on tooth coverage similar to the variants of fixed mandibular protruding devices described by Herbst [22]. The MARA is a two-part appliance with a maxillary and mandibular component that encourages the patient to reposition the mandible forward to bring their anterior teeth together. A horizontal "arm" extends laterally from a stainless steel crown on the lower first molar. A vertical "elbow" on an upper first molar crown that guides the lower jaw forward into the desired position when the patient attempts to close their mouth.

Progressive advancement of the mandible may be achieved by adding a shim of varying size to the maxillary component that forces the mandible to close in a progressively more anterior position (Fig. 5.29). As with the Herbst appliance, stepwise advancement has been recommended with the same spurious suggestion that an enhanced growth effect observed in a rat model may be realised in the human [26].

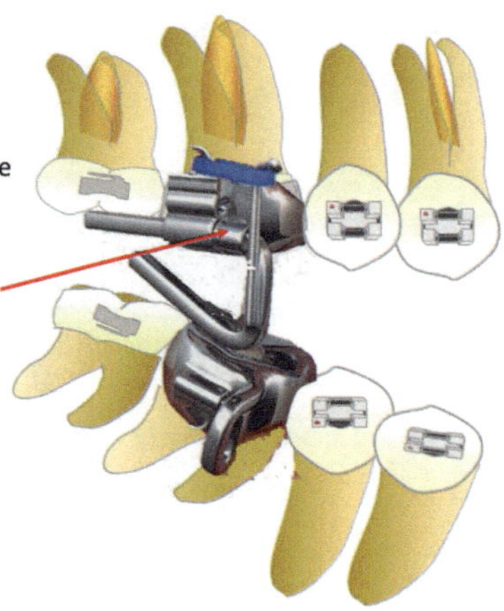

Fig. 5.29 The MARA (Mandibular Anterior Repositioning Device) is a two-part appliance with a maxillary and mandibular component that encourages the patient to reposition the mandible forward to bring their anterior teeth together. A horizontal "arm" extends laterally from a stainless steel crown on the lower first molar. A vertical "elbow" on an upper first molar crown that guides the lower jaw forward into the desired position

The similar advantage of the MARA together with the Forsus™ module enables the clinician to simultaneously align and level the arches whilst correcting the class II relationship. The clinical effects of the MARA appliance are similar to and again provide no significant benefit when compared to analogous fixed class II correctors [62, 63]. The MARA may also be considered in the mixed dentition, leaving alignment issues for a second phase of treatment. Caution must also be taken when treating class II problems in the early mixed dentition with questions related to stability and significant observed relapse [19, 64]. Moreover, the reduced bulk and visibility of the appliance affords the patient an improved aesthetic impact when compared to the larger analogous class II correctors [62].

The disadvantage of the MARA appliance relates to the bulk of the molar crowns and the vertical opening of the occlusion and increased mobility of the lower molar. Moreover, the cost of the MARA appliance is similar to the Herbst appliance and the efficacy of using this appliance must be carefully considered when applied to early treatment in the mixed dentition.

5.13 Magnoglide Appliance

The Magnoglide appliance (Macono Orthodontic Lab, Sydney, Australia) is a fixed functional appliance consisting of maxillary and mandibular right and left-bonded acrylic resin blocks [65]. A series of magnets are located in the blocks to facilitate mandibular posture into a class I relationship (Fig. 5.30). Bonding the appliance addresses any compliance issues and breakages are minimised because of lack of moving parts. The magnetic system eliminates friction, excludes material fatigue with predictable force levels over long periods of time, and no need for direct contact [66, 67].

The clinical effects of the Magnoglide appliance are consistent with changes described following the Herbst appliance with a combination of maxillary incisor retraction and lower incisor proclination (Fig. 5.31). However, in the short term, there appears to be a reduction in vertical

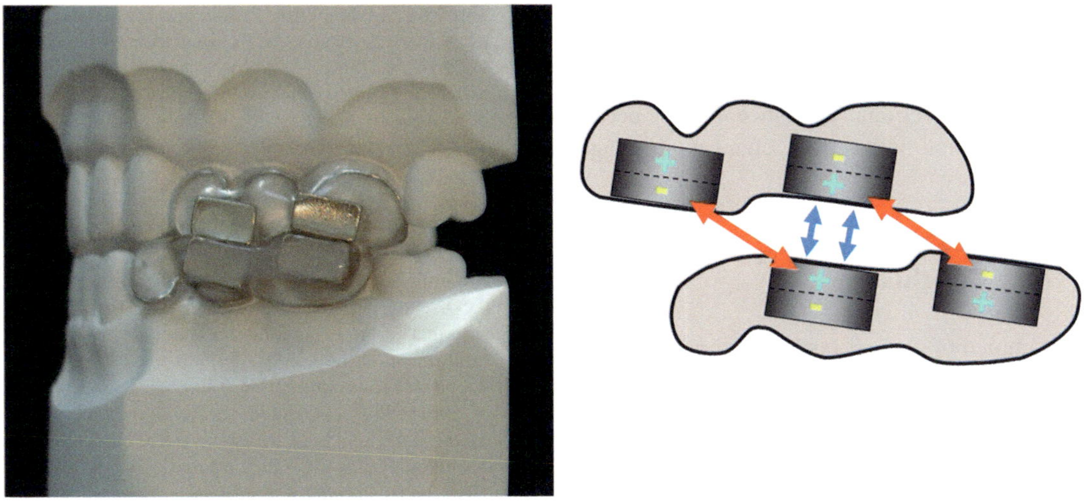

Fig. 5.30 The Magnoglide appliance was developed as a non-compliance class II corrector that is bonded to the upper and lower teeth, effectively acting as a fixed twin block appliance. The attraction of magnets, strategically placed maintains the mandible in a protrusive relationship. (Courtesy of Professor Ali Darendelier, Drs Paul Taylor and Emma McKenzie)

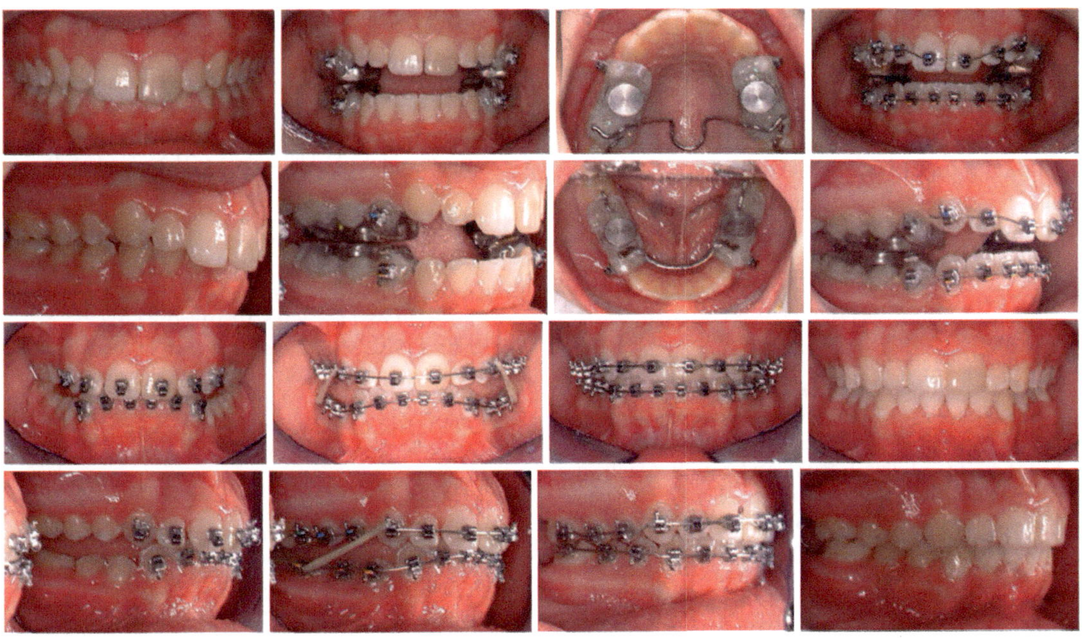

Fig. 5.31 An 11-year-old female presented with a class II division 2 type malocclusion with increased overbite and overjet. A bonded magnetic mandibular advancement device and partial fixed edgewise appliances were placed for 6 months followed by full fixed edgewise appliances and class II elastics for an additional 16 months. (Courtesy of Professor Ali Darendelier, Drs Paul Taylor and Emma McKenzie)

skeletal development. As with most class II correctors, it is expected that the patient will probably realise their original vertical dimension during the post-treatment growth period.

The reported disadvantages of the Magnoglide appliance include the inability to reactivate the appliance, with the indication for a possible second appliance for large overjet corrections, as the magnets could be too far apart to produce a significant force to posture the mandible forward. Moreover, expansion must be performed before or after the functional appliance therapy because any expansion will effect changes in magnet alignment.

5.14 Conclusion

The choice of class II corrector should be based on the realisation of specific goals. These goals are often complex and should be carefully considered with the patient and parents. If the goals include compensation of the upper and lower teeth within the biological constraints and the patient is growing, then any of the multitude of removable or fixed functional appliances will have the same chance of satisfactorily treating most patients. The choice therefore becomes a practice management issue. If the patient or parents desire a significant change to the chin position, then combined surgery and orthodontics should be considered. If the goals of treatment are directed at retraction of the maxillary dentition then either extractions or an upper arch distalising strategy are indicated.

References

1. Festa RS, Tamaroff MH, Chasalow F, Lanzkowsky P. Therapeutic adherence to oral medication regimens by adolescents with cancer. I Laboratory assessment. J Pediatrics. 1992;120(5):807–81.
2. Bos A, Hoogstraten J, Prahl-Andersen B. On the use of personality characteristics in predicting compliance in orthodontic practice. Am J Orthod and Dentofacial Orthopedics. 2003;123(5):p568–70.
3. Al-Mograbi D, Colonia Salazar F, Pandis N, Fleming PS. Compliance with removable orthodontic appliances and adjuncts: a systematic review and meta-analysis. Am J Orthod Dentofacial Orthop. 2017;152(1):17–32.
4. Proffit WR, Fields HW, Moray LJ. Prevalence of malocclusion and orthodontic treatment need in the United States: estimates from the NHANES III survey. Int J Adult Orthodon Orthognath Surg. 1998;13(2):97–106.
5. Brunelle JA, Bhat M, Lipton J. Prevalence and distribution of selected occlusal characteristics in the US population, 1988–1991. J Dent Res. 1996;75:706–13.
6. Tod MA, Taverne AR. Prevalence of malocclusion traits in an Australian adult population. Aust Orthod J. 1996;15(1):16–22.
7. Mills LF. Epidemiologic studies of occlusion IV. The prevalence of malocclusion in a population of 1,455 school children. J Dent Res. 1964;45(2):332–6.
8. Lam R, Mustac S, Goonewardene MS. A clinically based review of patient and treatment characteristics in Western Australian private orthodontic practice. Aust Orthod J. 2020;36:9–19.
9. Annemieke B, Hoogstraten J, Prahl-Andersen B. On the use of personality characteristics in predicting compliance in orthodontic practice. Am J Orthod Dentofacial Orthop. 2003;122:568–70.
10. Pacha MM, Fleming PS, Johal A. A comparison of the efficacy of fixed versus removable functional appliances in children with class II malocclusion: a systematic review. Eur J Orthod. 2016;38(6):621–30.
11. Chadwick SM, Banks P, Wright JL. The use of myofunctional appliances in the UK: a survey of British orthodontists. Dent Update. 1998;25(7):302–8.
12. Bahar AD, Kamarudin Y, Chadwick S. A national survey of orthodontists in Malaysia and their use of functional appliances for class II malocclusions. Aust Orthod J. 2021;37(2):217–26.
13. Johnston LE. Let's pretend. Sem Orthod. 2014;20:249–52.
14. Johnston LE. Growing jaws for fun and profit. In: McNamara Jr JA, editor. Monograph 35, Craniofacial growth series. Ann Arbor, MI: Center for Human Growth and Development, The University of Michigan; 1999.
15. Perinetti G, Primozic J, Franchi L, Contardo L. Treatment effects of removable functional appliances in pre-pubertal and pubertal class II patients: a systematic review and meta-analysis of controlled studies. PLoS One. 2015;10(10):e0141198.
16. Bishara SE. Mandibular changes in persons with untreated and treated class II division 1 malocclusion. Am J Orthod Dentofacial Orthop. 1998;113(6):661–73.
17. Solow B. The dentoalveolar compensatory mechanism: background and clinical implications. Br J Orthod. 1980;7(3):145–61.
18. Jakobsson SO. Cephalometric evaluation of treatment effect on class II, Division I malocclusions. Am J Orthod. 1967;53(6):446–57.
19. Wieslander L. Long-term effect of treatment with the headgear-Herbst appliance in the early mixed dentition. Stability or relapse? Am J Orthod Dentofacial Orthop. 1993;104(4):319–29.
20. Batista KB, Thiruvenkatachari B, Harrison JE, O'Brien KD. Orthodontic treatment for prominent upper front teeth (class II malocclusion) in children and adolescents. Cochrane Database Syst Rev. 2018;3:CD003452.
21. Peck S. Dentist, artist, pioneer : orthodontic innovator Norman Kingsley and his Rembrandt portraits. J Am Dent Assoc. 2012;143(4):393–7.

22. Herbst E. Atlas and Grundriss der Zahnärztlichen Orthopädie. s: J.F.Lehmann; 1910.
23. Rogers AP. Henry albert baker. Am J Orthod. 1958;44(12):940–2.
24. Armstrong MM. Controlling the magnitude, direction, and duration of extraoral force. Am J Orthod. 1971;59(3):p217–43.
25. Pancherz H. Treatment of class II malocclusions by jumping the bite with the Herbst appliance. A cephalometric investigation. Am J Orthod. 1979;76(4):423–42.
26. Purkayastha SK, Rabie AB, Wong R. Treatment of skeletal class II malocclusion in adults: stepwise vs single-step advancement with the Herbst appliance. World J Orthod. 2008;9(3):233–43.
27. Von Bremen J, Bock N, Ruf S. Is Herbst-multibracket appliance treatment more efficient in adolescents than in adults? Angle Orthod. 2009;79(1):173–7.
28. Ruf S, Pancherz H. Orthognathic surgery and dentofacial orthopedics in adult Class II Division 1 treatment: mandibular sagittal split osteotomy versus Herbst appliance. Am J Orthod Dentofacial Orthop. 2004;126(2):140–52.
29. Pancherz H, Bjerklin K. The Herbst appliance 32 years after treatment. J Clin Orthod. 2015;49(7):442–51.
30. Von Bremen J, Pancherz H. Efficiency of class II division 1 and class II division 2 treatment in relation to different treatment approaches. Semin Orthod. 2003;9:87–92.
31. O'Brien K, Wright J, Conboy F, et al. Effectiveness of treatment for class II malocclusion with the Herbst or twin-block appliances: a randomized, controlled trial. Am J Orthod Dentofacial Orthop. 2003;124(2):128–37.
32. Schioth T, von Bremen J, Pancherz H, Ruf S. Complications during Herbst appliance treatment with reduced mandibular cast splints: a prospective, clinical multicenter study. J Orofac Orthop. 2007;68(4):321–7.
33. Kanuru RK, Bhasin V, Khatri A, et al. Comparison of complications in removable mandibular acrylic splint and cantilever Herbst for management of class II malocclusion: a retrospective study. J Contemp Dent Pract. 2017;18(5):363–5.
34. Windmiller EC. The acrylic-splint Herbst appliance: a cephalometric evaluation. Am J Orthod Dentofacial Orthop. 1993;104:73–84.
35. Burstone CJ. Diagnosis and treatment planning of patients with asymmetries. Semin Orthod. 1998;4:153–64.
36. Janson G, de Lima KJ, Woodside DG, Metaxas A, de Freitas MR, Henriques JF. Class II subdivision malocclusion types and evaluation of their asymmetries. Am J Orthod Dentofacial Orthop. 2007;131:57–66.
37. Sanders DA, Rigali PH, Neace WP, Uribe F, Nanda R. Skeletal and dental asymmetries in class II subdivision malocclusions using cone-beam computed tomography. Am J Orthod Dentofacial Orthop. 2010;138(542):e1–20.
38. Janson G, Dainesi EA, Henriques JF, de Freitas MR, de Lima KJ. Class II subdivision treatment success rate with symmetric and asymmetric extraction protocols. Am J Orthod Dentofacial Orthop. 2003;124:257–64. quiz 339
39. Janson G, Baldo T, Garib D, Barros SE, Silva Poletto R, Bittencourt Dos Santos P. Efficiency of class II subdivision malocclusion treatment with 3 and 4 premolar extractions. Am J Orthod Dentofacial Orthop. 2016;150(3):499–503.
40. Cassidy SE, Jackson SR, Turpin DL, Ramsay DS, Spiekerman C, Huang GJ. Classification and treatment of class II subdivision malocclusions. Am J Orthod Dentofacial Orthop. 2014;145:443–51.
41. Mayes JH. Improving appliance efficiency with the Cantilever Herbst: a new answer to old problems. Clin Impressions. 1994;3(2–5):17–9.
42. Keim RG, Gottlieb EL, Nelson AH, Vogels DS. 2002 JCO study of orthodontic diagnosis and treatment procedures: part 1, results and trends. J Clin Orthod. 2002;36:553–68.
43. Mayes JH. The single-appointment preattached cantilever. Clin Impressions. 1996;5:14–23.
44. Moro A, Janson G, de Freitas MR, Henriques JFC, Petrelli NE, Lauris JRP. Class II correction with the cantilever bite jumper. Angle Orthod. 2009;79(2):221–9.
45. Coelho Fılho CM. The mandibular protraction appliances for class II treatment. J Clin Orthod. 1995;29:319–36.
46. Coelho Fılho CM. The mandibular protraction appliance no.3. J Clin Orthod. 1998;32:379–84.
47. Jasper JJ, McNamara JA. The correction of interarch malocclusions using a fixed force module. Am J Orthod Dentofacial Orthop. 1995;108(6):641–50.
48. Stucki N, Ingerval B. The use of the jasper jumper for correction of class II malocclusion in young permanent dentition. Eur J Orthod. 1998;20:271–81.
49. Weiland F, Bantleon HP, Droschl H. Initial effects of treatment of class II malocclusion with Herren activator, activator-headgear combination, and Jasper jumper. Am J Orthod. 1997;112:19–27.
50. Weiland F, Bantleon HP. Treatment of class II malocclusion with the Jasper jumper appliance-a preliminary report. Am J Orthod. 1995;108:341–50.
51. DeVincenzo JP. The Eureka spring: a new interarch delivery system. J Clin Orthod. 1997;31:454.
52. Guimarães CH Jr, Henriques JFC, Janson G, Almeida MR, Araki J, Cançado RH, et al. Prospective study of dentoskeletal changes in class II division malocclusion treatment with twin force bite corrector. Angle Orthod. 2012;83(2):319–26.
53. Altug-Atac AT, Dalci ON, Memikoglu UT. Skeletal class II treatment with twin force bite corrector: case reports. World J Orthod. 2008;9:e7–17.
54. Chhibber A, Upadhyay M, Uribe F, Nanda R. Long-term stabilityof class II correction with the twin force bite corrector. J Clin Orthod. 2010;44:363–76.
55. Zymperdikas VF, Koretsi V, Papageorgiou SN, Papadopoulos MA. Treatment effects of fixed func-

tional appliances in patients with class II malocclusion: a systematic review and meta-analysis. Eur J Orthod. 2016;38(2):113–26.
56. Aidar LA, Abrahao M, Yamashita HK, Dominguez GC. Herbst appliance therapy and temporomandibular joint disc position: a prospective longitudinal magnetic resonance imaging study. Am J Orthod Dentofacial Orthop. 2006;129(4):486–96.
57. Aras A, Ada E, Saracoglu H, et al. Comparison of treatments with the Forsus fatigue resistant device in relation to skeletal maturity: a cephalometric and magnetic resonance imaging study. Am J Orthod Dentofacial Orthop. 2011;140(5):616–25.
58. Hanoun A, Al-Jewair TS, Tabbaa S, et al. A comparison of the treatment effects of the Forsus fatigue resistance device and the twin block appliance in patients with class II malocclusions. Clin Cosmet Investig Dent. 2014;6:57–63.
59. Karacay S, Akin E, Olmez H, et al. Forsus nitinol flat spring and Jasper jumper corrections of class II division 1 malocclusions. Angle Orthod. 2006;76(4):666–72.
60. Aslan BI, Kucukkaraca E, Turkoz C, Dincer M. Treatment effects of the Forsus fatigue resistant device used with miniscrew anchorage. Angle Orthod. 2014;84(1):76–87.
61. Flores-Mir C, Barnett G, Higgins DW, Heo G, Major PW. Short-term skeletal and dental effects of the Xbow appliance as measured on lateral cephalograms. Am J Orthod Dentofacial Orthop. 2009;136(6):822–32.
62. Kulbersh VP, Berger JL. Treatment effects of the mandibular anterior repositioning appliance on patients with class II malocclusion. Am J Orthod. 2003;123:286–95.
63. Siara-Olds NJ, Pangrazio-Kulbersh V, Berger J, Bayirli B. Long-term dentoskeletal changes with the Bionator, Herbst, twin block, and MARA functional appliances. Angle Orthod. 2010;80:18–29.
64. Pancherz H. The nature of class II relapse after Herbst ap-pliance treatment: a cephalometric long-term investigation. Am J Orthod Dentofacial Orthop. 1991;100:220–33.
65. Phelan A, Tarraf NE, Taylor P, Hönscheid R, Drescher D, Baccetti T, Darendeliler MA. Skeletal and dental outcomes of a new magnetic functional appliance, the Sydney Magnoglide, in class II correction. Am J Orthod Dentofacial Orthop. 2012;141(6):759–72.
66. Darendeliler MA, Darendeliler A, Mandurino M. Clinical application of magnets in orthodontics and biological implications: a review. Eur J Orthod. 1997;19:431–42.
67. Noar JH, Evans RD. Rare earth magnets in orthodontics: an overview. Br J Orthod. 1999;26:29–37.

6 Molar Distalization: Bad English, Good Practice

S. Jay Bowman

6.1 Introduction

Although the term, molar distalization, is actually a neologism and perhaps an example of bad use of *The King's English*, the actual orthodontic biomechanic concept may be an exemplar of "good practice." In fact, the idea of pushing maxillary molars "distally" or posteriorly has been promoted as one method of correcting Class II malocclusion that has been around for nearly as long as orthodontics has been a specialty. Interestingly enough, Fowlers' guide to English usage was not published until 6 years after the birth of orthodontia in 1900. Unfortunately, the term "distalization" occasionally is confused (possibly by a few tipplers) with the technique used by bootleggers during the U.S. Prohibition (1920–31) to "distill" their spirits. Notwithstanding, the terms distalization and distalizing have been adopted into the common orthodontic vernacular and these terms will be belabored throughout this communication.

At the outset, it is important to note that there have been seemingly innumerable publications in our specialty's history describing various mechanisms to produce "molar distalization" (as the late Tony Gianelly described some as the latest "gimmicks, gizmos, and gadgets"), accompanied by their respective "management and effects" [1–41]. This chapter will not feature recipes or "how to" distalize molars (those types of things can be easily gleaned by reading publications describing their clinical applications [1–41]). Rather, it is more important to discuss how the Class II correction occurs. The point of the present message is to simply reiterate that there are very little (if any) differences in the final effects of any of the different methods of correcting Class II relationships for patients that are still experiencing facial growth [42, 43]. A previously used analogy is that All Class II roads lead to Rome: push the upper jaw or teeth, yank on the lower jaw or teeth, and you get to the same destination. You pick [44].

6.2 Getting Even with Overjet

Ever since Edward Hartley Angle defined and categorized the Classes of malocclusion for orthodontia [45], practitioners of our art and science have quested to position first permanent molars (and canines) squarely into so-called Class I relationship (and after the advent of cephalometry, maxillary molars were thought necessary to be oriented under the "key ridge"). Although demonstrable health benefits of this occlusal arrangement may not be substantial, the resolution of other

S. J. Bowman (✉)
Saint Louis University-CADE, St. Louis, MO, USA

The University of Michigan, Ann Arbor, MI, USA

Case Western Reserve University,
Cleveland, OH, USA
e-mail: info@kalamazooorthodontics.com

M. T. Cobourne (ed.), *Orthodontic Management of Class II Malocclusion*,
https://doi.org/10.1007/978-3-031-57530-3_6

associated alignment issues (crowding, spacing, crossbite, overbite, overjet, and the like) all often fall-in-line when molars are fitted together appropriately. Consequently, our raison d'être.

6.3 Hold Up! What's the Deal with Class II Correction?

Before delving into a discussion of molar distalization for the correction of Class II malocclusion, let's tap the brakes and delineate some terms, specifications, and definitions. First off, orthodontics is a service, based in science, that has been demonstrated to be useful in treating patients at nearly any age, but mostly adolescents and adults. That implies that a significant number of people using these services are themselves in the business of growing (including their faces) and then there are others that aren't growing much anymore.

Considering that one of the major issues in diagnosing Class II malocclusion is that there is often a skeletal growth component mismatch (upper, lower, or both jaws). Then, it is likely important if a patient seeking treatment may yet provide some possibly favorable growth to assist in the correction (i.e., pre-adults). It might also be useful to know when the maximum growth potential for an individual is going to occur (e.g., some sort of growth prediction: statural height, age, or some other "sciency-sounding" elaborate scheme, often involving irradiating the patient). As such, discussions regarding best treatments and timing for Class II cases have gotten very messy and argumentative over the past century with name-calling and testy interchanges in print and at professional meetings with little sign of consensus. At best, we know for certain that Things Go Better with Growth.

6.4 Interruption of Dentoalveolar Compensation

What the heck is the dentoalveolar compensation mechanism (DCM)? In 1980, Solow [46] described the background and clinical implications. Simply put (sarcasm intended), DCM is defined as "a system which attempts to maintain normal interarch relationships under varying jaw relationships." Continuing, "the differences in the interarch relationships of subjects with Class I, II, and III malocclusions are probably not directly due to differences in skeletal morphology, but rather to the fact that in the Class I group, in contrast to Class II and III subjects, the variation in jaw relationship has been compensated for by the dentoalveolar compensatory mechanism." So, the dental relationship has been compensated for by the compensatory mechanism? Wait, let's try this: The coordination of the development of the upper and lower arches is not always *perfect*. Some mechanism is therefore needed to coordinate the eruption and position of the teeth relative to their jaw bases in order for a normal relationship between the upper and lower dental arches to be achieved and maintained. DCM. Clear as mud.

In pre-adolescents, the maxilla is generally outgrowing the mandible, yet Class I remains Class I; Class IIs remain Class IIs (i.e., the old adage: them that has, gets more). In adolescents, the mandible outgrows the maxilla, yet Class II does not spontaneously improve, and Class Is are not likely to become Class IIs. The unfortunate Class III doesn't benefit in either regard.

There is often a mismatch in skeletal development, yet the DCM results in virtually the same classification of dental occlusion throughout growth, although there may be some variations such as tipping and crowding of incisors and the like. What if you desire to change that dental occlusion arrangement? Then interrupting, altering, or changing that dental occlusion is likely to artificially permit or allow the underlying skeletal development to occur (carrying the dentoalveolus along), precluding compensation, ending with a new dental relationship result [47–50]. However, this is only reasonable for the growing patient. When done growing, then orthodontists are generally left with simply moving teeth around: Class II correction with molar distalization in adults is primarily due to pushing the maxillary dentition. If using "functional devices" in adults, then upper and lower teeth are just pushed around (although there could be some "postural" positioning or condylar remodeling at work).

If you're moving teeth, then the dentoalveolus housing is changing. It is quite doubtful that we're substantially moving basal bone, unless involved with some type of sutural change. As both the upper and lower dentoalveolus are altered during years of growth and remodeling, it requires some type of interruption to affect antero-posterior changes during that time. Then it follows that just about anything that provides that interruption may result in some antero-posterior change for pre-adult patients. However, to be clear, we aren't "growing bone;" specifically, mandibles during orthodontics [47–50].

After the teenage years, you can push and pull on the dentoalveolus for change, but those changes are not of the same nature as those seen with those pre-adults. In simpler terms, growth does what it does, behind the scenes during pre-adult orthodontics. But for adults, orthodontics does what it does to the teeth and underlying dentoalveolus, but without "much, if any" growth.

6.5 Dentition Marching in Lockstep

An illustration featuring marching band members in lockstep with a quote from Lysle Johnston may be helpful [42] (Fig. 6.1). "As has been noted, it is usual for the mandible to outgrow the maxilla in both Class I and Class II malocclusions. This pattern, although 'favorable,' would have no effect on the occlusion, thanks to the phenomenon of dentoalveolar compensation." (a) The large arrows indicate a Class I adolescent is exhibiting jaw growth of both the maxilla and mandible with the mandible outgrowing the maxilla. The marching "molars" are in lockstep in Class I relationship due to the dentoalveolar compensation mechanism from the occlusion. (b) In Class IIs, although the upper molars and lower molars are mismatched, mandibular growth will not correct that lock-step Class II relationship due to that same compensation mechanism. (c)

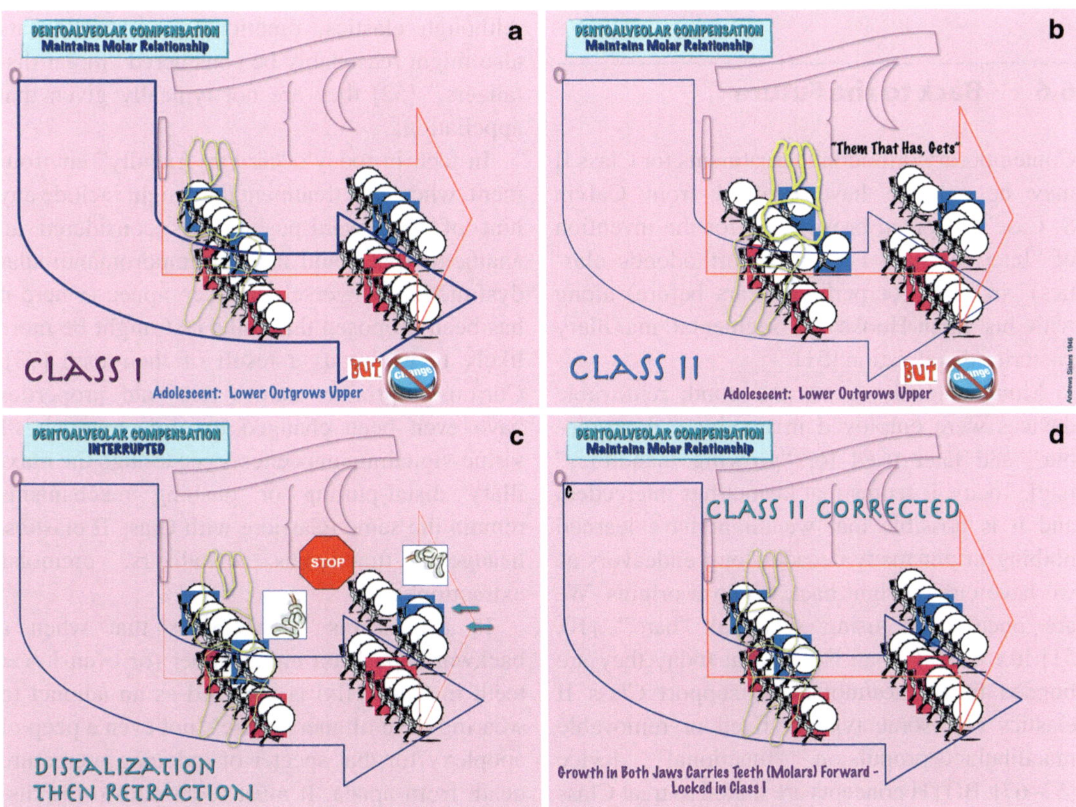

Fig. 6.1 Graphic representation of the effects of interrupting dentoalveolar compensation on Class II correction with the analogy of lock-step marching band percussionists as molars and incisors in growing jaws

Orthodontic mechanisms are used to interrupt the compensation by separating the occlusion; possibly holding the mandible forward, and/or pushing or holding the maxillary dentition posteriorly. (d) Once the dentition is in Class I and overjet is reduced, then *both* upper and lower jaws continue on their course of remaining growth. The difference is that both jaws now advance with Class I molars. It is like a command to the band members: "change step, march!" This may be accomplished by a "stutter-step" by the upper percussionists, interrupting their forward movement to match the lower. Subsequently, both the upper *and* lower molars are carried forward by continuing facial growth. This led to an old trepidation that after distalization, the upper molars ended-up more forward than where they started out originally: "didn't we just lose all the distal movement we worked to get?" No, in a pre-adult undergoing any type of Class II treatment, this would be completely expected—quite simply, both jaws are still growing, downwards and forwards; so all molars are carried forward.

6.6 Back to the Future

Contemporary orthodontic treatments for Class II may be said to have evolved from Calvin S. Case's disputed provenance for the invention of "Intermaxillary Force (i.e., orthodontic elastics)" in 1904 (or perhaps years before) along with his Span-Hooks for segmental maxillary posterior distalization [51].

Simultaneously across the pond, removable devices were employed in treating "glossoptopia," and later used for "growing mandibles" [sic]. Today, it seems that kismet has interceded, and it is possible that we might have learned nothing in our many decades-long endeavors as we have circled right back to those origins. We are once again using sectional "bars," [10, 51] like Case's Span-Hooks, but today they are bonded to canines/molars, to support Class II elastics *OR,* some type of fixed or removable mandibular propulsion "functional" device [52–67]. BOTH concepts are touted to treat Class IIs, TMD, and sleep apnea.

Take for instance the question of Phase I or early treatment for Class II. It would seem the evidence produced in substantial trials and other sundry studies have demonstrated that this type of treatment costs more, takes longer, and does not provide any added benefits [68–70]. Yet, there are those still wishing to impeach all research results in preference of their favorite "flavor-of-the-month" appliances, including clear aligners, as though they offer some new twist on an old tale. This is almost as absurd as the occasional resurrection of the defrocked Functional Matrix Hypothesis of "spaces (e.g., airway) growing faces" [71].

Meanwhile, two other major modes of treatments besides elastics and functionals have also been used throughout our history for Class II, namely: the headgear [72] and molar distalization. The headgear has been one of the most successful and time-tested, evidence-based devices, yet has fallen out of favor in the past 40 years due to a rise in methods not as dependent upon compliance for success (e.g., distalizers, functionals). Although elastics, functionals, and headgears also might reasonably be considered "molar distalizers," [52] they are not typically given that appellation.

In fact, in today's "airway friendly" environment, where any treatment that might include any hint of "backward-pushing" is considered an anathema that could induce temporomandibular dysfunction or worse yet, sleep apnea (where it has been proposed that folks just might be more likely to expire as a result of their use) [73]. Curiously, product names and said properties have even been changed to project an air of virtue-signaling innocence, even though the maxillary distal-pulling or pushing mechanisms remain the same (Carriere with Class II elastics, headgear, functionals, distalizers, premolar extractions).

It also seems disingenuous that when a backwards-push on either upper (or even lower teeth in Class IIIs) is involved as an adjunct to wearing clear aligners, there's not even a peep of apoplexy for that specter of inducing premature death from apnea. It must seem odd to the discerning skeptic that attempting to pull forward on the maxilla in the pre-adult Class III population often yields much the same results as pushing on the lower teeth with elastics and bonded bars; but in some circles, one is verboten and the other is championed. How is the conscientious and evidence-based clinician to square all these perplexing conundrums? What is a discriminating orthodontist to do?

6.7 How Can We Know What Works and How?

Considering the various ideas still perpetually recycling out there: Who do we trust? How do we know? Is there a market for evidence? Perhaps, more importantly, will the patients ever know? Lysle Johnston [74] has opined, "There's a real market for straight teeth, but not for straight thought." In other words, what is the value of the work-product of the academic if the results are so quickly ignored when they might not square with what you do in your own practice, or that of your favorite guru?

If one wishes to determine the difference in results from various methods of correcting Class IIs, the first critical discriminator is whether the selection of samples to evaluate are from pre-adults OR "non-growers" to offer a fair playing field. Since nearly any method or mechanism that has been introduced in the past 100 years to correct Class IIs has proven a modicum of success [75], perhaps then some tacit stipulation could be agreed upon. Unfortunately, there have been strongly held "beliefs" that there must be a difference in the results from the use of fixed and removable functional appliances in contrast to other options. In other words, pushing and holding the mandible in a protracted position has been thought to somehow create *accentuated* horizontal growth—or "mandibular enhancement [76]." It certainly often seems that our treatment choices may have more to do with clinical utility or profitability than optimal patient care (i.e., what's easy, popular, and pays the bills?) when it seems even easier to be dismissive of opposing evidence [75].

6.8 Class II Correction: A Battle with Compliance and Anchorage Loss

It is readily apparent that fixed and removable functional appliances have a long history of success in correcting Class IIs, but not without documented side-effects and missteps along the path. Originally thought to stimulate mandibular growth, then turning to a "headgear effect," "condylar remodeling," and even now, in a twist of fate, maxillary distalization has been used to explain how they work [52]. Unfortunately, none of these descriptions seem to adequately provide the complete answer. Examining contemporary Class II treatments and their favorability seems to hinge upon an ongoing clinical battle between patient compliance with treatment along with some level of resulting iatrogenic anchorage loss attending each method (i.e., there is no free lunch).

As patient cooperation seems to have significantly diminished starting in about the 1970s with reticence in wearing headgears, elastics, and removable devices, orthodontists were perplexed by their patients shunning the mechanisms crucial for fixing their bites. This led to the resurrection of the Herbst appliance, followed by a hundred offshoots; all intending to hold the mandible in a protracted position, much like removable functional devices. The one key difference: these fixed devices were not dependent on patient adherence to wearing a chunk or two of plastic. However, with all mechanisms applying any direct or reciprocal force on the lower dentition, they caused untoward flaring, tipping, or labial movement of the lower anterior teeth (also characterized as "anchorage loss") [62–65]. Besides negative changes in the lower lip, the amount of Class II correction possible can be compromised as labial tipping of lower incisors closes the "gap" of overjet; perhaps ahead of any change coming through mandibular development (via interruption of the compensation mechanism): robbing Peter to pay Paul.

Long before the advent of skeletal anchorage in orthodontics, the issue of anchorage was always in hot debate. The predictability of tooth movement was subject to innumerable schemes to control it [77]. “Ganging-up” big molars, bundled together with braces against other teeth, tipping them way back to “prepare” anchorage, elaborate frameworks across the palate, tipping auxiliaries, combinations of devices [40, 41], and adding headgears and elastics to shore-up support are just some examples.

If, however, some compressed spring-type mechanism were added to move molars, there is a price to pay: anchorage loss due to the typical reciprocal force on the anterior teeth. In that historic milieu of spring-loaded mechanisms, there was the thought that if the molars were simply moved posteriorly first (in contrast to distal maxillary *en masse* movement) [33, 38, 39], then maybe the cost of anchorage loss in the anterior would be less; hence, the idea of molar distalization was born. While reducing reliance upon patient cooperation, distalization unfortunately can still suffer from anchorage loss. The probable solution (for either lower or upper flaring) appeared in the form of skeletal anchorage support, primarily with plates or miniscrews [77–90]. As Watson [91] astutely recognized in 2006, the real key to Class II distalization is not the fact that the molars are moved back or even to what degree, but rather, what happens afterward (i.e., retraction of the remaining maxillary teeth, the effects of interrupting compensation, maintaining the new, distal molar position, finishing the occlusion, etc.) [92, 93].

Ah, but wait, detractors opined that you are addressing the wrong arch with mechanisms focused on the maxilla! After all, isn’t Class II a disease of small mandibles? Might it not be important to know what also happens to the mandible during treatments featuring maxillary distalization in pre-adults and how that might compare to other Class II treatment methods considered to be “mandible-friendly?”

6.9 Mandibular Response. What Gives?

Entering the discussion of the contribution of mandibular response during different treatments, it would be quite useful to review Lysle Johnston’s Pitchfork Cephalometric Analysis [94] (Fig. 6.2). This is a “cost accounting” method to evaluate the contributions of orthodontic and skeletal components to correction, based on cephalometric superimpositions on the “functional occlusal plane” (i.e., where the “action is” in orthodontic correction). With this method, the effects of growth, molar movement, incisor changes, “headgear effect on the maxilla” and mandibular

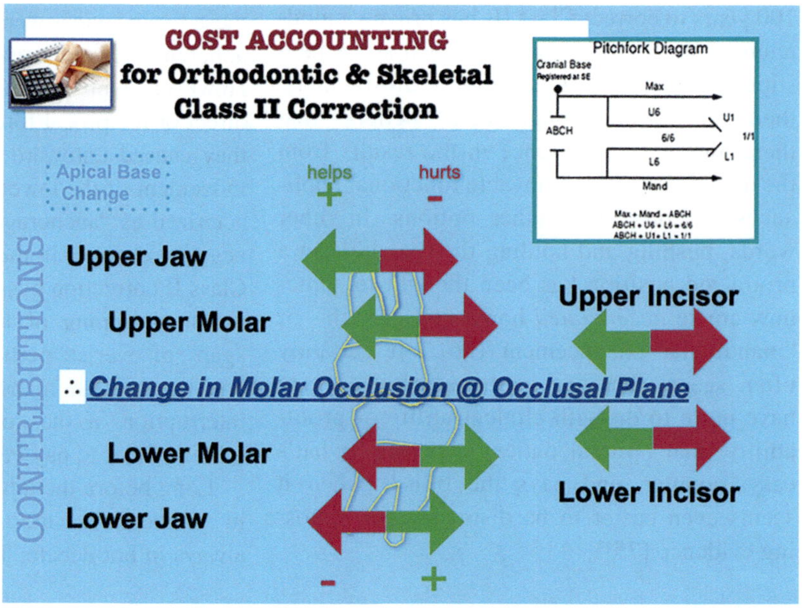

Fig. 6.2 Lysle E. Johnston’s Pitchfork Analysis [94] is a “cost accounting” technique to determine the skeletal and dental contributions for Class II correction

response during treatment can be delineated: "an algebraic sum of facial skeletal growth and tooth movement relative to basal bone" [94].

So as a primer, we have adapted a selection of studies on a variety of functional appliances, simply assessing the "mandibular response" measured for each (Fig. 6.3) [54–61]. It appears in this group, the largest amount measured was 4.7 mm for a sample of 30 patients who were treated for 32 months [54]. The most important caveat was that these were "cherry-picked" as those patients that demonstrated the most "favorable treatment response" with the Activator appliance. Interestingly enough, Livieratos and Johnston [68] (Fig. 6.4) found the same mandibular response for a sample of 40 treated for 24 months with a Bionator followed by Edgewise appliances. Even more curious was the 4.2 mm of mandibular response reported by Phaerukkakit [95] for a group of 50 Class IIs treated for

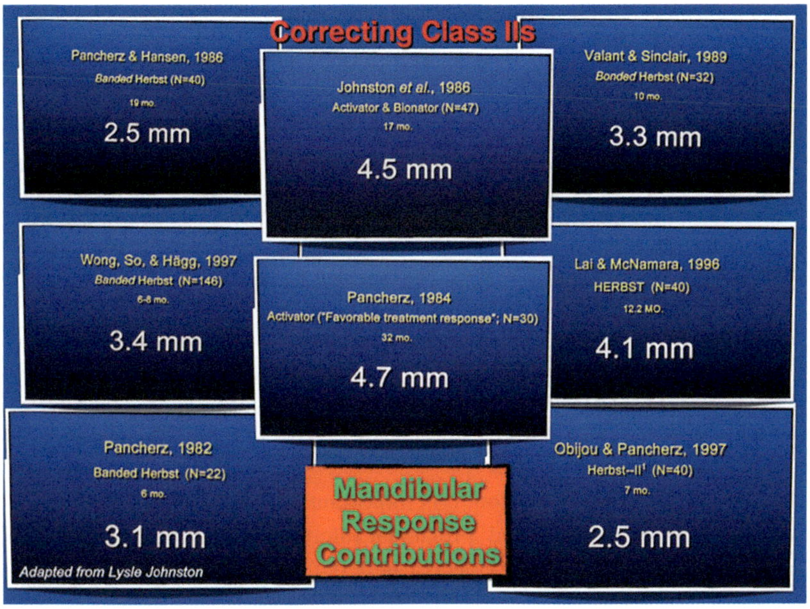

Fig. 6.3 The contribution of mandibular response to a variety of Class II corrections [54–61]

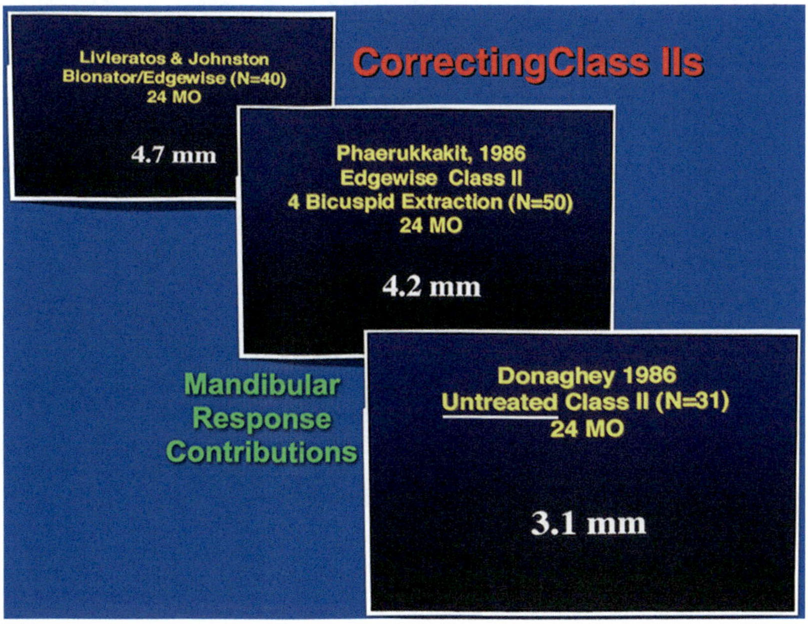

Fig. 6.4 Comparing the mandibular response from functional and braces, extraction and braces, and no treatment at all [68]. It appears that Class II treatments might offer only 1.6 mm of added "mandibular response"

24 months with Edgewise appliances employing the "dreaded" extraction of four dental units and no functionals. So, there's a half millimeter difference in mandibular response between the best in functionals and removing teeth in standard braces Class II treatment?

Now, wait just a second! The mandible has been growing along with all these different treatments, but how much would it have grown without any intervention at all? Donaghey [96] evaluated a sample of 31 Class IIs, also over a 24-month period, but they were untreated. The amount of unfettered normal mandibular response was an uncanny 3.1 mm (Fig. 6.4). It would seem quite apparent and logical to conclude the orthodontic Class II treatments may at best offer only about 1.6 mm of additional mandibular response compared to doing no treatment.

Growth Does What It Does While Working in the Background—Lysle E. Johnston, Jr.

6.10 How Does Molar Distalization Compare with Other Methods?

At the outset of this discussion, it is important to note that the author once had a financial interest in a distalization gadget over a decade ago, but no longer and, in fact, has utilized in practice, every mechanism described in this chapter.

As both distalization and functional appliances gained popularity to reduce reliance upon patient compliance, both suffered from side effects of anchorage loss seen in the anterior dentition. Likely that the enquiring clinician might find it useful to determine if both methods' final effects are different. This question was answered by Burkhart, McNamara, and Baccetti [76] in 2003 in an investigation comparing the effects of molar distalization versus "mandibular enhancement" (this term, used in their article, appeared to signal that the authors anticipated a "special effect" might occur in treatment addressing the lower jaw). Specifically, they evaluated three Class II samples: 30 Steel Crown Herbst, 30 Acrylic Herbst, and 30 Pendulum patients (Fig. 6.5). Total treatment times were within 4 months of each other, and these patients were treated by recognized clinical experts with these devices. The most intriguing result was the noted mandibular response contribution for each approach. The Herbst/Edgewise patients experienced 28 months of treatment with 3.7 mm of mandibular response while the Pendulum/Edgewise sample resulted in 3.1 mm in 32 months. Although there were different treatment mechanisms, addressing different jaws, the

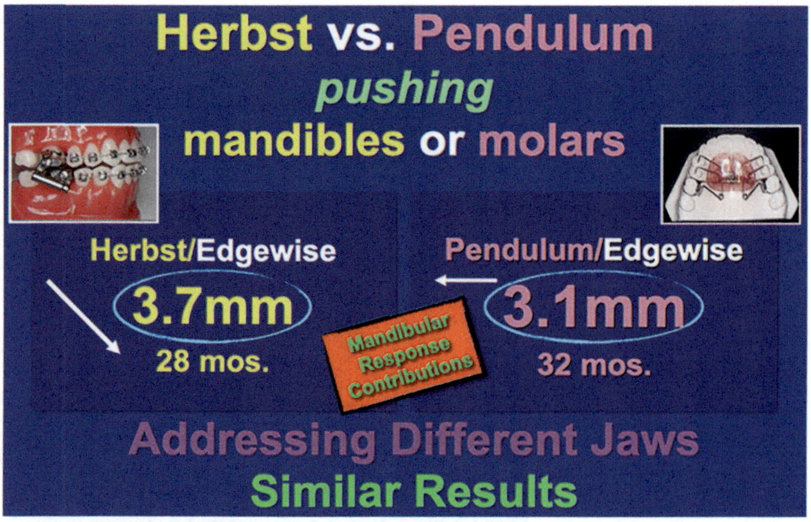

Fig. 6.5 Burkhardt, McNamara, and Baccetti [76] reported that there was only 0.6 mm more mandibular response from patients treated with the Herbst compared to the Pendulum. Different Jaws, Similar Results

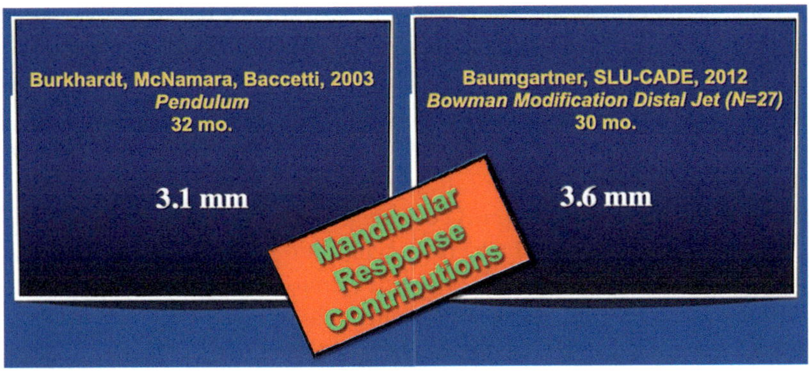

Fig. 6.6 Baumgartner [85] measured 3.6 mm of mandibular response with the Distal Jet, only 0.5 mm more than Burkhardt et al. [76] found with the Pendulum and curiously, nearly the same amount as the Herbst. Addressing Different Jaws, Similar Results

results were quite similar. Push the mandible forward or maxillary teeth posteriorly, similar deal—give or take 0.6 mm in mandibular response. Same Thing, Only Different?

In 2012, Baumgartner [85] (Fig. 6.6) evaluated the results from a different molar distalizer (Distal Jet) with a sample of 27 treated in 30 months. Remarkably, this sample exhibited 3.6 mm of mandibular response—nearly identical to the previously evaluated Herbst samples. Look, even if we consider Class II might be due to "small mandibles," jacking them forward doesn't appear to produce any different result than by leaning on maxillary teeth.

In a subsequent study by Mellion [89], a group of 63 patients was treated with an alternative fixed functional (i.e., Forsus) for 28 months, yielding 3.4 mm of mandibular response; just a bit less (0.3 mm) than the Herbst noted previously. This sample was also compared with a collection of 47 patients treated with a miniscrew-supported version of the Distal Jet (Horseshoe Jet). The intent of adding skeletal anchorage was to eliminate any anterior anchorage loss during distalization. The results in 30 months with the Horseshoe Jet were 2.0 mm of mandibular response. It is surmised that the miniscrew support reduced maxillary incisor flaring; thereby, producing a bit more molar distalization, and consequently, less mandibular change was needed to correct to a Class I occlusion. The difference between the two approaches was only 1.4 mm more for the mandible pushing; once again about the same as noted previously in other studies.

6.11 Can We Draw Conclusions?

Might we conclude that all types of Class II treatments for pre-adults (including most of those discussed within the pages of this tome) likely produce no more than about 1.6 mm of additional "mandibular enhancement" when compared to applying *no treatment at all*? Many decades ago, a cigarette company advertised that their product had a unique 101 mm length: "Well, it's one better. A silly millimeter longer." Therefore, Class II correction is mostly about interrupting dentoalveolar compensation, whatever the mechanism used—with a silly millimeter or so longer "mandibular enhancement" if you shove on the mandible. Wonder how that works out for those claiming to be able to "develop the maxilla" even further forward with plastic devices and then, somehow "growing" the mandible out to meet it (i.e., absurdly named "orthotropics")?

A little inaccuracy saves a world of explanation.—C.E. Ayres

Johnston [42] reported, "Lager (1967) was the first to propose a version of this argument when he argued that functional appliances serve as bite planes that would allow the normal pattern of facial growth to change the occlusion by preventing maxillary dentoalveolar compensation." In 2022, workers at the Bauru Dental School Department of Orthodontics in Brazil concluded [52], "The Forsus and MARA associated with fixed appliances, effectively corrected the Class II malocclusion, mostly using dentoalveolar changes and maxillary growth restriction." It has become curiouser and curiouser that after nearly a century of pushing on mandibles that the focus has now turned to the other arch.

It would seem then that the selection of a treatment method (e.g., headgear, elastics, functional, distalizer, *en masse* retraction; extractions or not) appears, on average, to be a practice management issue, not a biological one. In the battle with compliance and anchorage loss, one must determine the arch where you can afford to lose anchorage: upper or lower, or NOT! Since "mandibular enhancement" contributes minimally *res ipsa loquitur*, Tsourakis and Johnston [97] concluded, "The 'take-home' message is simple: from the standpoint of prevention and correction of Class II malocclusion, *the maxilla is the right jaw*."

References

1. Gianelly AA, Vaitas AS, Thomas WM. The use of magnets to move molars distally. Am J Orthod Dentofacial Orthop. 1989;96:161–7.
2. Bondemark L, Kurol J. Distalization of maxillary first and second molars simultaneously with repelling magnets. Eur J Orthod. 1992;14:264–72.
3. Locatelli R, Bednar J, Deitz VS, Gianelly AA. Molar distalization with superelastic NiTi wire. J Clin Orthod. 1992;26:277–9.
4. Muse DS, Fillman MJ, Emmerson WJ. Molar and incisor changes with Wilson rapid molar distalization. Am J Orthod Dentofacial Orthop. 1993;104:556–65.
5. Cetlin NM, Ten Hoeve A. Nonextraction treatment. J Clin Orthod. 1996;17:396–413.
6. Jones R, White J. Rapid class II molar correction with an open-coil jig. J Clin Orthod. 1992;26:661–4.
7. Runge ME, Martin JT, Bukai F. Analysis of rapid maxillary molar distal movement without patient cooperation. Am J Orthod Dentofacial Orthop. 1999;115:153–7.
8. Brickman CD, Sinha PK, Nanda RS. Evaluation of the Jones Jig appliance for distal molar movement. Am J Orthod Dentofacial Orthop. 2000;118:526–34.
9. Walde KC. The simplified molar distalizer. J Clin Orthod. 2003;37:616–9.
10. Carrière L. A new class II distalizer. J Clin Orthod. 2004;38:224–31.
11. Maino G, Mariani L, Bozzo I, Maino G, Caprioglio A. Maxillary molar distalization with MGBM-system in class II malocclusion. J Orthod Sci. 2013;2(3):101–8.
12. Hilgers JJ. The pendulum appliance for class II non-compliance therapy. J Clin Orthod. 1992;26:700–13.
13. Byloff FK, Darendeliler MA. Distal molar movement using the pendulum appliance. Part I: clinical and radiological evaluation. Angle Orthod. 1997;67:249–60.
14. Kinzinger G, Fuhrmann R, Gross U, Diedrich P. Modified pendulum appliance including distal screw and uprighting activation for non-compliance therapy of class-II malocclusion in children and adolescents. J Orofac Orthop. 2000;61(3):175–90.
15. Bussick TJ, McNamara JA Jr. Dentoalveolar and skeletal changes associated with the pendulum appliance. Am J Orthod Dentofacial Orthop. 2000;177:333–43.
16. Chaqués-Asensi J, Kalra V. Effects of the pendulum appliance on the dentofacial complex. J Clin Orthod. 2001;35:254–7.
17. Kinzinger GSM, Fritz UB, Sander FG, Diedrich RP. Efficiency of a pendulum appliance for molar distalization related to second and third molar eruption stage. Am J Orthod Dentofacial Orthop. 2004;125:8–23.
18. Kinzinger GS, Wehrbein H, Diedrich PR. Molar distalization with a modified pendulum appliance: in vitro analysis of the force systems and in vivo study in children and adolescents. Angle Orthod. 2005;75(4):558–67.
19. Angelieri F, de Almedia RR, Almeida MR, Fuziy A. Dentoalveolar and skeletal changes associated with the pendulum appliance followed by fixed orthodontic treatment. Am J Orthod Dentofacial Orthop. 2006;129:520–7.
20. Caprioglio A, Beretta M, Lanteri C. Maxillary molar distalization: Pendulum and Fast-Back, comparison between two approaches for Class II malocclusion. Prog Orthod. 2011;12(1):8–16.
21. Chiu PP, McNamara JA Jr, Franchi L. A comparison of two intraoral molar distalization appliances: distal jet versus pendulum. Am J Orthod Dentofacial Orthop. 2005;128:353–65.
22. Bowman SJ. Upper-molar distalization and the distal jet. J Clin Orthod. 2016;50(3):159–69.
23. Carano A, Testa M. The distal jet for upper molar distalization. J Clin Orthod. 1996;30:374–80.
24. Ghosh J, Nanda RS. Evaluation of an intraoral maxillary molar distalization technique. Am J Orthod Dentofacial Orthop. 1996;110:639–46.
25. Bowman SJ. Modifications of the distal jet. J Clin Orthod. 1998;32:549–56.
26. Huerter G. A retrospective evaluation of maxillary molar distalization with the distal jet appliance. Master's Thesis. St. Louis, MO: Saint Louis University, Center for Advanced Dental Education; 2000.
27. Ngantung V, Nanda R, Bowman S. Post-treatment evaluation of the distal jet appliance. Am J Orthod Dentofacial Orthop. 2001;120:178–85.
28. Ngantung V, Nanda RS, Bowman SJ. Author's response. Am J Orthod Dentofacial Orthop. 2001;120:14A–5A.

29. Carano A, Testa M, Bowman S. The distal jet: simplified and updated. J Clin Orthod. 2002;36:586–90.
30. Bolla E, Muratore F, Carano A, Bowman S. Evaluation of maxillary molar distalization with the distal jet. Angle Orthod. 2002;72:481–94.
31. Maginnis JJ. Treatment effects of the distal jet with 180 gram and 240 gram springs. Masters degree thesis. St. Louis, MO: Saint Louis University, Center for Advanced Dental Education; 2002.
32. Nishii Y, Katada H, Yamaguchi H. Three-dimensional evaluation of the distal jet appliance. World J Orthod. 2002;3:321–7.
33. Ferguson DJ, Carano A, Bowman SJ, Davis EC, Guiterrez Vegas ME, Lee SH. A comparison of two maxillary molar distalizing appliances with the distal jet. World J Orthod. 2005;6:382–90.
34. Carano A, Bowman S. Non-compliance class II treatment with the distal jet. In: Papadopoulos MA, editor. Orthodontic treatment for the class II noncompliant patient: current principles and techniques. Elsevier, Mosby: Edinburgh; 2006. p. 265–89.
35. Kinzinger GSM, Diedrich PR. Biomechanics of the distal jet. Angle Orthod. 2008;78:676–81.
36. Cali L. Comparing two method of non-compliance class II therapy: the distal jet and the SMD (Frog). Master's Thesis. St. Louis, MO: Saint Louis University, Center for Advanced Dental Education; 2011.
37. Kaplan NL. Comparison of effects of the distal jet appliance, upper premolar extraction, and headgear in patients with class II malocclusion., Master's Thesis. St. Louis, MO: Saint Louis University, Center for Advanced Dental Education; 2012.
38. Flores-Mir C, McGrath L, Heo G, Major PW. Efficiency of molar distalization associated with second and third molar eruption stage. Angle Orthod. 2013 Jul;83(4):735–42.
39. Papadopoulos MA, Mavropoulos A, Karamouzos A. Cephalometric changes following simultaneous first and second molar distalization using a non-compliance intraoral appliance. J Orofac Orthop. 2004;65:123–36.
40. Bowman SJ. Class II combination therapy: molar distalization and fixed functionals to reduce reliance upon compliance for predictable case completion. J Clin Orthod. 1998;32:611–20.
41. Bowman SJ. Class II combination therapy: molar distalization and fixed functionals. In: Nanda R, Kapila S, editors. Current therapy in orthodontics. St. Louis, MO: Elsevier, Mosby; 2009. p. 115–36.
42. Johnston LE Jr. Let's pretend. Semin Orthod. 2014;20:249–52.
43. Johnston LE Jr. A comparative analysis of class II treatment methods. In: McNamara Jr JA, Carlson DS, Vig PS, Ribbens KA, editors. Science and clinical judgment in orthodontics, Craniofacial Growth Series. Ann Arbor, MI: The University of Michigan; 1986. p. 103–48.
44. Bowman SJ. All roads Lead to Rome: new directions for class II. Semin Orthod. 2014;20(4):247–342.
45. Angle EH. The treatment of malocclusion of the teeth. 7th ed. Philadelphia, PA: SS White; 1907.
46. Solow B. The dentoalveolar compensatory mechanism: background and clinical implications. Br J Orthod. 1980;7:145–61.
47. Johnston LE Jr. Functional appliances: A mortgage on mandibular position. Aus Orthod J. 1996;14:154–6.
48. Johnston LE Jr. Growth and the class II patient: rendering unto Caesar. Semin Orthod. 1998;4:59–62.
49. Johnston LE Jr. Growing jaws for fun and profit: A modest proposal. In: McNamara Jr JA, editor. What works, what doesn't, and why, Monograph 35, craniofacial growth series. Ann Arbor, MI: Center for Human Growth and Development, The University of Michigan; 1998. p. 63–86.
50. Johnston LE Jr. If wishes were horses: functional appliances and growth modification. Prog Orthod. 2005;6:36–47.
51. Case CS. A practical treatise on the technics and principles of dental orthopedia and prosthetic correction of cleft palate. Chicago, IL: C.S. Case Company; 1921.
52. Nogueira CQ, Chiqueto KFG, Fernandes TMF, Henriques JFC, Janson G. Effects of the Forsus fatigue-resistant device and mandibular anterior repositioning appliance in class II malocclusion treatment. Am J Orthod Dentofacial Orthop. 2022;162:814–23.
53. Lai M. Molar distalization with the Herbst appliance. Semin Orthod. 2000;6:119–28.
54. Pancherz H. A cephalometric analysis of skeletal and dental changes contributing to class II correction in activator treatment. Am J Orthod. 1984;85:125–34.
55. Pancherz H, Hansen K. Occlusal changes during and after Herbst treatment: a cephalometric investigation. Eur J Orthod. 1986;8:215–8.
56. Wong G, So L, Hägg U. A comparative study of sagittal correction with the Herbst appliance in two different ethnic groups. Eur J Orthod. 1997;19:195–204.
57. Pancherz H. The mechanism of class II correction in Herbst appliance treatment. A cephalometric investigation. Am J Orthod. 1982;82:104–13.
58. Johnston LE Jr. A comparative analysis of class II treatments. In: Vig PS, Ribbens KA, editors. Science and clinical judgment in orthodontics. Ann Arbor, MI: Center for Human Growth and Development; 1986. p. 103–48.
59. Valant JR, Sinclair PM. Treatment effects of the Herbst appliance. Am J Orthod Dentofacial Orthop. 1989;95:138–47.
60. Lai M, McNamara JA Jr. An evaluation of two-phase treatment with the Herbst appliance and preadjusted edgewise therapy. Semin Orthod. 1998;4:46–58.
61. Obijou C, Pancherz H. Herbst appliance treatment of class II, division 2 malocclusions. Am J Orthod Dentofacial Orthop. 1997;112:287–91.

62. May PW, Chada J, Ledoux WR, Weinberg P, Block MS, McMinn RW. Skeletal and dental changes using a Jasper Jumper appliance. J Dent Res. 1992;71(suppl):1645.
63. Hansen K, Koutsonas TG, Pancherz H. Long-term effects of Herbst treatment on the mandibular incisor segment: a cephalometric and biometric investigation. Am J Orthod Dentofacial Orthop. 1997;112:92–103.
64. Ruf S, Hansen K, Pancherz H. Does orthodontic proclination of lower incisors in children and adolescents cause gingival recession? Am J Orthod Dentofacial Orthop. 1998;114:100–6.
65. Nalbantgil D, Arun T, Sayinsu K, Isik F. Skeletal, dental and soft-tissue changes induced by the Jasper Jumper appliance in late adolescence. Angle Orthod. 2005;75:426–36.
66. Rothenberg J, Campbell ES, Nanda R. Class II correction with the twin force bite corrector. J Clin Orthod. 2004;38:232–40.
67. Aslan BI, Kucukkaraca E, Turkoz C, Dincer M. Treatment effects of the Forsus fatigue resistant device used with miniscrew anchorage. Angle Orthod. 2014;84:76–87.
68. Livieratos FA, Johnston LE Jr. A comparison of one- and two-stage non-extraction alternatives in matched class II samples. Am J Orthod Dentofacial Orthop. 1995;108:118–31.
69. Bowman SJ. One-stage versus two-stage treatment: are two really necessary? Am J Orthod Dentofacial Orthop. 1998;113(1):111–6.
70. Johnston LE Jr. Early treatment 2005—Déjà vu all over again. Am J Orthod Dentofacial Orthop. 2006;129(Suppl. 1):S45–6.
71. Johnston LE Jr. The functional matrix hypothesis: reflections in a jaundiced eye. In: McNamara Jr JA, editor. Factors affecting the growth of the midface, vol. 399. Ann Arbor, MI: Center for Human Growth and Development; 1976. p. 131–68.
72. Graber TM. Extraoral force-fact and fallacies. Am J Orthod. 1955;41:490–505.
73. Gulleminault C. Lecture. AAO conference on obstructive sleep apnea: consensus and guidance. January 30, 2019.
74. Sichtermann L. The conscience of orthodontics. Practice profiles Orthodontic Products. Oct 5, 2012. https://orthodonticproductsonline.com/practice-management/practice-profiles/the-conscience-of-orthodontics/.
75. Johnston LE Jr. When everything works and nothing matters. World J Orthod. 2002;3:92–3.
76. Burkhardt DR, McNamara JA Jr, Baccetti T. Maxillary molar distalization or mandibular enhancement: a cephalometric comparison of comprehensive orthodontic treatment including the pendulum and the Herbst appliances. Am J Orthod Dentofacial Orthop. 2003;123:108–16.
77. Melsen B, Bosch C. Different approaches to anchorage: A survey and an evaluation. Angle Orthod. 1997;67:23–30.
78. Kircelli BH, Pektaş ZO, Kircelli C. Maxillary molar distalization with a bone-anchored pendulum appliance. Angle Orthod. 2006;76(4):650–9.
79. Escobar SA, Tellez PA, Moncada CA, Villegas CA, Latoree CM, Oberti G. Distalization of maxillary molars with the bone-supported pendulum: A clinical study. Am J Orthod Dentofacial Orthop. 2007;131(4):545–9.
80. Kinzinger GS, Diedrich PR, Bowman SJ. Upper molar distalization with a miniscrew-supported distal jet. J Clin Orthod. 2006;40(11):672–8.
81. Kinzinger GS, Gülden N, Yildizhan F, Diedrich PR. Efficiency of a skeletonized distal jet appliance supported by to anchorage for noncompliance maxillary molar distalization. Am J Orthod Dentofacial Orthop. 2009;136(4):578–86.
82. Oberti G, Villegas C, Ealo M, Palacio JC, Baccetti T. Maxillary molar distalization with the dual-force distalizer supported by mini-implants: a clinical study. Am J Orthod Dentofacial Orthop. 2009;135(3):282.e1–5; discussion 282–3
83. Wilmes B, Drescher D. Application and effectiveness of the Benesider: a device to move molars distally. World J Orthod. 2010;11:331–40.
84. Fudalej P, Antoszewska J. Are orthodontic distalizers reinforced with the temporary anchorage devices effective? Am J Orthod Dentofacial Orthop. 2011;139:722–9.
85. Baumgartner KM. Evaluation of final effects of conventional versus implant supported distal jet followed by comprehensive orthodontic treatment. Master's Thesis. St. Louis, MO: Saint Louis University, Center for Advanced Dental Education; 2012.
86. Bowman SJ. Settling the score with class IIs using miniscrews. In: Kim KB, editor. Temporary skeletal anchorage devices: A guide to design and evidence-based solutions. Berlin: Springer; 2014. p. 55–70.
87. Bowman SJ. The evolution of the horseshoe jet. In: Papadopoulos MA, editor. Skeletal Anchorage in orthodontic treatment of class II malocclusion: contemporary applications of orthodontic implants, miniscrew implants and miniplates. St. Louis, MO: Mosby Elsevier; 2014. p. 168–70.
88. Fotakidou E. Comparison of soft tissue and dentoalveolar effects of the TAD-supported distal jet versus upper premolar extractions. Master's Thesis. St. Louis, MO: Saint Louis University, Center for Advanced Dental Education; 2015.
89. Mellion TH. Comparisons of the horseshoe jet versus the Forsus appliance. Master's Thesis. St. Louis, MO: Saint Louis University, Center for Advanced Dental Education; 2015.
90. Bowman SJ. The effect of vibration on molar distalization. J Clin Orthod. 2016;50(11):683–93.
91. Watson WG. Distal jet versus pendulum appliance. Letter to the editor. Am J Orthod Dentofacial Orthop. 2006;129:3.
92. Bowman SJ. Alternatives after molar distalization. Am Orthod Good Pract. 2000;1:2–3.

93. Bolla E, Doldo T, Giorgetti R. Distal movement of maxillary canines and premolars with sectional mechanics following distal jet application to molars. Prog Orthod. 2004;5:72–89.
94. Johnston LE Jr. Balancing the books on orthodontic treatment: an integrated analysis of change. Br J Orthod. 1996;23(2):93–102.
95. Phaerukkakit S. The relative effects of growth and tooth movement in the correction of class II division 1 malocclusion. Thesis. St. Louis, MO: Saint Louis University Department of Orthodontics; 1985.
96. Donaghey JB. A cephalometric evaluation of tooth movement and growth of the jaws in untreated individuals, ages 11–15. Master's Thesis. St. Louis, MO: Saint Louis University; 1986.
97. Tsourakis AK, Johnston LE Jr. Class II malocclusion: The aftermath of a "perfect storm". Semin Orthod. 2014;20(1):59–73.

7 Fixed Appliance Treatment in the Management of Class II Malocclusion

Sercan Akyalcin

7.1 Introduction

The anteroposterior discrepancy between the maxillary and mandibular arches that leads to a Class II malocclusion should typically be addressed during the active growth period. Since more than two-thirds of Class II malocclusions originate from mandibular deficiency, growth plays an integral part in managing the problem. However, most treatment changes are of dentoalveolar origin, even with growth modification protocols, and require clinically significant tooth movement.

The extent of tooth movement observed to achieve Class II correction is usually a combination of maxillary teeth moving backward and mandibular teeth moving forward. While the anteroposterior limits of the dentition will significantly affect how much correction can realistically be achieved, vertical control and eruption changes are equally important to account for at the beginning of treatment. During average growth and development, the estimated annual eruption rate of maxillary and mandibular first molars is 1.2 mm and 0.9 mm, respectively; with the molars also erupting mesially at about 0.5 mm per year [1]. Throughout orthodontic treatment, which usually lasts about 2 years, these numbers can dramatically impact on treatment, especially if absolute anchorage is employed with mini-screws. Limiting vertical eruption of the maxillary molars and perhaps both maxillary and mandibular molars when 2–2.5 mm annual changes are expected in vertical development of the posterior ramus and mandibular condyle would inevitably result in mandibular autorotation and Class II correction. While this may be a fair strategy to follow in individuals with a steep mandibular plane angle, low angle cases or forward rotators may not benefit from limiting the amount of vertical eruption of teeth.

A better protocol for individuals with upward mandibular rotation is to optimize the dentition's anteroposterior movement within the jaws' physical confines. From a clinical treatment planning approach, the mandibular symphysis's buccal and lingual cortical plates define the limits of orthodontic tooth movement that can rationally be expected. Since the cortical plates provide a physical boundary for tooth movement that cannot be exceeded without expecting deleterious effects, they were defined as "orthodontic walls" [2]. Based on traditional orthodontic training and classic cephalometric studies [3–5], definitive position and angulation of the mandibular incisor within the symphysis is regarded as a key to diagnosis, treatment planning, long-term stability, and esthetics. It has been argued that exceeding a 2 mm advancement in the mandibular incisors creates potential stability concerns due to

S. Akyalcin (✉)
Department of Developmental Biology, Harvard School of Dental Medicine, Boston, MA, USA
e-mail: sercan_akyalcin@hsdm.harvard.edu

M. T. Cobourne (ed.), *Orthodontic Management of Class II Malocclusion*,
https://doi.org/10.1007/978-3-031-57530-3_7

increased pressure from the lips and also, periodontal limitations [6]. Keeping mandibular incisors upright is an important element when considering treatment planning and has been regarded as a diagnostic guide for many clinicians. However, it should be noted that modern orthodontic treatment philosophies consider maxillary incisor position as the main reference for achieving harmonious profile and smile esthetics [7–10]. In this sense, mandibular arch and final position of the mandibular incisors remain a primary element from the perspective of diagnosis and stability [11].

Considering backward movement of the maxillary teeth, if no extractions are planned, the maxillary tuberosity area and how much space exists in this area will determine the success of this treatment approach. Secondly, appliance choice is critical. Extraoral appliances are practical for distalizing teeth, but they are not favored in contemporary practice as many patients reject using them. There are now many intraoral distalization appliances and techniques. However, anchorage loss, such as excessive maxillary incisor proclination and other side effects, including but not limited to excessive distal tipping of the molars and bite opening, are significant concerns associated with their use [12]. The most efficient way to distalize teeth is to use absolute anchorage via the palate or the zygomatic process.

Another approach for Class II correction is to move the teeth differentially in the maxillary and mandibular arches via tooth extraction spaces. Extracting premolars can be helpful in eliminating arch discrepancies such as the curve of Spee, crowding, midline issues, and optimizing the incisor positions. In Class II correction, it is essential to determine how much of the space will be used for the dental discrepancy as opposed to the differential tooth movement required for anteroposterior correction. As indicated before, change in the maxillary incisor position is of tremendous importance for providing optimum esthetics. The timing of extractions is also an essential consideration because taking out teeth early for retracting the maxillary incisors might potentially limit the changes in the mandibular position from growth. There are many different extraction schemes that could help with camouflaging Class II cases. It could be a combination of four premolars, maxillary premolars only, maxillary premolars, and a lower incisor and maxillary second molars to facilitate the distal movement of the maxillary arch. Careful planning and utilizing appropriate treatment mechanics are essential from facial balance, long-term stability, and periodontal health perspectives.

The following sections in this chapter are intended to elaborate on the fixed appliance treatment mechanics for Class II correction within the scope of current evidence and clinical limitations.

7.2 Non-extraction Treatment Mechanics

Comprehensive fixed appliance therapy for the correction of Class II malocclusion requires adequate space in the dental arches for differential movement of maxillary and mandibular teeth. Figure 7.1 demonstrates a perfect example of consolidating existing spaces for anteroposterior correction. This is a case where torque control on the mandibular incisors should also assist with molar correction. When uprighting the mandibular incisors via the utilization of existing spaces, the addition of positive torque or flipping the (−) torque incisor brackets upside down should add more demand to the posterior anchorage. Space closure with chain elastics will upright the incisor crowns and because of the additional resistance from the lingually torquing roots posterior teeth will move forward a lot easier. This is a particularly important concept when the mesial movement of the posterior teeth could contribute to the Class II correction. Having sufficient space is a critical issue unless the treatment is provided following or during a growth modification protocol. In that case, the remaining growth of the individual determines the feasibility of the case for the non-extraction protocol. As a practical rule, a Class II case with a full-step molar relationship and limited growth potential is not an ideal candidate for non-extraction therapy.

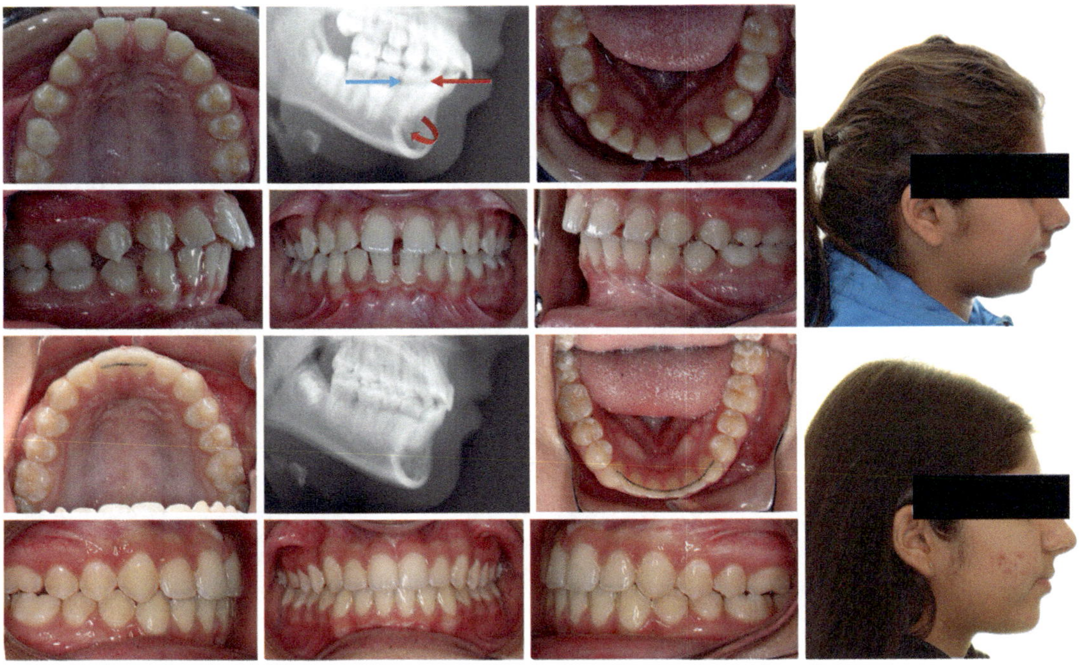

Fig. 7.1 Before and after records of a 12-year-old female patient with bilateral end-on Class II molar relationships. The treatment protocol included 0.022″-slot MBT appliances, Class II elastics, and space consolidation via power-chain elastics. Utilizing (+) torque in the mandibular incisor area helps increase the uprighting efforts with power-chain elastics because this type of labial retraction force (red arrow) would normally create a lingual tipping effect on the mandibular incisors. But when rectangular wires interact with the bracket slots, the resulting clockwise moment (red arrow) would prevent the labial tipping of the roots and create an additional demand on the posterior anchorage (blue arrow) that makes the Class II mechanics more efficient. Post-treatment radiographic image displays the uprighting of the mandibular incisors within the mandibular symphysis and mesial movement of the posterior teeth in relation to the developing third molar germs

7.2.1 Protraction of Mandibular Teeth

If Class II correction is achieved via appliances such as functional appliances or Class II correctors and elastics, the goal of the fixed appliance therapy would be to maintain the correction and to correct the position of the teeth after they were exposed to some possible side effects. For instance, following removable or fixed-functional treatment the mandibular incisors are most likely inclined forward because of the mesially directed pressure from the appliance. Figure 7.2 demonstrates a 12-year-old male treated initially with a twin-block appliance for 11 months and was immediately bonded with fixed appliances. Please note that the mandibular incisor position was kept virtually stable. Among the strategies to maintain the mandibular incisor inclination in this case are:

- Case selection (late mixed dentition/early permanent dentition/good grower).
- Capping the mandibular incisors with acrylic during the twin-block use.
- Patient compliance with the appliance and no heavy reliance on Class II elastics during fixed-appliance therapy.
- Bonding the case with −6 ° (negative) torque brackets in the mandibular incisors.
- Interproximal enamel reduction (IPR) and subsequent uprighting with rectangular wires in place with bend-backs and power-chain space closure.

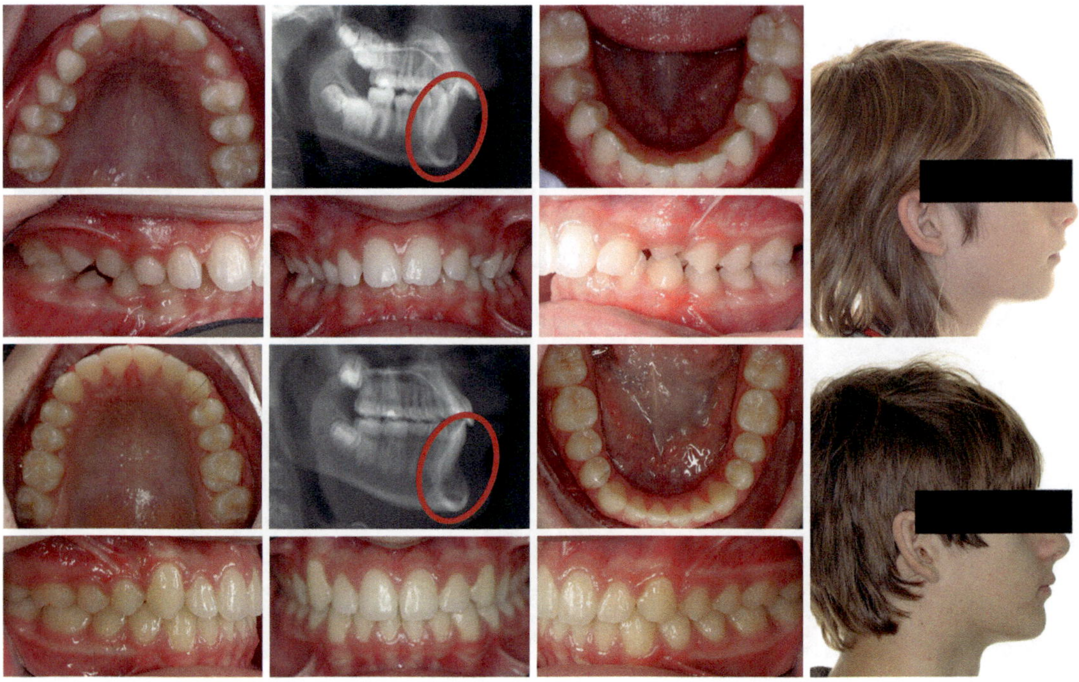

Fig. 7.2 Before and after records of a 12-year-old male patient who is about to experience peak height velocity. The patient was treated with a twin-block appliance initially and was bonded with 0.022″-slot MBT appliances. Incisor mandibular plane angle remained virtually the same (T1: 99 ° T2: 98 °) using the clinical strategies defined above

There is no point in utilizing a growth modification appliance in cases where the growth is almost complete. Using Class II elastics or Class II correctors in the permanent dentition in conjunction with fixed appliance therapy is more logical. A study comparing Class II intermaxillary elastics with Forsus FRD concluded that the two treatment alternatives are interchangeable [13]. In general terms, Forsus FRD is a good substitute for Class II elastics, especially for noncompliant patients. However, it may be essential to note that the Forsus FRD may bring about more mandibular incisor proclination compared to the Class II elastics [13].

In general, maxillary and mandibular molars erupt vertically in patients treated with Class II elastics and Class II correctors, and mandibular incisors are proclined. However, with Class II mechanics, a more considerable portion of the molar correction is likely due to increased apical base growth for patients within their peak growth period instead of those in the post-peak group [14]. This observation does not mean that changes captured by rapid growth would continue to be relevant upon long-term follow-up. Indeed, during the detailing/finishing stage, there were no significant differences between pre-peak and post-peak patients treated with Forsus FRD [14]. It is also important to note that Class II correctors are not designed to work as "rigid functional" appliances because they are comprised of springs that increase the elasticity of the force application. Not surprisingly, the increase in mandibular length in growing children has differing ranges for Class II correctors (1.3–3.7 mm) and removable functional appliances (3.7–6.6 mm). However, there is no sufficient evidence to differentiate between fixed and removable appliances in the long term when looking at skeletal, dental, and patient-reported outcomes [15].

When there is minimal or no growth remaining, the entire mandibular arch may have to be protracted with Class II correctors. The addition of negative (−) torque should be helpful if the mandibular symphysis would allow the labial movement of the roots. However, the width of the symphysis is a critical issue and should be carefully evaluated. Suppose the posttreatment position of the mandibular incisors would not compromise the bone support around the mandibular incisors. In that case, the forward movement of the incisors could be kept under the physiologically defined limits, and the resultant treatment outcomes might be deemed reasonable. In patients with limited remaining growth, mesial movement of the mandibular incisors is inevitable. However, clinicians should do their best to keep this effect to a minimum (Fig. 7.3).

When utilizing Class II correctors or elastics, the significant factors to control are vertical eruption of the posterior and excessive mesial inclination of the mandibular incisor teeth. Figure 7.4 demonstrates the adverse effects of Class II elastics clinically. Remaining growth is an essential element of success considering the vertical effects. While posterior extrusion of posterior teeth via Class II elastic traction may help open the bite and level the curve of Spee in deep-bite cases, the absence of remaining growth could complicate the situation as the mandible would inevitably rotate backward and downward (Fig. 7.5). Backward rotation of the mandible is counterproductive and is not helpful with the sagittal correction. Long-term use of Class II elastics (exceeding 3–4 months) is not recommended. Vertical control plays a more influential role in correcting the molar relationship in high-angle patients. Extrusive mechanics should be avoided at all costs.

Torque expression in straight-wire appliances with orthodontic wires is critical before installing Class II correctors to prevent excessive tipping of

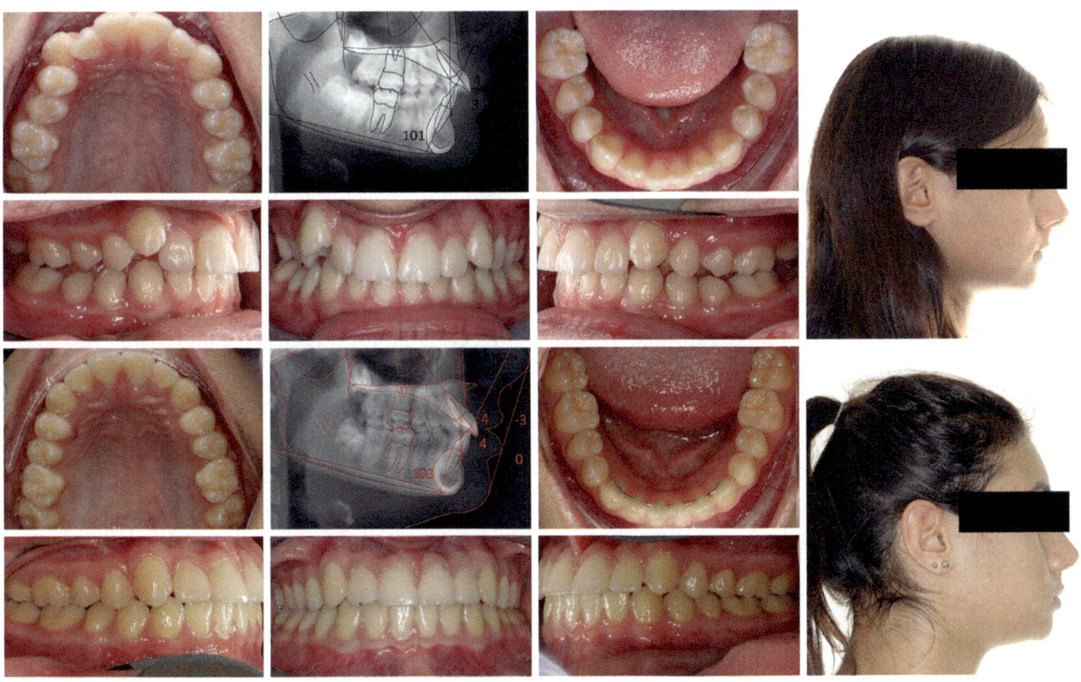

Fig. 7.3 The 14-year-old female patient demonstrated in this compilation presented with bilateral end-on Class II molar relationship. The patient was treated with expansion in the maxillary arch and a Class II corrector with 0.022-slot MBT appliances. In cases with limited/no growth, forward movement of the incisors is inevitable. However, the clinician should minimize this effect. In this case, a combination of −6 ° torque brackets and IPR was used, and the mandibular incisor proclination was limited to a 1 mm (2 °) change in the incisor mandibular plane angle. Please note that the width of the mandibular symphysis and the presence of available bone surrounding the incisors following the treatment make these cases feasible to treat with Class II correctors

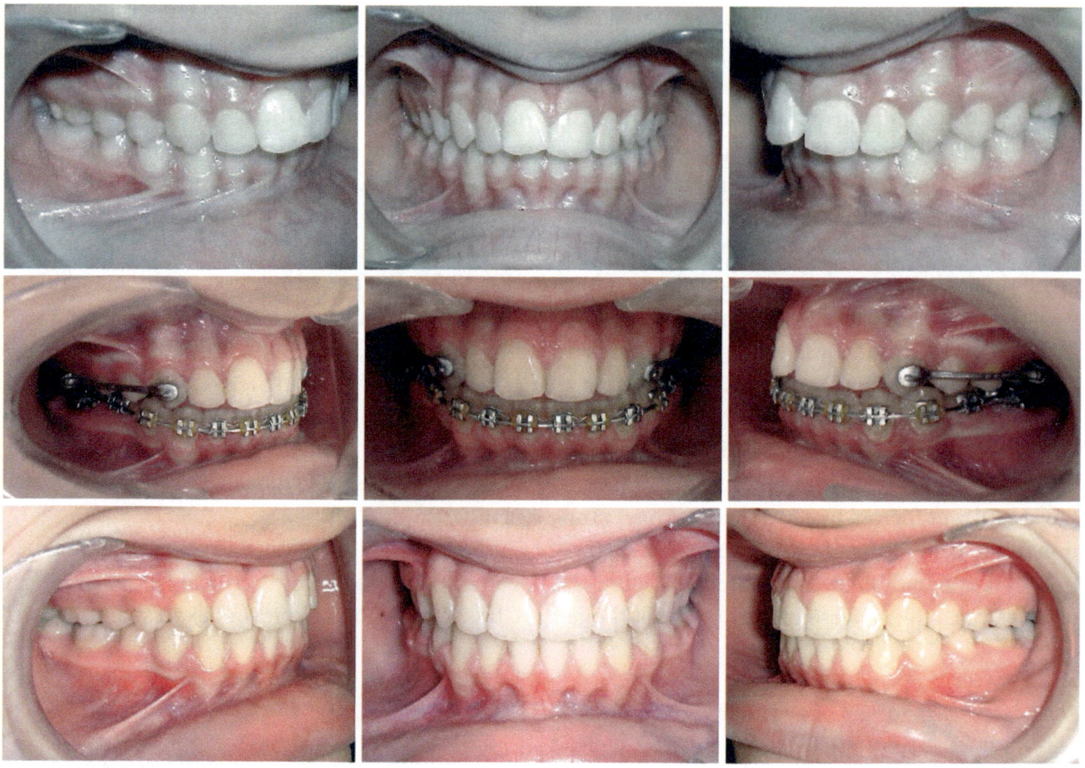

Fig. 7.4 A 13-year-old girl presenting with bilateral end-on Class II and 4.5 mm overjet is treated with full-bonding of the mandibular arch (0.018″-slot pure edgewise appliances), Carriere® Motion™ appliance and Class II elastics. ¼″ medium to heavy (4–6 ounces) Class II elastics were used once the lower arch was stabilized with a 0.017 × 0.025-in. SS arch wire with negative torque bend added in the incisor region. Even though Class I molar and canine relationships were achieved after 4 months of Class II elastic use, extrusion of posterior teeth and proclination of the mandibular incisors caused opening of the bite. Case was finished with interproximal enamel reduction, space consolidation, vertical seating elastics and detailing bends

the mandibular incisors. Ideally, full-size wires, such as 0.019 × 0.025-inch (in.) or 0.021 × 0.025-in. stainless steel (SS) in a 0.022-in. slot or 0.017 × 0.02-in. SS in an 0.018-in. bracket slot are recommended for full control and dimensional stability. Besides adequate torque control, interproximal enamel reduction and other clinical measures such as adding temporary anchorage devices to limit the anterior expansion of incisors in the mandible are beneficial for success. Several attempts have been made to prevent excessive proclination of mandibular incisors and increase the skeletal response by adding mini-screws [16, 17] and mini plates [18] in clinical trials with Class II correctors. However, as outlined in a systematic review and meta-analysis, adding temporary anchorage devices (TADs) to Class II correctors is not effective in increasing the sagittal skeletal response to treatment. However, utilizing TADs is conceivably a good clinical measure to prevent the excessive tipping of the mandibular incisors [19].

There are several ways to incorporate TADs in the treatment mechanics. Figure 7.6 demonstrates a patient with an end-on Class II molar relationship treated with a combination of Class II elastics, Carriere® Motion™ appliance, and full-fixed appliances anchored by mini-screws between the first and second molars in the mandibular arch. Figure 7.7 shows another Class II patient with increased mandibular divergence and vertical overlap of the incisors with no contact treated with Class II elastics, Carriere® Motion™ appliance, and a lower lingual holding arch anchored by mini-screws. In both cases, the overjet was limited, and there was not much room for mandibular incisor proclination. The addition of mini-screws proved helpful with mandibular incisor inclination and vertical management. As a result, the maxillary teeth were distalized and spaces opened in the maxillary anterior region. When contrasting these changes to the patient in Fig. 7.4, it is clear that TADs virtually managed the initial overjet and overbite better. Management of incisors and the bite is an excellent clinical feature during the retraction phase because the incisors would not be coupling prematurely due to the excessive tip.

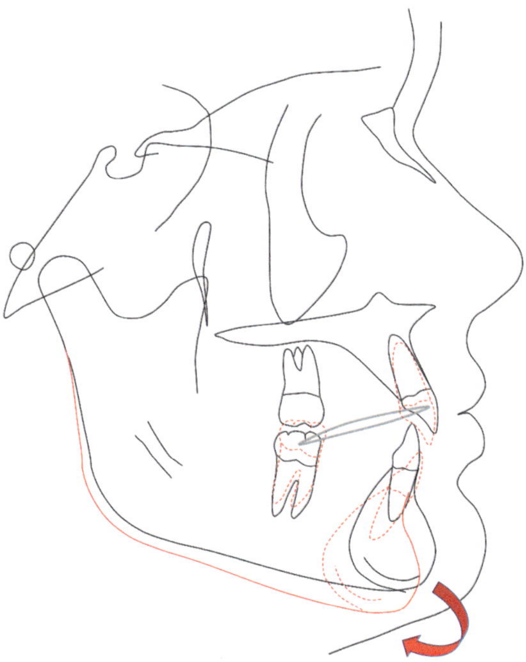

Fig. 7.5 In non-growing individuals and in cases where molar extrusion and vertical alveolar development are not adequately compensated by condylar and ramus growth, use of Class II elastics rotates the mandible backward. This treatment effect is particularly unacceptable for high-angle patients and jeopardizes the progress in anteroposterior correction

Class II correctors and elastics work efficiently in Class II subdivision cases as well. It was reported that it took a significantly shorter treatment time with Forsus FRD than Class II elastics [20]. Extrusion and palatal tipping of maxillary incisors and clockwise rotation of the occlusal plane were some of the side effects in the elastics group that were not observed with the Forsus FRD. Figure 7.8 demonstrates the treatment of a 12-year-old female patient presenting with deep-bite and a full-step Class II molar relationship on the left and a Class I molar relationship on the right. The upper midline is on with the facial midline, and the lower midline has deviated about 3 mm to the patient's left. The treatment involved expanding the maxillary arch with a Haas-type expander with thickened acrylic in the anterior maxillary area serving as an anterior bite plane. The appliance was used for 5 mm arch expansion and held in place for 6 months to facilitate the leveling of the curve of Spee. After carefully assessing the remaining growth potential of the patient, bilateral Forsus FRD appliances were installed after the placement of 0.019 × 0.02-in. SS wires in both arches. No activations were planned for the right side. However, the left side was activated incrementally to correct the molar relationship and the midline. Selective interproximal enamel reduction was utilized to achieve asymmetric tooth movement.

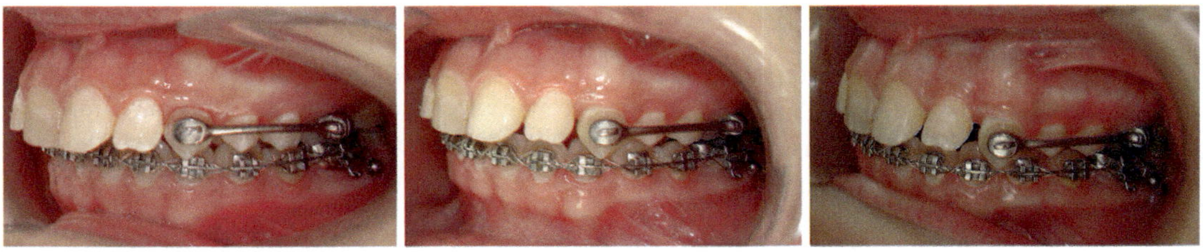

Fig. 7.6 The mandibular arch was stabilized with 0.017 × 0.025-in. SS wires in 0.018-in. edgewise brackets. Mini-screws were placed distal to the first molars to anchor the mandibular arch. ¼-in. medium to heavy Class II elastics was used between the mandibular arch and the Class II corrector

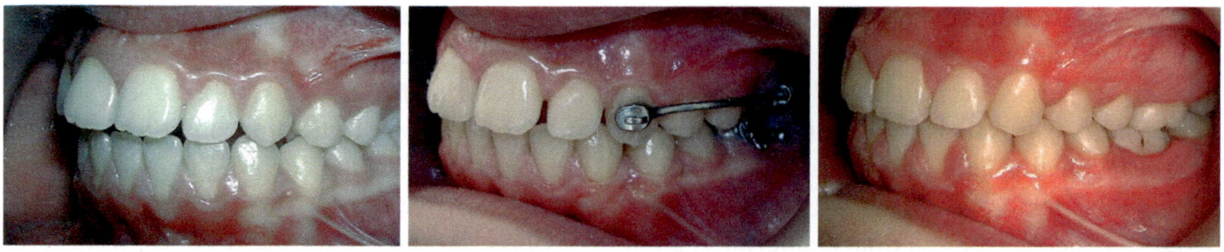

Fig. 7.7 The mandibular arch was stabilized with a lower lingual holding arch. Mini-screws were placed distal to the first molars to anchor the mandibular arch and tied to the first molar bands with heavy steel ligatures. ¼-in. medium to heavy Class II elastics was used between the mandibular arch and the Class II corrector. Despite the lack of initial overjet and the open bite tendency, posterior maxillary teeth were distalized efficiently via the TAD-anchored Class II elastics

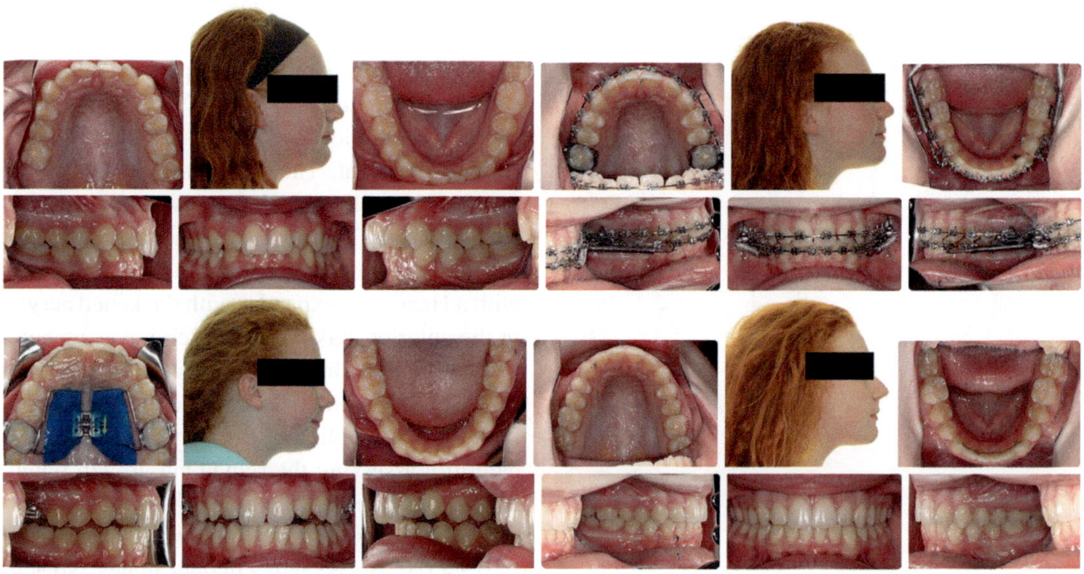

Fig. 7.8 A 12-year-old female presenting with a Class II subdivision was treated with asymmetric activation of the Forsus FRD appliance. The photographs represent the initial, post-expansion, installation of Forsus FRD, and the posttreatment outcome phases

7.2.2 Distal Movement of Maxillary Teeth

Distal repositioning of the maxillary molars can create extra space to correct the Class II relationship with headgear, intra-oral distalizing appliances, and temporary anchorage devices. Headgear may be a simplistic approach in the mixed dentition to aid in restricting excess maxillary growth and distalizing molars. The main advantages of headgear are the biomechanical versatility and the synchronous use with fixed appliances while allowing clinicians to make necessary adjustments during treatment. The significant drawbacks of headgear are compliance, social issues, and safety. For example, suppose growth modification is not the primary objective of the treatment plan, and heavy orthopedic forces are not required to restrict the maxillary growth. In that case, maxillary molars can also be distalized by intra-oral appliances, which typically consist of heavy palatal arches, an acrylic pad in the anterior palate for anchorage, and spring attachments to the molars.

There are many types of distalizing appliances in the literature. However, anchorage reinforcement, mainly in the anterior palatal area, is insufficient to resist the reciprocal mesial force generated by the appliance. Typically, anchorage loss will appear in the form of maxillary incisor proclination and protrusion. Forward movement of maxillary teeth may be tolerated in patients with upright maxillary incisors. However, it is not desirable in patients with lip protrusion and increased overjet from an esthetic perspective. Furthermore, retracting the incisors into the spaces created by molar distalization will provoke round tripping and additional demand on the posterior anchorage. Headgear or distalization appliances also tip and rotate the maxillary molars backward and may cause the opening of the bite via unwanted extrusion if not administered properly (Fig. 7.9). Lack of vertical growth during the Class II correction causes long-term stability concerns as bite-opening mechanics are prone to relapse and failure because of the musculature.

Another important aspect of molar distalization to be discussed is the availability of space in the maxillary tuberosity area. After all, bodily distalization of posterior teeth may not be viable in individuals with lack of bone support in the posterior maxilla. From the growth and development perspective, this is an area that shows bone apposition—a mechanism to facilitate the eruption of posterior teeth. However, in non-developing patients the amount of bodily movement in the distal direction is questionable. It has been argued that without vertical growth and elongation of the maxillary teeth, it is difficult to achieve more than 2–3 mm of distalization [6]. Attempts were made to utilize TADs for distalization. TADs could potentially increase the amount of distalization with no anchorage concerns. However, space behind the molars continues to be a limitation with TAD-supported distalization techniques.

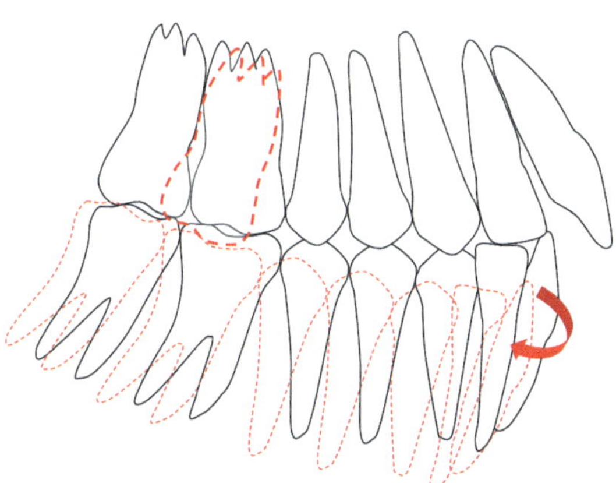

Fig. 7.9 Excessive distal tipping of the molars via headgear or distalization appliances is not ideal and should be carefully evaluated in patients with minimum growth potential

Considering that vertical management of the case does not create any immediate issues, correcting the axial inclinations of the significantly tipped back molars could be a concern in the lack of space. The case demonstrated in Fig. 7.10 was treated with a TAD-supported Pendulum appliance during the root development of the third molars. Successful distalization was achieved as expected since the effect of maxillary second and third molar eruption stage on molar distalization is minimal [21]. However, suppose third molars cannot be extracted to allow root uprighting—as was the case with the patient in Fig. 7.10. In that case, lack of leveling marginal ridges during fixed appliance therapy may take away from the clinical excellence regardless of the occlusal outcome. For this reason, early removal of third molars is recommended in cases when second molars are fully erupted and need to be distalized as well. If significant distalization (4–6 mm) is targeted as part of the treatment, some clinicians also suggest removing the second molars and replacing them with the erupting third molars.

According to a meta-analysis [22] average molar distalization equals to 3.34 mm with conventional anchorage and 5.10 mm with skeletal anchorage. Another systematic review and meta-analysis concluded that the conventional and skeletal anchorage devices were not significantly different in terms of the amount of molar distalization/tipping [23]. In light of the current evidence, we can conclude that both anchorage systems are effective. However, both reports [22, 23] underlined the advantage of TADs for preventing anchorage loss particularly when used as

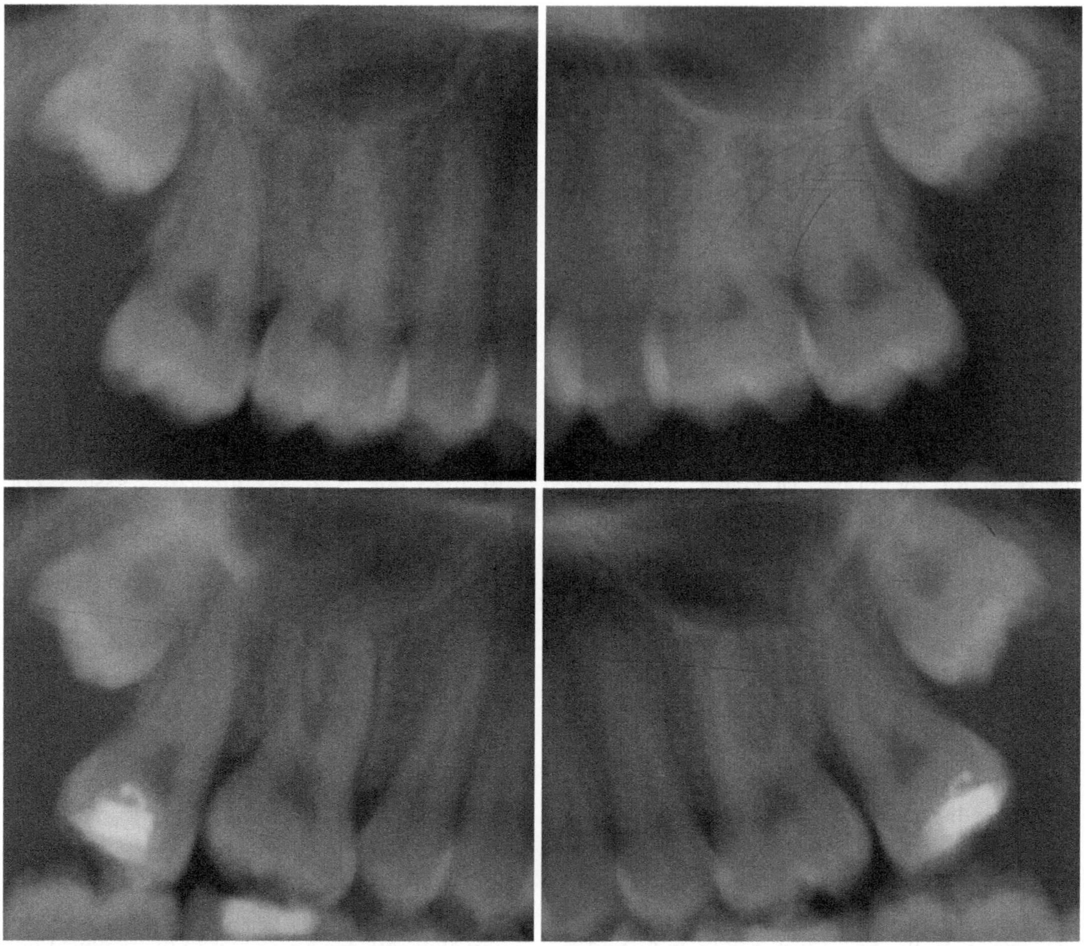

Fig. 7.10 Pre- and post-treatment radiographs of a 15-year-old female who was treated with a Pendulum appliance. Post-treatment radiographs demonstrate the residual distal tip in the posterior teeth after the fixed appliances were removed. Developing third molars usually complicate the uprighting of the roots in molar distalization cases

direct anchorage. In terms of treatment timing, it was shown that correction of a half-to-full cusp Class II molar relationship with intraoral distalizers could be achieved in an average of 8.3 months in another meta-analysis [24]. Furthermore, the time spent for distalization with skeletal vs. conventional anchorage was deemed practically identical.

From a biomechanical point of view, force application for distalization should be performed on the buccal aspect of the first molars. This is because maxillary first molar teeth usually have a mesial rotation in Class II malocclusion and should be de-rotated to gain more space for the bicuspids. Inserting mini-plates or longer infrazygomatic screws above the roots may be acceptable in some cases that require significant distalization. However, based on the available evidence from the literature demonstrating no significant differences between conventional and skeletal anchorage, it should be questioned whether “the means justify the ends” for these kinds of applications. There are also proponents of using the palate in molar distalization that offers more room for the insertion of TADs. However, keeping the orthodontic force on the buccal aspect of the first molars is more desirable.

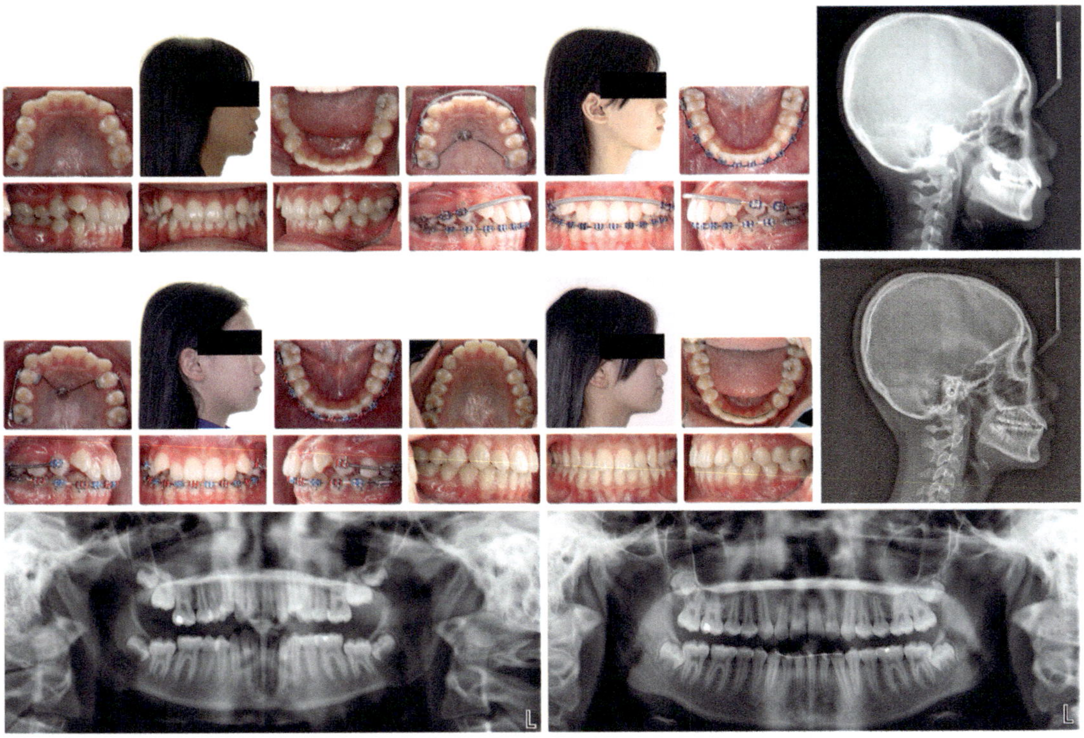

Fig. 7.11 Pre-treatment, progress, and post-treatment photos of a 12-year-old female that was treated with a mini-screw supported distalization protocol in conjunction with fixed appliances. The patient had good facial ratios with a normal mandibular divergence. Distalization was accomplished on 0.017 × 0.025-in. SS sectional wires via the first bicuspids anchored to the mini-screw. The same mini-screw was utilized to hold the maxillary first molars during incisor retraction and space closure

Figure 7.11 shows a sample case that illustrates the best of both worlds. A single mini-screw was placed 1 mm paramedian to the mid-palatal suture slightly distal to the third rugae (1.7 × 8 mm, OrthoEasy, Forestadent, Pforzheim, Germany). A mini-screw-supported transpalatal arch (TPA) design was placed to hold the U4s in AP, transverse, and vertical planes. Maxillary posterior quadrants were then aligned to eventually accommodate a 0.017 × 0.025-in. SS archwire. Nickel-titanium (NiTi) open coil springs with 2 mm incremental activations were placed at each visit between the maxillary first premolars and first molars on each side. Bodily molar distalization was achieved in nearly 6 months. Once distalization was complete, another TPA was designed from the same mini-screw to hold the maxillary first molars. The rest of the maxillary teeth were bonded, and maxillary canine and premolars were retracted with maximum anchorage by sliding mechanics on 0.020-in. SS archwire. Incisor retraction was carried out by active tiebacks on 0.019 × 0.025-in. posted SS archwires.

Because of the limitations discussed in this section not every case should be treated with non-extraction protocols via skeletal or conventional anchorage. The following section details the value and role of extractions in Class II correction with modern fixed appliances.

7.3 Extraction-Based Treatment Mechanics

As briefly explained in the non-extraction treatment section, there should be adequate space in dental arches for differential movement of maxillary and mandibular teeth. The presence of space plays a vital role from the view of the physical limitations of tooth movement. In addition, when considering a patient's chief concerns, the orthodontist should decide whether the upper lip is in a harmonious relationship with the rest of the face or not. In most Class II cases, upper lip position does not seem to be a concern. And, if the upper lip position is esthetically pleasing, minimum or no change should be planned for the maxillary incisors. However, protrusion of the maxilla and maxillary incisors should be evaluated carefully. Orthopedic intervention with headgear or distalization may resolve the concerns in some select cases.

Extractions may be necessary in some other cases (Fig. 7.12). It is essential to assess the vertical characteristics of the patients as a hyperdivergent skeletal profile may not be suitable for distalization or any other non-extraction option. Increased divergence of the mandible worsens the sagittal discrepancy as the mandible would rotate backward and downward. The limited evidence in the literature shows that the apical base sagittal relationship may not be reduced with the non-extraction approach. But the two-maxillary and four-premolar extractions Class II treatments decrease the ANB angle by 1.8 and 2.5 °, respectively [25]. In addition to the increased mandibular divergence, the patient in Fig. 7.12 also had an impacted maxillary right maxillary cuspid and mesially tipped second molars. Non-extraction treatment of such a patient with additional treatment discrepancies and the increased overjet may

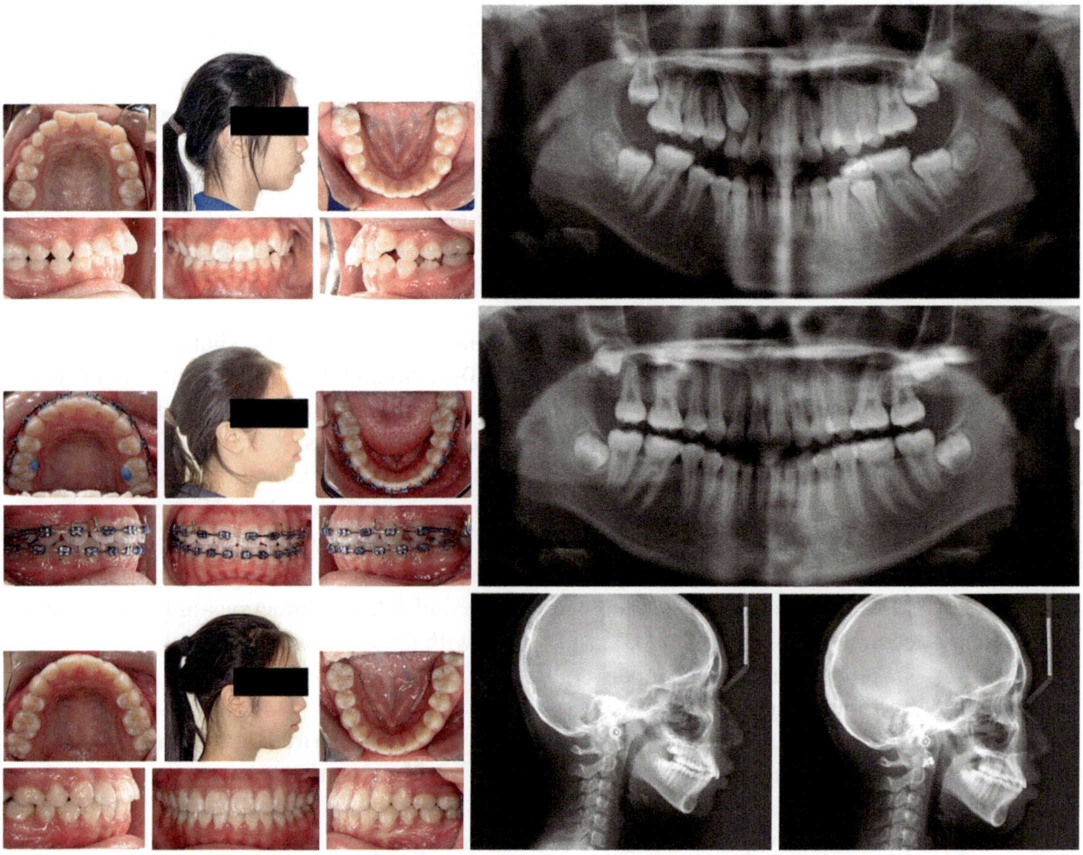

Fig. 7.12 Pre-treatment, progress, and post-treatment photos of a 12-year-old female that was treated with maxillary first bicuspid extractions. Maxillary bicuspid extractions versus distalization were preferred in this case due to additional treatment complexities such as increased mandibular divergence, impacted right cuspid, maxillary posterior crowding in addition to increased overjet

increase the skeletal divergence and affect the lip position negatively and therefore may cause an undesired protrusion of the upper lip profile. Some clinicians may choose to extract four bicuspids in these types of cases. According to a systematic review [26], when Class II patients with increased overjet are treated with premolar extractions, the nasolabial flattens because of incisor retraction. However, the lower lip retraction is less with the 2-maxillary premolar extraction protocol than with the four-premolar extraction protocol. Therefore, one can appreciate that the case presented in Fig. 7.13 did not require any lower lip changes.

The position of the upper teeth also affects the lower lip esthetically. Figure 7.13 demonstrates a high-angle, skeletal Class II patient with proclined maxillary incisors and increased overjet. Extractions of upper bicuspids and adequately managing the vertical plane improved the facial appearance of this patient. When extracting the first bicuspids and finishing in the Class II molar relationship, certain adjustments should be made to the maxillary first molars. In MBT prescription, maxillary first molar bands or buccal tubes have a 10 ° distal offset. The addition of distal offset rotates the maxillary first molar in the transverse plane due to its rhomboidal morphol-

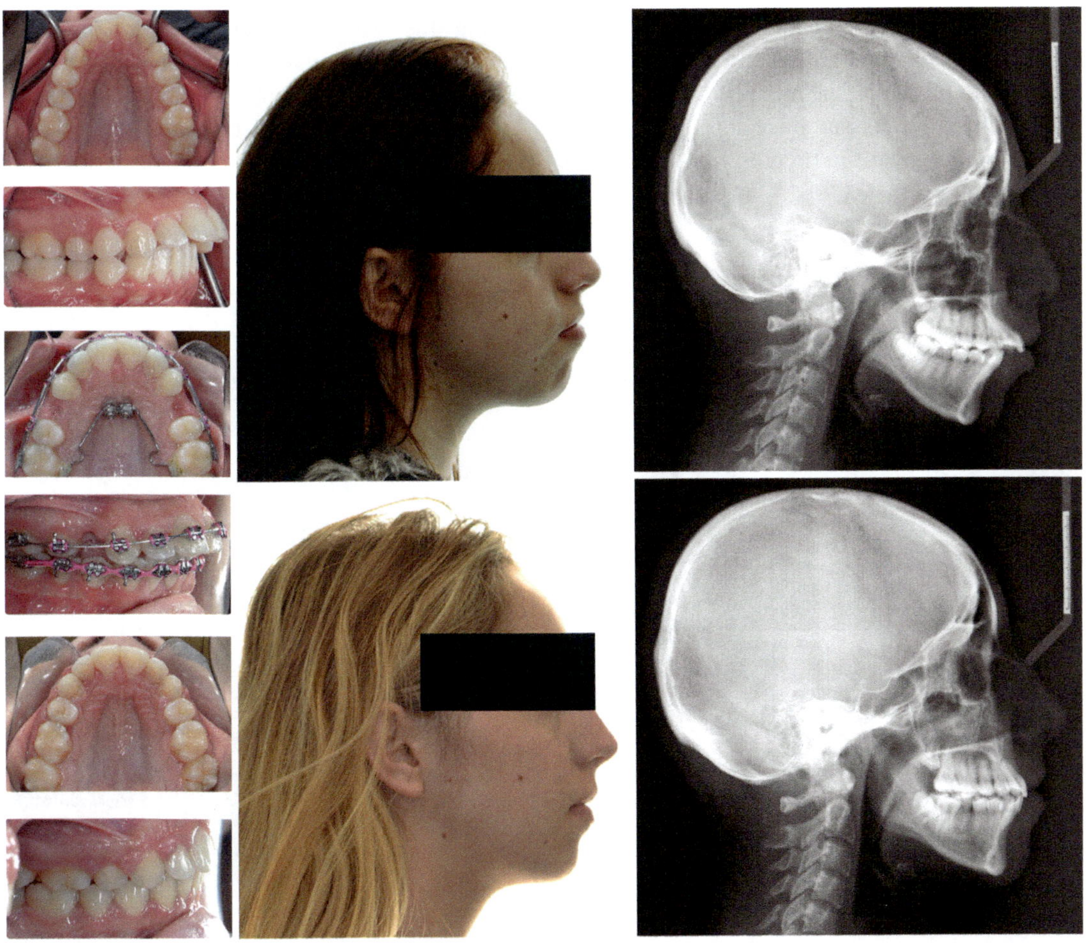

Fig. 7.13 Pre-treatment, progress, and post-treatment photos of a young adult female who presented with a high-angle skeletal Class II pattern. Maxillary incisor proclination is causing a soft tissue profile concern including the lower lip position. Intrusion and vertical control with TADs and uprighting of the maxillary incisors were instrumental in achieving a balanced facial outcome

ogy, which is analogous to the molar offset bend in the edgewise ideal wire. The first-degree adjustment is helpful for the achievement of proper overjet and Class I molar occlusion. However, when finishing in Class II molar relationship, the maxillary first molar occludes between the mandibular first molar and the second premolar and may not need rotation control. Otherwise, there will be excess overjet in this section. A helpful pearl to counteract this clinical issue is replacing the upper first molar buccal tubes with the lower first molar buccal tubes with "zero" rotation. The mandibular right buccal tube should be flipped and placed on the maxillary left first molar, and the mandibular left buccal tube should be flipped and placed on the maxillary right first molar. The mandibular buccal tubes will produce a similar negative torque when flipped and placed on the maxillary arch, and the tip should not be an issue since none of these buccal tubes have a built-in tip prescription.

Vertical management is imperative in high-angle skeletal Class II patients. And it is essential when dealing with patients with remaining vertical growth. When considering the annual eruption changes of posterior teeth, it may be good to hold the maxillary and mandibular molars in the vertical plane during the incisor retraction phase. Mini-screws aid with anteroposterior anchorage reinforcement. However, inserting mini-screws for the vertical management of hyperdivergent patients with remaining growth brings excellent clinical results (Fig. 7.14). According to Buschang et al. [1], the annual eruption rate of maxillary and mandibular first molars totals about 2 mm. Therefore, limiting the vertical eruption of maxillary and mandibular molars during the vertical development of posterior ramus and mandibular condyle should be helpful with mandibular autorotation and Class II correction. However, it should be noted that without active intrusion or holding the posterior teeth

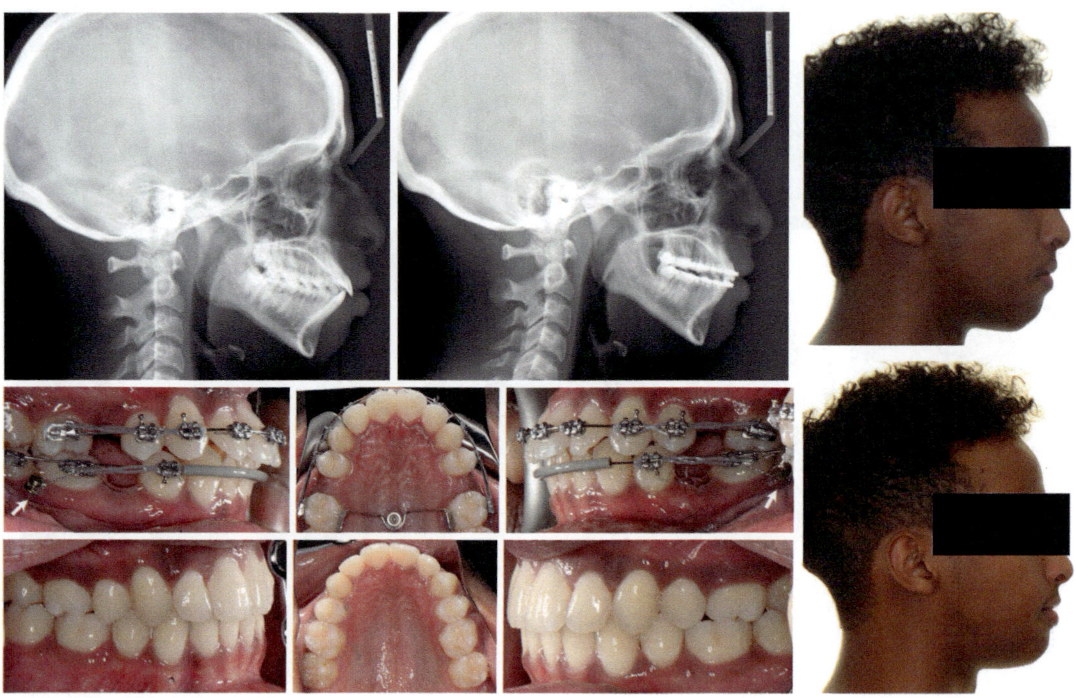

Fig. 7.14 A 15-year-old male patient presenting with skeletal Class II, bimaxillary protrusion, and a hyperdivergent mandible was treated with extraction of second bicuspids. A palatal mini-screw-supported palatal bar anchored the maxillary first molars for both A-P anchorage and vertical control. Two mini-screws were placed distal to the mandibular first molars for vertical control and to help with mandibular incisor retraction

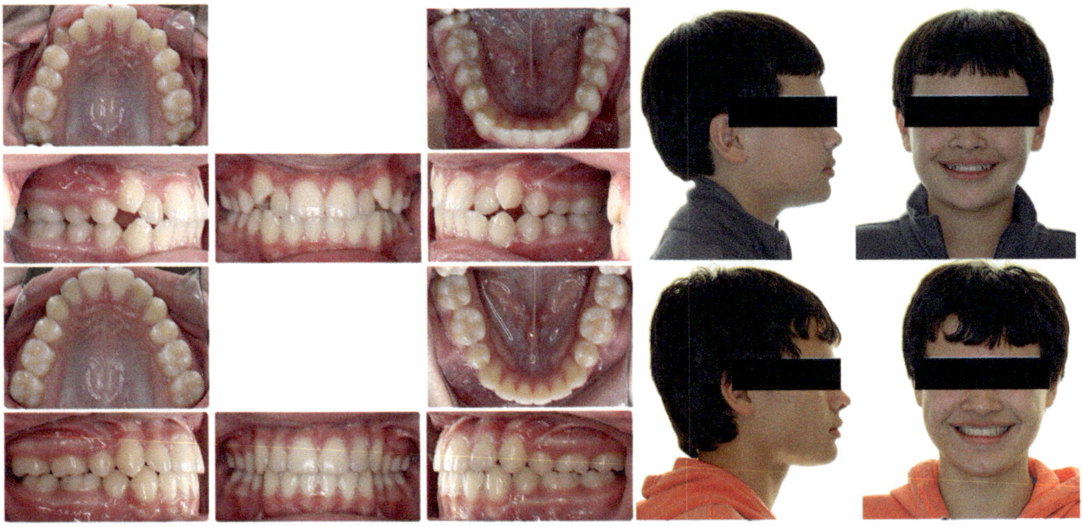

Fig. 7.15 A 14-year-old male patient presenting with Class II, maxillary incisor protrusion, and a flattened smile arc was treated with maxillary first and mandibular second bicuspid extractions via moderate anchorage. Extractions of mandibular second bicuspids were essential in achieving a Class I molar relationship and helping with space creation to retract the maxillary incisors for the smile arc development

during growth period, merely extracting teeth would not reduce or control the vertical dimension. It was shown that a four-premolar extraction treatment has no specific effect on the skeletal vertical dimension [27].

Ideal positioning of the maxillary incisor is essential from the profile perspective and for planning a better smile arc relationship. Figure 7.15 presents an 11-year-old male patient with a skeletal Class II patient with bilateral end-on molar relationships, proclined maxillary incisors, and moderate crowding in the maxillary arch. His treatment included the extractions of maxillary first and mandibular second bicuspids with moderate anchorage in both arches. Improvement of the pretreatment flattened smile arc was possible upon retracting and relatively extruding the maxillary central incisors, which would not have been possible without extractions. Many clinicians are concerned about facial profile flattening in extraction cases. However, as we explained elsewhere [11], targeted tooth movement in carefully planned cases targeting the optimum positioning of the maxillary incisors would not compromise the facial esthetics and instead would improve the outcome. Interestingly, there seems to be no sound evidence from clinical trials to discourage the choice of extraction or non-extraction treatment even in children with Class II Division 2 malocclusions [28].

7.4 Summary

In light of current evidence, there is no preformulated way of treating Class II malocclusions with fixed appliances. Therefore, the clinician must thoroughly assess the individual case needs and adjust the mechanotherapy with the patient's facial form and physiological requirements. Growth pattern, presence of available space, bone support, and the final positioning of the incisors seem to be the keywords in Class II correction. In addition, as we tried to describe in this chapter, fixed appliance therapy should be modified and supplemented adequately with adjunctive appliances and methods to optimize tooth movement to manage Class II cases successfully.

References

1. Buschang PH, Roldan SI, Tadlock LP. Guidelines for assessing the growth and development of orthodontic patients. Semin Orthod. 2017;23:321–35.
2. Handelman CS. The anterior alveolus: its importance in limiting orthodontic treatment and its influence on the occurrence of iatrogenic sequelae. Angle Orthod. 1996;66:95–110.
3. Tweed C. The Frankfort-mandibular incisor angle in orthodontic diagnosis, treatment planning and prognosis. Angle Orthod. 1954;24:121–69.
4. Steiner CC. Cephalometrics in clinical practice. Angle Orthod. 1959;29:8–29.
5. Ricketts CM. Cephalometric synthesis. Am J Orthod Dentofacial Orthop. 1960;46:647–73.
6. Proffit WR, Fields HW, Larson B, Sarver DM. Contemporary orthodontics. 6th ed. Philadelphia, PA: Elsevier; 2019.
7. Sarver DM. The importance of incisor positioning in the esthetic smile: the smile arc. Am J Orthod Dentofacial Orthop. 2001;120:98–111.
8. Isiksal E, Hazar S, Akyalcin S. Smile esthetics: perception and comparison of treated and untreated smiles. Am J Orthod Dentofacial Orthop. 2006;129:8–16.
9. Akyalcin S, Hazar S, Guneri P, Gogus S, Erdinc AM. Extraction versus non-extraction: evaluation by digital subtraction radiography. Eur J Orthod. 2007;29:639–47.
10. Hayashida H, Ioi H, Nakata S, Takahashi I, Counts AL. Effects of retraction of anterior teeth and initial soft tissue variables on lip changes in Japanese adults. Eur J Orthod. 2011;33:419–26.
11. Akyalcin S. Chapter 60: facial esthetics-oriented treatment planning with dental VTOs and TADs. In: Park JH, editor. Temporary anchorage devices in clinical orthodontics. 1st ed. Hoboken, NJ: John Wiley & Sons, Inc.; 2020. p. 661–74.
12. Oncag G, Akyalcin S, Arikan F. The effectiveness of a single osteointegrated implant combined with pendulum springs for molar distalization. Am J Orthod Dentofacial Orthop. 2007;131:277–84.
13. Jones G, Buschang PH, Kim KB, Oliver DR. Class II non-extraction patients treated with the forsus fatigue resistant device versus intermaxillary elastics. Angle Orthod. 2008;78:332–8.
14. Servello DF, Fallis DW, Alvetro L. Analysis of class II patients, successfully treated with the straight-wire and Forsus appliances, based on cervical vertebral maturation status. Angle Orthod. 2015;85(1):80–6.
15. Pacha MM, Fleming PS, Johal A. A comparison of the efficacy of fixed versus removable functional appliances in children with class II malocclusion: a systematic review. Eur J Orthod. 2016;38:621–30.
16. Elkordy SA, Abouelezz AM, Fayed MM, Attia KH, Ishaq RA, Mostafa YA. Three-dimensional effects of the mini-implant anchored Forsus fatigue resistant device: a randomized controlled trial. Angle Orthod. 2016;86:292–305.
17. Eissa O, El-Shennawy M, Gaballah S, El-Meehy G, El Bialy T. Treatment outcomes of class II malocclusion cases treated with miniscrew-anchored Forsus fatigue resistant device: a randomized controlled trial. Angle Orthod. 2017;87:824–33.
18. Elkordy SA, Abouelezz AM, Fayed MMS, Aboulfotouh MH, Mostafa YA. Evaluation of the miniplate-anchored Forsus fatigue resistant device in skeletal class II growing subjects: a randomized controlled trial. Angle Orthod. 2019;89:391–403.
19. Liu L, Zhan Q, Zhou J, Kuang Q, Yan X, Zhang X, Shan Y, Lai W, Long H. A comparison of the effects of Forsus appliances with and without temporary anchorage devices for skeletal class II malocclusion. Angle Orthod. 2020;91:794–803.
20. Aras I, Pasaoglu A. Class II subdivision treatment with the Forsus fatigue resistant device vs intermaxillary elastics. Angle Orthod. 2017;87:371–6.
21. Flores-Mir C, McGrath L, Heo G, Major PW. Efficiency of molar distalization associated with second and third molar eruption stage. Angle Orthod. 2013;83:735–42.
22. Grec RH, Janson G, Branco NC, Moura-Grec PG, Patel MP, Castanha Henriques JF. Intraoral distalizer effects with conventional and skeletal anchorage: a meta-analysis. Am J Orthod Dentofacial Orthop. 2013;143:602–15.
23. Soheilifar S, Mohebi S, Ameli N. Maxillary molar distalization using conventional versus skeletal anchorage devices: a systematic review and meta-analysis. Int Orthod. 2019;1:415–24.
24. Bellini-Pereira SA, Pupulim DC, Aliaga-Del Castillo A, Henriques JFC, Janson G. Time of maxillary molar distalization with non-compliance intraoral distalizing appliances: a meta-analysis. Eur J Orthod. 2019;41:652–60.
25. Janson G, Castillo AA, Niederberger A. Changes in apical base sagittal relationship in class II malocclusion treatment with and without premolar extractions: a systematic review and meta-analysis. Angle Orthod. 2017;87:338–55.
26. Janson G, Mendes LM, Junqueira CHZ, Garib DG. Soft tissue changes in class II malocclusion patients treated with extractions: a systematic review. Eur J Orthod. 2016;38:631–7.
27. Kouvelis G, Dritsas K, Doulis I, Kloukos D. Gkantidis N (2018) effect of orthodontic treatment with 4 premolar extractions compared with nonextraction treatment on the vertical dimension of the face: a systematic review. Am J Orthod Dentofacial Orthop. 2018;154:175–87.
28. Goldstein B, Veitz-Keenan A. Extraction or non-extraction treatment for class II division 2 malocclusion? Evid Based Dent. 2018;19:88–9.

Class II Correction with Clear Aligners

8

Eugene Chan and M. Ali Darendeliler

8.1 Introduction

Orthodontic Class II correction is complex due to its multifactorial cause and its different phenotypical expression. The skeletal and dental implications further complicate the diagnosis and hence, the treatment plans. Successful Class II correction could be age-related, which means early consultations and early identification of problems are of paramount importance. The knowledge of the growth potential and biology of dental movements influences the appliance of choice, design and staging patterns, and the need to incorporate auxiliaries such as TADs and elastics, as well as the need for any interdisciplinary collaboration.

8.2 Age-Related Class II Planning

When children are treated orthodontically during a phase of active growth, there is an opportunity to harness growth to achieve correction of the differential jaw growth and harmonize dental relationships [1–4]. Correction outside of such premise will mostly be dental in nature. For adolescents or young adult patients with little or unfavourable future jaw and dento-alveolar growth, treatment is more likely to be either repositioning the teeth to camouflage the skeletal discrepancy or, for the more severe and/or older patient, surgical correction. Even though the goals of these alternative treatment approaches may be the same, namely improved aesthetics and a stable functional pattern with long-term dental health, the timing of treatment, mechanics used, and direction of tooth movement are substantially different [5].

The Burlington growth studies [6] evaluated the various growth time points of growing male subjects and their related height growth, to growth of the sutures and condyles. They correlated the parameters and noted a similar peak growth at approximately 14 years (Fig. 8.1a). It has also been reported that in comparison, girls mature and hit their peak growth approximately 2 years before boys [7] (Fig. 8.1b). It would then be logical to be guided by these growth estimates when planning Class II-related treatment.

E. Chan · M. A. Darendeliler (✉)
Faculty of Medicine and Health, Department of Orthodontics, Sydney Dental Hospital, University of Sydney, Sydney, NSW, Australia
e-mail: eugene.chan@sydney.edu.au; ali.darendeliler@sydney.edu.au

M. T. Cobourne (ed.), *Orthodontic Management of Class II Malocclusion*,
https://doi.org/10.1007/978-3-031-57530-3_8

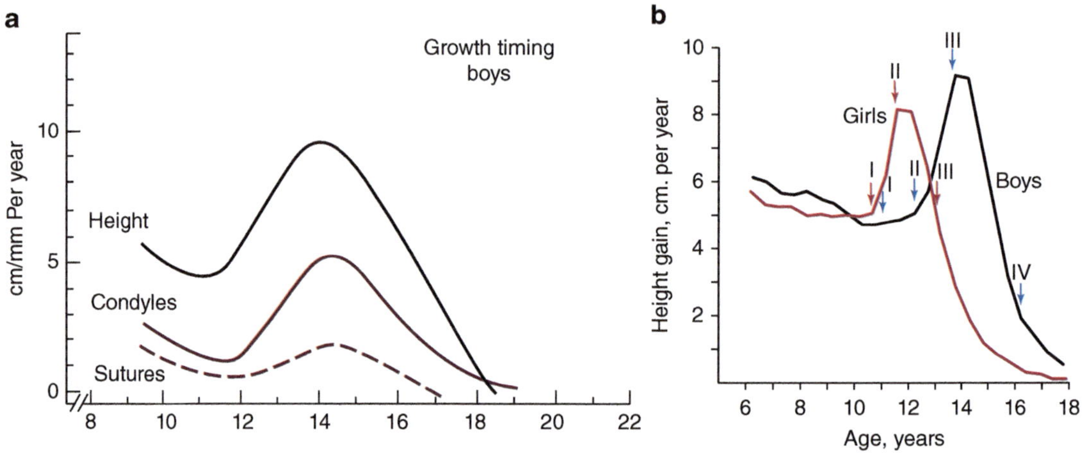

Fig. 8.1 (**a**) Burlington growth studies looking at various growth time points of boys and related height growth to growth of sutures and condyles. (**b**) Peak height growth differences between boys and girls from 6 to 18 years old

8.3 Pre-adolescent Class II Correction

Early interceptive orthodontic treatment is usually indicated under several conditions. These conditions may commonly include supernumerary teeth disrupting routine dental eruption, disparity in jaw growth, the presence of parafunctional habits that may have disturbed the equilibrium of dental positioning, missing or the early loss of deciduous teeth leading to the loss of space, anterior and/or posterior crossbites that may hinder the symmetrical dento-alveolar development. Other indications may also include trauma, soft tissue abnormalities, variations in dental anatomy, obstructive sleep apnoea, or transpositioned teeth.

Traditionally, we associate orthodontic treatment in pre-adolescence with removable or fixed expanders, used with the collaboration of fixed appliances where appropriate. The clinician never had the option to consider clear aligners as another treatment modality until recently. Clear aligner treatment in the pre-adolescent treatment has its own unique criteria.

The Invisalign First ™ appliance is typically indicated for the early mixed dentition ranging from the age of approximately 6–10 years old. However, it is reserved for cases where the permanent first molars have sufficiently erupted, and with at least 2 incisors that are at least two-thirds erupted. The case should also have at least 2 non-mobile primary teeth (C, D, or E), or a partially erupted permanent tooth (3, 4, or 5) per quadrant in at least 3 quadrants.

Successful phase 1 treatment usually takes between 12 and 18 months [8] and the primary dentition present needs to be firm enough throughout this duration in order to allow the clear aligners to have sufficient engagement of the dentition, to fully express their mechanics. The deciduous teeth C's, D's, and E's exfoliate at approximately between 9 and 12 years old (Fig. 8.2). If active phase 1 treatment takes between 12 and 18 months, treatment needs to commence between the ages of 7.5 and 10.5 years old in order to prevent the exfoliation of these teeth during treatment. The key to perfect timing of treatment commencement is to ensure you consult the patient early. It is essential to examine a current OPG (ortho-pantomogram) radiograph carefully. The child grows very quickly and OPG radiographs should not be older than 3–6 months. If the child is not ready for an immediate treatment start, place them on a periodic recall and review them again in approximately 3–6 months' time to avoid missing the window of opportunity for treatment.

Fig. 8.2 Estimated eruption and shedding timing of upper and lower deciduous dentition

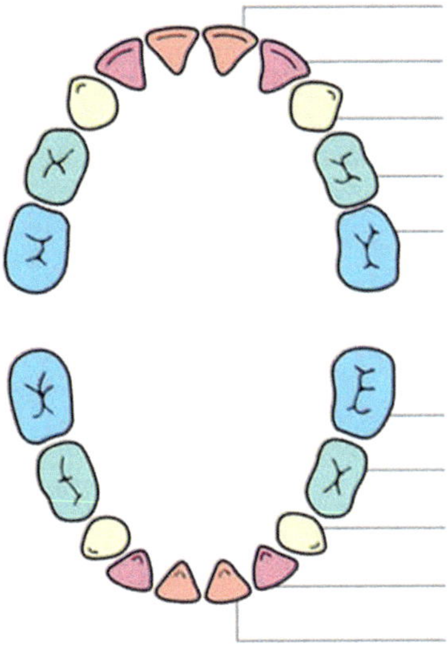

Upper Teeth	Erupt	Shed
Central incisor	8-12 mos.	6-7 yrs.
Lateral incisor	9-13 mos.	7-8 yrs.
Cuspid (canine)	16-22 mos.	10-12 yrs.
First molar	13-19 mos.	9-11 yrs.
Second molar	25-33 mos.	10-12 yrs.

Lower Teeth	Erupt	Shed
Second molar	23-31 mos.	10-12 yrs.
First molar	14-18 mos.	9-11 yrs.
Cuspid (canine)	17-23 mos.	9-12 yrs.
Lateral incisor	10-16 mos.	7-8 yrs.
Central incisor	6-10 mos.	6-7 yrs.

One of the early contributors to a Class II malocclusion is the loss of the maxillary "E" space during the mixed dentition phase. The early loss of the upper second deciduous molar, usually due to decay, encourages the distally placed first molar to drift mesially, tipping into the eruption space of the second premolar (Fig. 8.3a). The OPG radiograph shows the potential impaction of tooth #15 with the mesial tipping of tooth #16 into the "E" space in quadrant one (Fig. 8.3b). Clear aligners using the Invisalign First ™ appliance was used to regain the "E" space by distalizing the #16 (Fig. 8.3c).

Treatment in mixed dentition may be tricky. Often with multiple deciduous teeth previously exfoliated, and the succedaneous ones not, or insufficiently erupted, there might be insufficient anchorage to hold the aligners in place. During the process of ClinCheck treatment planning, ensure the placement of sufficient "attachments" on the dentition (Fig. 8.3d, e). The appliance can also be designed to support the use of Class II elastics. This is required to support the #16 distalization, regaining the "E" space, as well as to retract the increased overjet.

Most early Class II correction may also require some dental arch expansion. This 8-year 11-month-old Class II div 2 male patient presented with moderate degrees of dental crowding, a deep dental overbite, with rather constricted upper and lower dental archforms (Fig. 8.4a, b). The Invisalign First ™ appliance allowed simultaneous dental arch expansion (Fig. 8.4c), dental alignment, bite opening as well as sagittal correction. Computer-aided designed, optimized attachments were placed on dentition that did not show signs of exfoliation. An eruption "compensator" or "tooth pontic" is designed over the erupting #44 to allow the natural eruption of the tooth. Interproximal dental spaces ranging up to 0.6 mm are designed mesial and distal to the upper and lower deciduous canines in order to accommodate the larger succedaneous permanent canines when they erupt through. "Precision cuts" allowed the use of Class II elastics clinically, and activated the sagittal correction as required (Fig. 8.4d). The clear aligners were changed weekly. Figure 8.4e shows the treatment progress after 31 weeks of active aligner wear. A progress OPG radiograph (Fig. 8.4f) was also taken at this stage when additional aligners were ordered with new intra-oral scans to determine our finishing movements. Figure 8.4g, h show the completed phase 1 treatment after 13 months of active clear aligner treatment with the Invisalign First ™ appliance. The three-dimensional correction has been evidently demonstrated. The dental arch expansion, overbite correction, sagittal change as

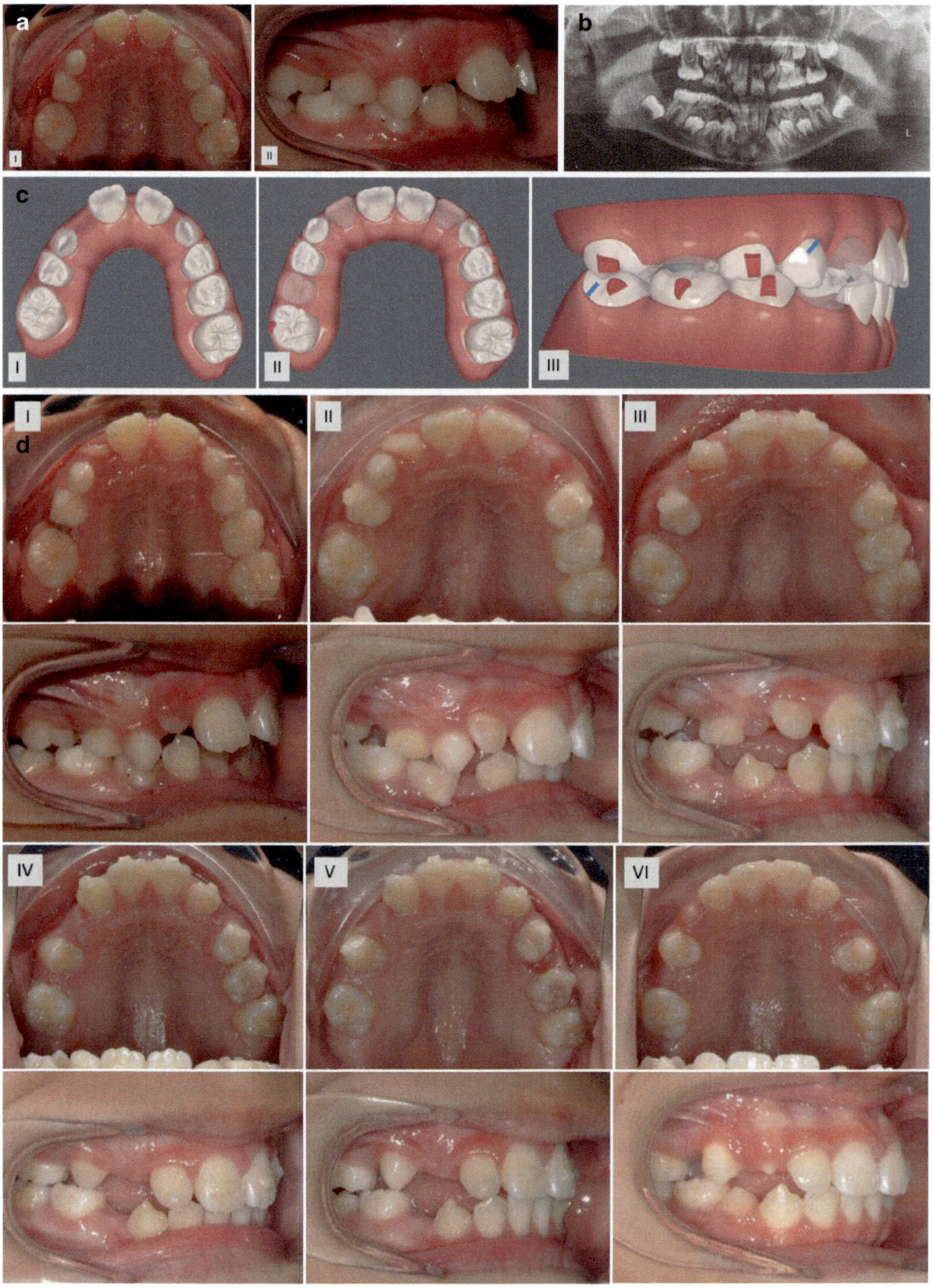

Fig. 8.3 (**a**) An 8-year-old male patient in mixed dentition was referred with regards to the early loss of #55 and mesial drifting of #16. (I) Maxillary view, (II) right buccal view show the increased dental overbite and overjet. (**b**) OPG radiograph of case showing the early loss of #55 and the mesial drifting of #16, and blocking the eruption of #15. (**c**) ClinCheck plans showing (I) pre-treatment, (II) predicted completion: maxillary occlusal view and (III) predicted completion: right buccal view. (**d**) Clinical images (I) to (VI) showing the regaining of the "E" space with molar distalization, correction of the deep overbite and increased overjet. (**e**) OPG radiograph at the end of phase 1 treatment

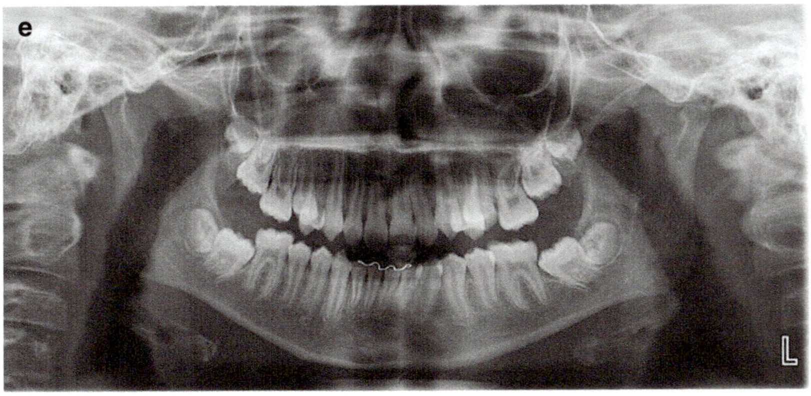

Fig. 8.3 (continued)

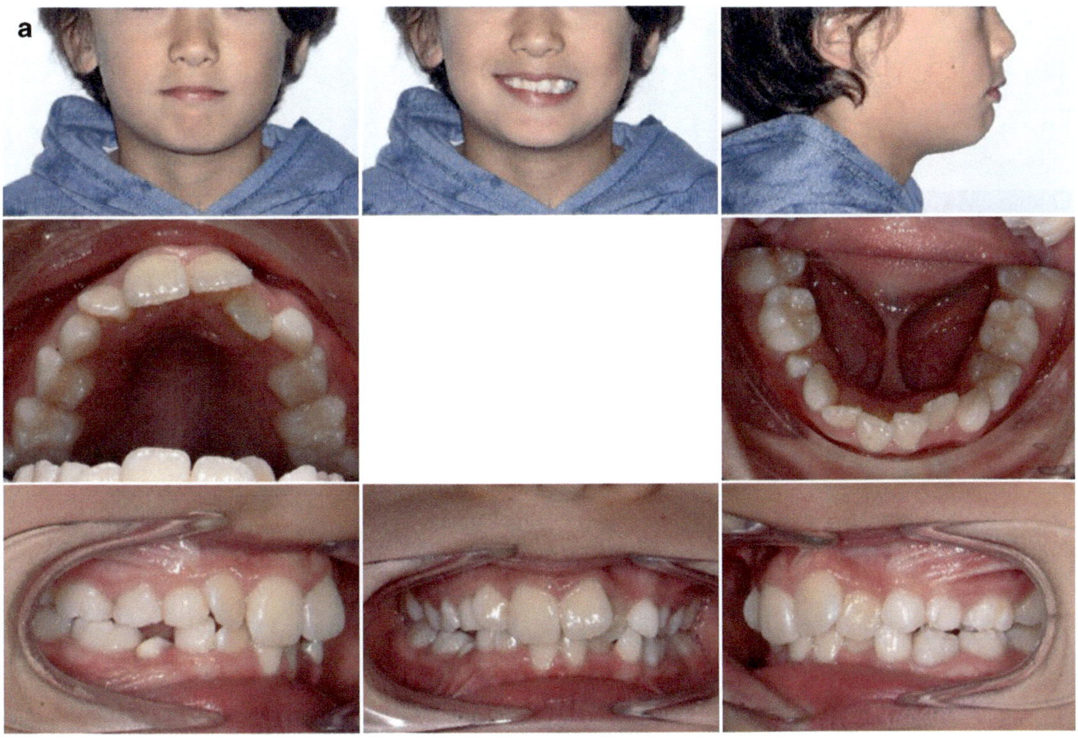

Fig. 8.4 (**a**) 8-year 11-month-old Class II div 2 male patient presented with moderate degrees of dental crowding, a deep dental overbite, with constricted upper and lower dental archforms. (**b**) Pre-treatment (I) OPG and (II) lateral cephalogram. (**c**) ClinCheck plans showing (I) pre-treatment maxillary occlusal view, (II) superimposition with dental expansion, and (III) predicted completion. (**d**) ClinCheck plans showing attachment and precision cut designs. (**e**) Treatment progress after 31 weeks of active aligner wear. (**f**) Progressive OPG taken at 31 weeks. (**g**) Completion of phase 1 treatment after 13 months of active treatment. (**h**) Completion OPG. (**i**) Comparison of before and after phase 1 treatment with Invisalign First™

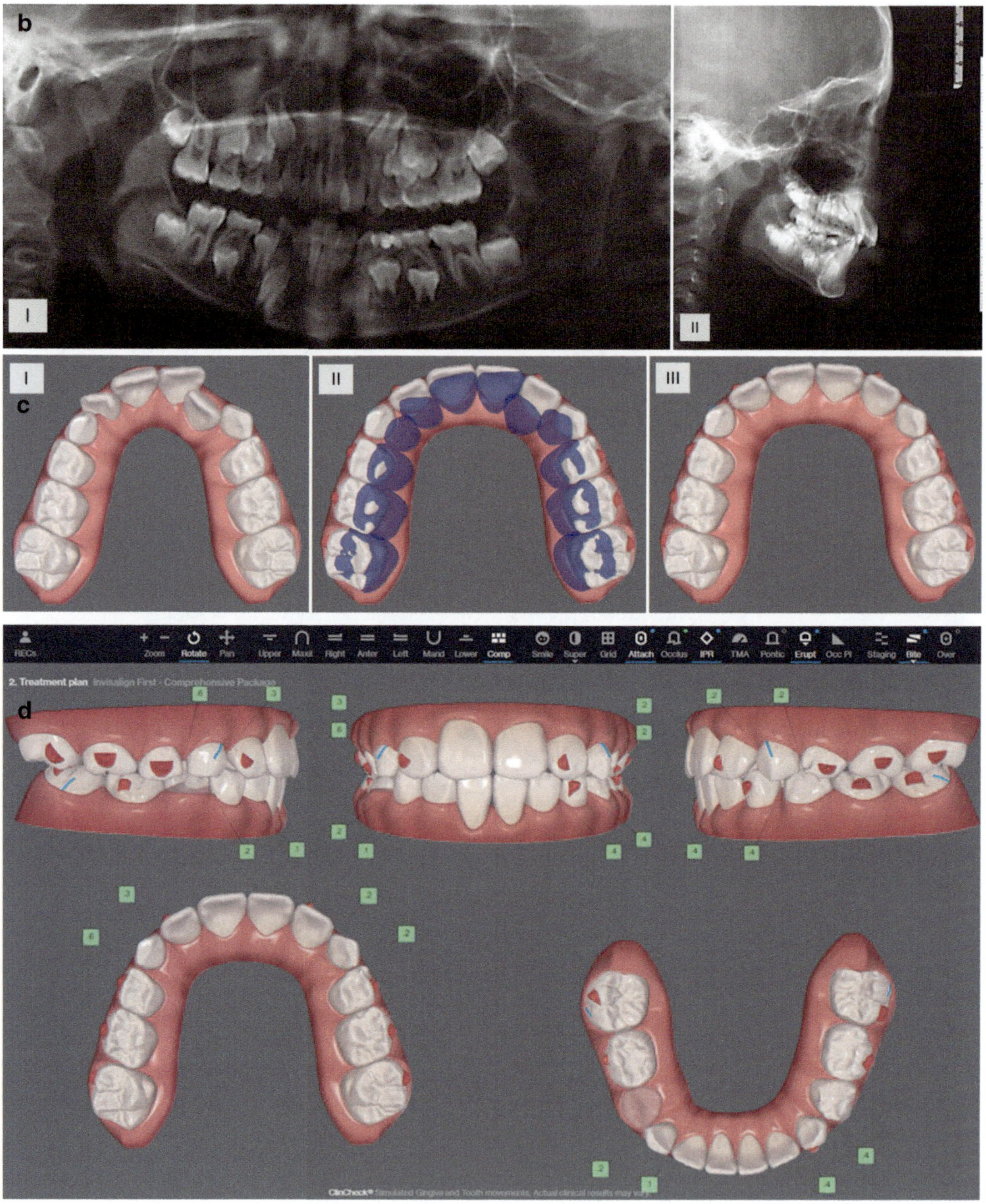

Fig. 8.4 (continued)

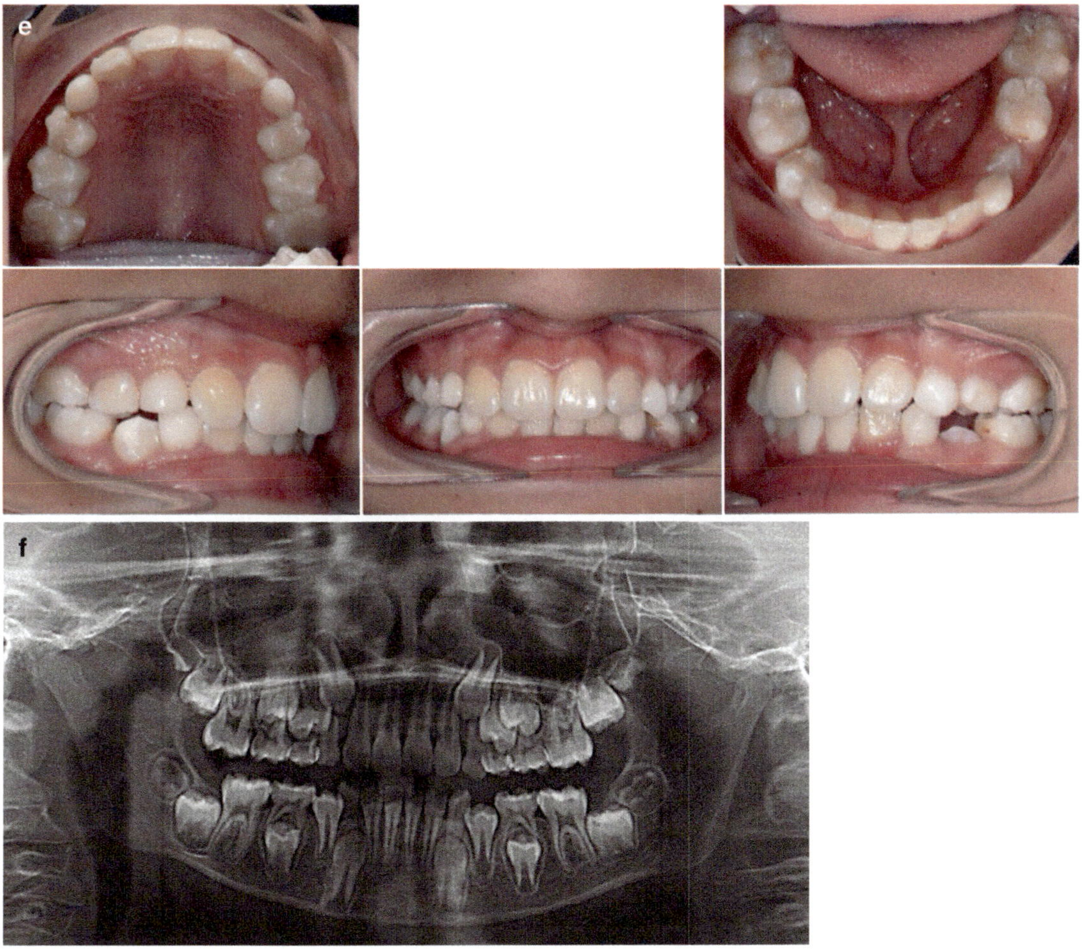

Fig. 8.4 (continued)

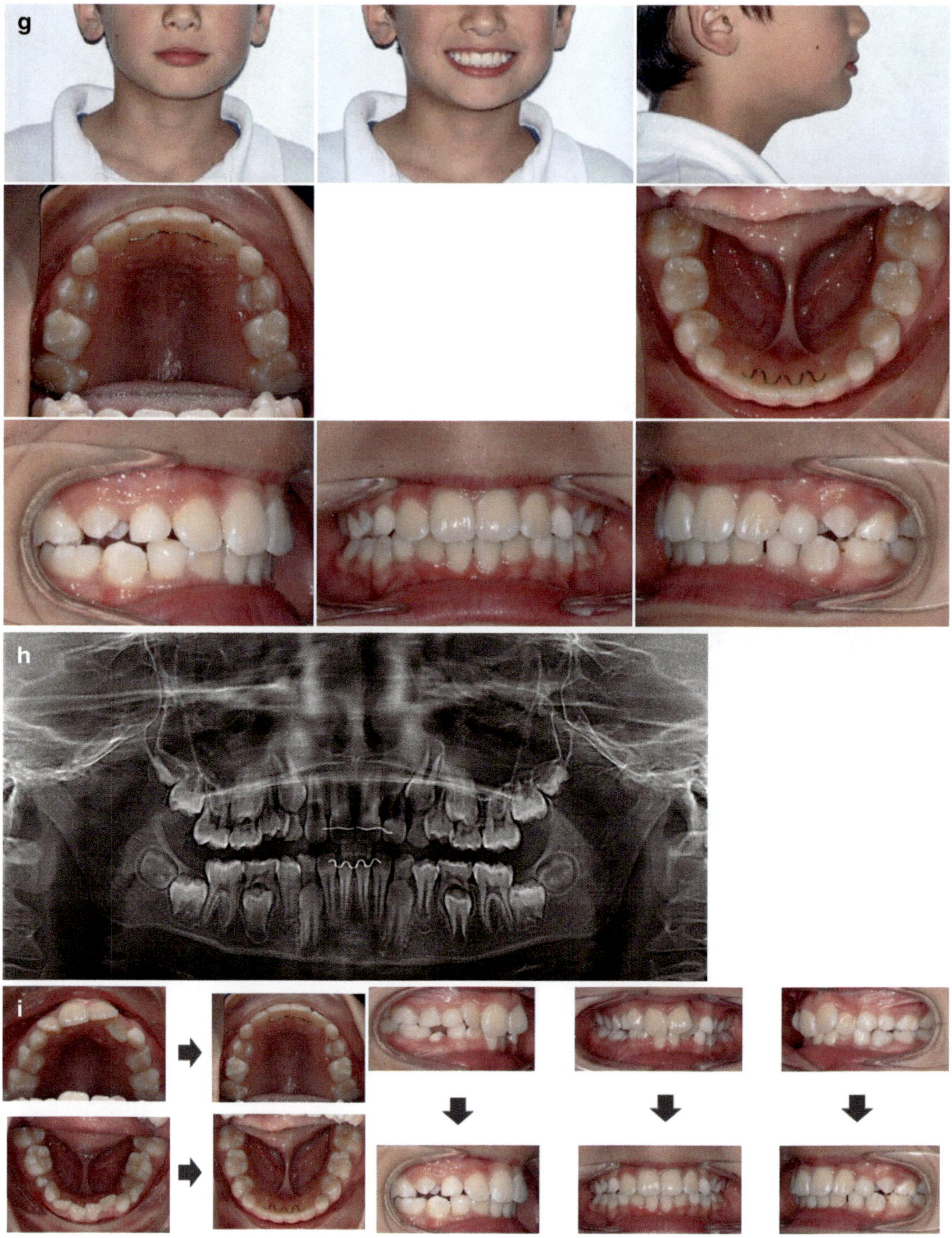

Fig. 8.4 (continued)

well as the dental spatial arrangement within the arch were well achieved (Fig. 8.4i). Upper and lower fixed retainers, and an upper Hawley-type removable retainer to be worn at night were prescribed to maintain the results of this phase 1 treatment. The patient was subsequently be placed on a periodic review to be checked every 3–6 months. The continued growth and dental development will be monitored until he transited into his full permanent dentition. The Hawley retainer may be trimmed and adjusted as required, as the remaining primary dentition exfoliates, and the permanent dentition erupts. Once the child has transited fully into the full permanent dentition, the clinician further assesses the case and determines if a phase 2 treatment will be required. Usually with successful phase 1 treatment, phase 2 treatment will be less complicated and has a potentially shorter treatment duration. In some rare cases, phase 2 treatment may not be required.

8.4 Functional Therapy in Class II Correction

Conventional functional therapy treatment in orthodontics includes removable appliances such as a Frankel, bionator or twin block. They all have a common feature in which when activated, the patients have their mandible perpetually positioned forwards in an edge-to-edge incisor relationship. This prolonged postured position, in patients with favourable growth, has purported dento-alveolar changes contributing to Class II dental and skeletal corrections.

The mandibular advancement (MA) features in the Invisalign appliance (Fig. 8.5a, b) and the MA features in the Angelalign A6 appliance (Fig. 8.6a, b) adopt this similar philosophy and have demonstrated promising results.

8.4.1 MA with Invisalign

The patient was 9 years 11 months old at presentation with a chief concern that "my front teeth stick out". She was diagnosed as a Class II div 1 dental malocclusion on a skeletal 2 base with a horizontal direction of growth (Fig. 8.7a). The ideal patient should be just about to hit their peak height growth [9, 10], this can be determined readily by studying the size of the third cervical vertebrae (CV3) in the lateral cephalometric radiograph (Fig. 8.7b) [11]. There was an upper median diastema, mild lower dental crowding, with an increased dental overjet of 8 mm, a deep dental overbite, with a recessive lower jaw.

The MA features in the Invisalign appliance and the Angelalign A6 appliance allow pre-MA phases whereby the clinician may choose to have certain dental movements prescribed prior to the mandibular advancement. These movements may include proclining the upper incisors of a Class II div 2 type malocclusion in order to allow the advancement of the lower jaw without the patient

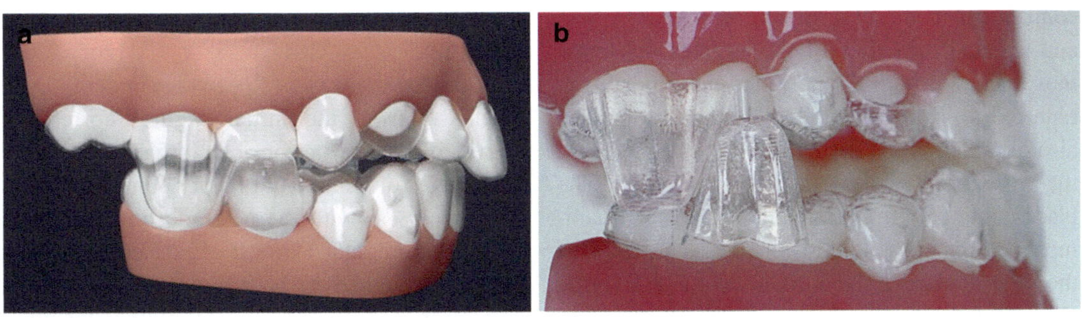

Fig. 8.5 (a) Mandibular advancement feature with the Invisalign appliance. (b) The Invisalign appliance with the "precision wings" on the buccal surfaces posturing the lower jaw forwards while activated

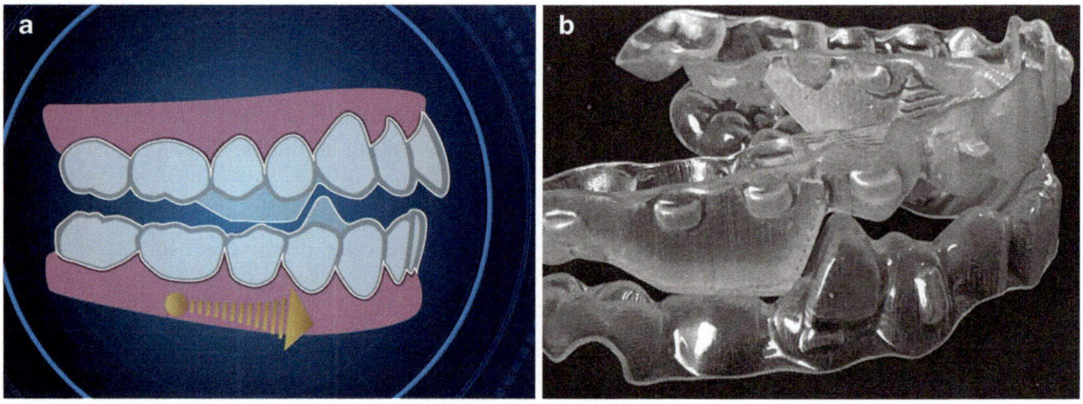

Fig. 8.6 (**a**) Mandibular advancement feature with the Angelalign A6 appliance. (**b**) The Angelalign A6 appliance with the "twin blocks" on the occlusal surfaces posturing the lower jaw forwards while activated

going into a negative overjet. Cases with a deep lower curve of Spee may also be levelled during this pre-MA phase.

One of the keys to the success of treatment with any clear aligners with the mandibular advancement feature is to ensure that the aligners fit and stay on the dentition well.

With the Invisalign aligner system, the ClinCheck plans showed attachments and the MA "precision wing" designs (Fig. 8.7c). When the mandibular advancement "precision wings" appear in the plan, usually after at least 4 stages of pre-MA aligners (if any pre-MA stages are planned), attachments cannot be placed on the buccal surfaces where the wings are. These are usually the upper and lower second premolars and first molars. When there are a lack of attachments on the posterior segments, the aligners do not retain well on the dentition. This often contributed to the ease of aligner dislodgement and negated the effect of the aligners on dental movements as well as the mandibular posturing required to achieve the Class II correction. This also often led to the flattening of the aligners and the "precision wings" during treatment. The placement of 5 mm horizontal rectangular attachments on the upper and lower lingual surfaces of the first molars helped to alleviate this issue (Fig. 8.7d).

With the Angelalign aligner system, the mandibular advancement features are designed to mimic the traditional "twin block" appliance. These features are designed on the occlusal and not the buccal surfaces of the aligners. Although it may increase the resting vertical dimension of the patient whilst in place, it allows the placement of attachments on the buccal surfaces to ensure good retention of the appliance (Fig. 8.6a, b). As such, the dislodgment of the aligners, flattening of the aligners and the MA features are a lot less likely.

The aligners were designed to be worn full time, at least 20–22 hours per day, and changed every week. The mandibular advancement "precision wings" may be designed to advance the mandible in a "step-wise" configuration, advancing 2 mm every 8 weeks (8 aligners). This "step-wise" advancement allows gradual posturing of the mandible to make the treatment progress more comfortable for the patient, and have potentially a greater effect in advancing the mandible as compared to a single-step maximum advancement [12].

If the lower curve of Spee was not completely levelled during the initial sagittal correction, there will be a posterior open bite evident in the later stages of treatment. Plan for continued Class II elastic wear with the new additional aligners order. A triangular Class II elastic configuration may be designed to both maintain the sagittal correction, as well as to assist with the closure of the posterior open bite (Fig. 8.7e). Figure 8.7f, g show the completion of the Class II correction after 23 months of active aligner treatment. The

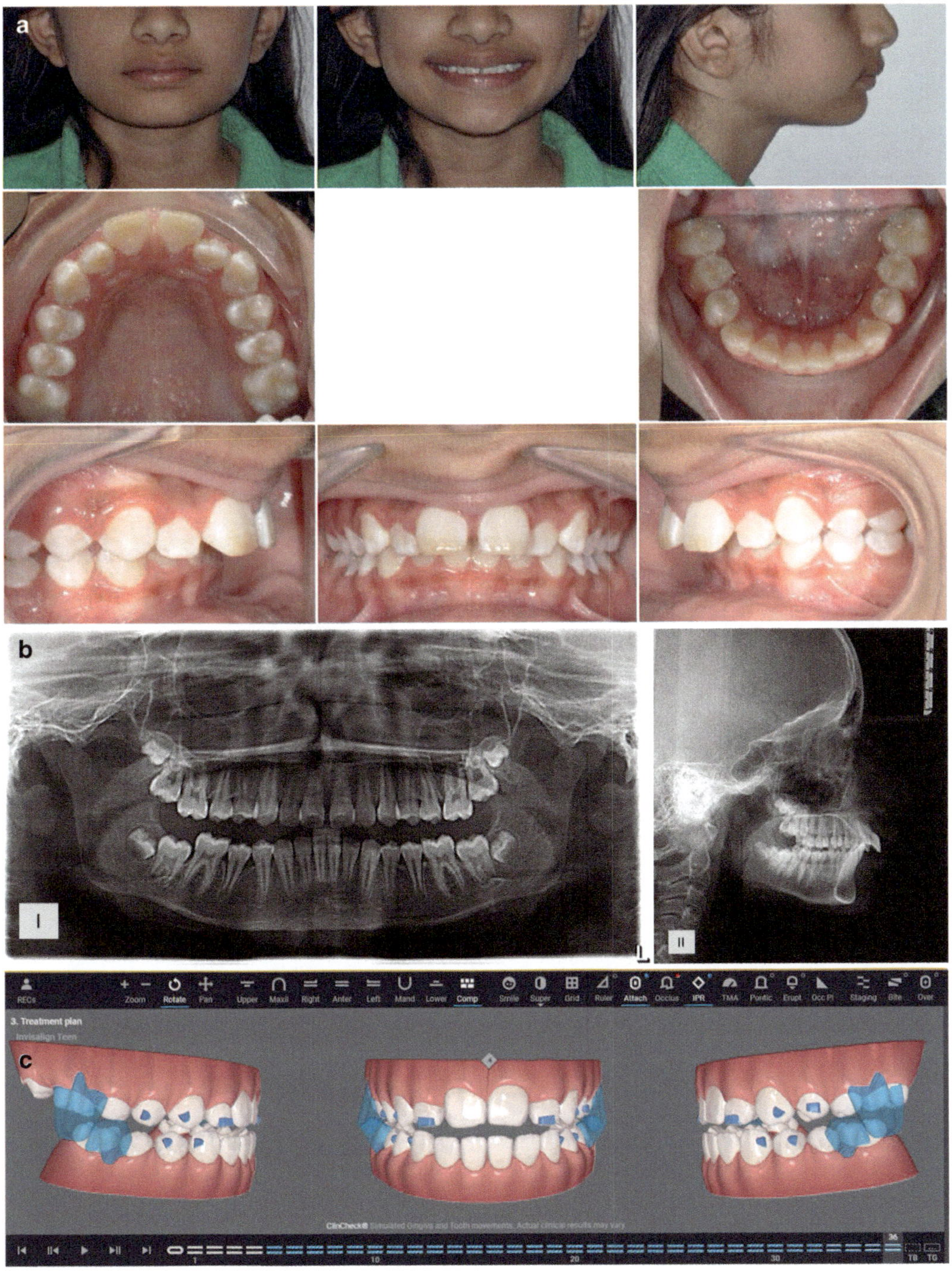

Fig. 8.7 (**a**) 9-years 11-month-old female patient: "my front teeth stick out". (**b**) Pre-treatment (I) OPG and (II) lateral cephalogram. (**c**) ClinCheck plans showing attachments placed to ensure the retention of the aligners. (**d**) The placement of 5 mm horizontal rectangular attachments on the upper and lower lingual surfaces of the first molars. (**e**) Triangular Class II elastic configuration designed to both maintain the sagittal correction, as well as to assist with the closure of the posterior open bite. (**f**) Completion of active treatment after 23 months. (**g**) Completion (I) OPG and (II) lateral cephalogram. (**h**) Comparison of (I) before and (II) after treatment with Invisalign MA appliance. (**i**) Superimposition tracing of before and after treatment. (**j**) Cephalometric changes with treatment compared with norms

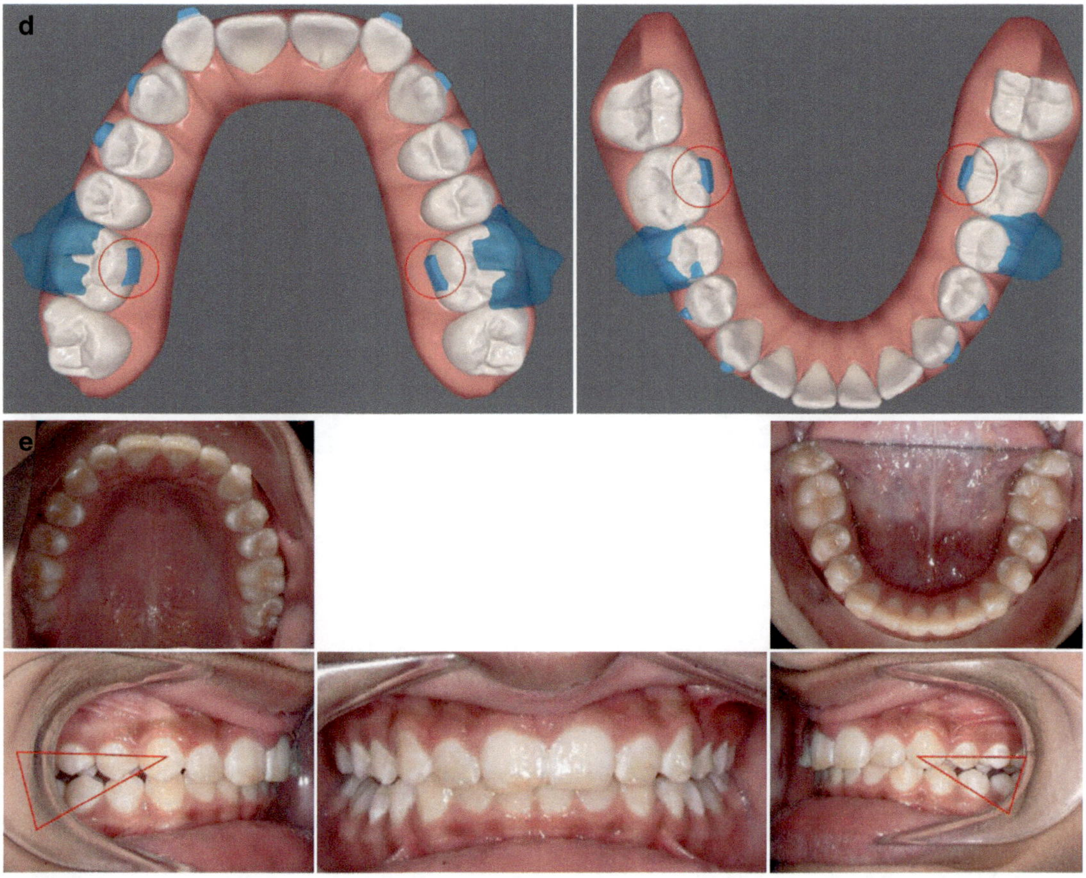

Fig. 8.7 (continued)

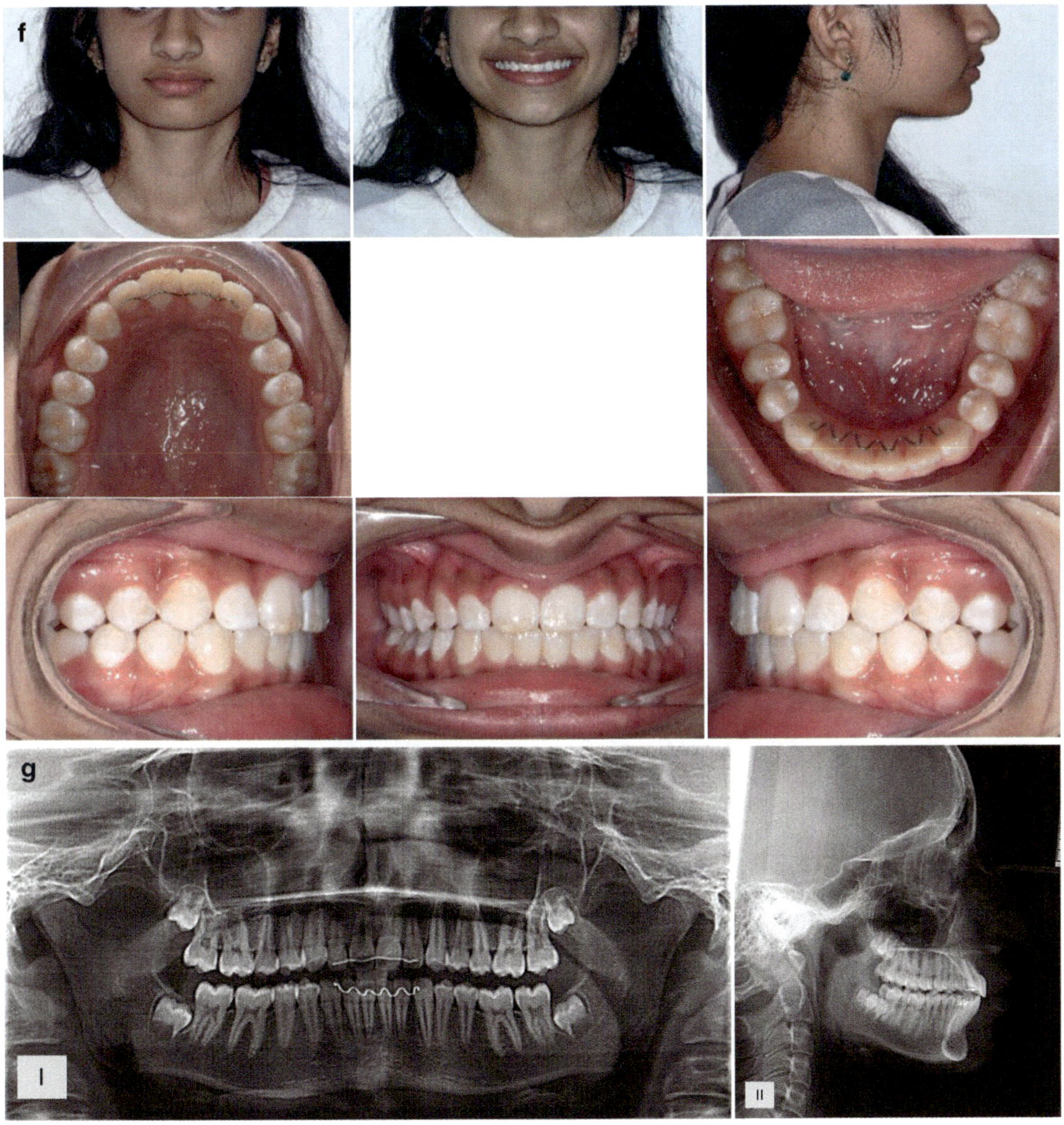

Fig. 8.7 (continued)

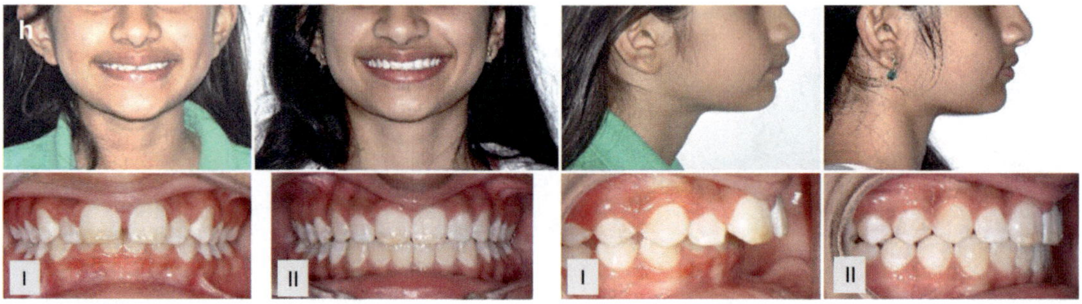

Superimposition

i

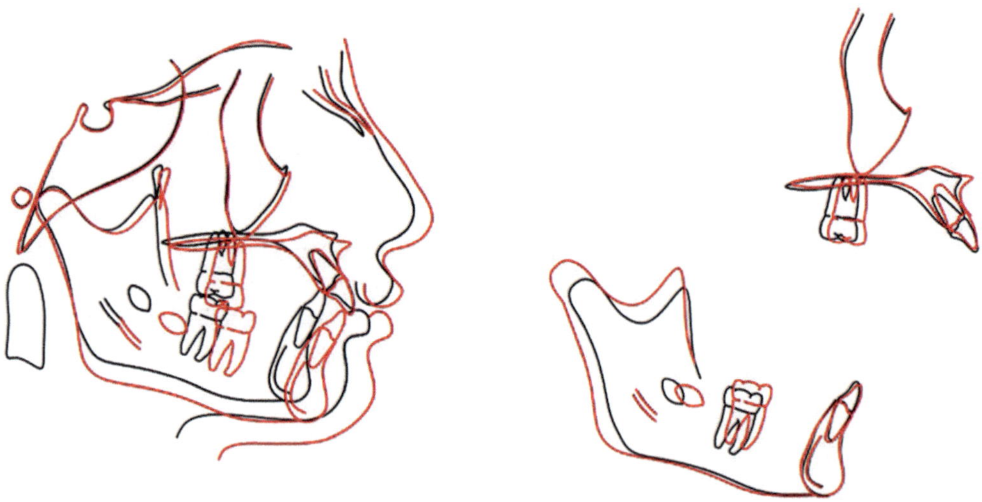

Fig. 8.7 (continued)

j

Sydney – Geneva Normas

Parameter	Norms	T1	T2
SNA	81 ± 3°	80.5°	81.4°
SNB	77 ± 3°	74.3°	77.5°
ANB	4 ± 2.6°	6.1°	3.9°
S-Go'/N-Me (J%)	61%	70.3%	72.7%
N-ANS	50 ± 3 mm	54.8 mm	56.8 mm
ANS - Me	60 ± 4 mm	56.3 mm	59.4 mm
N-ANS / ANS-Me	45%, 55%	49.3% 50.7%	48.9%, 51.1%
SN-PP	8 ± 2°	10.6°	11.3°
PP-MP	28 ± 5°	16.2°	13.6°
SN-MP	35 ± 5°	26.8°	24.9°
SN-OP	20 ± 4°	13.6°	14°
Gonial angle	127 ± 5°	122.7°	121.3°

Parameter	Norms	T1	T2
1/-SN	105 ± 6°	112.9°	106.8°
1/-PP	113 ± 7°	123.4°	118.1°
/1- MP	94 ± 7°	101.3°	107.4°
1 / 1	126 ± 10°	119.1°	120.9°
1/-N Pog	9 ± 33 mm	13.3 mm	8.1 mm
1/-A Pog	6 ± 3 mm	9.7 mm	5.7 mm
1/-A Pog	1 ± 3 mm	–0.5 mm	3.3 mm
OJ		9.4 mm	2.3 mm
OB		6 mm	1.1 mm

Sydney – Geneva Normas

Parameter	Norms	T1	T2
Y axis	68 ± 4°	67.3°	65.6°
Facial axis	90 ± 3°	91.5°	92.6°
S – N	73 ± 3 mm	73.4mm	75.4mm
SN / FH	7.8 ± 2.4°	9.5°	9.7°
SN – Ba	130 ± 4°	133.4°	133.3°
Wits	0 ± 2	7.5°	3.3°
Go' – Me	67 ± 4 mm	62.5 mm	67.6 mm
Co – Gn	106 ± 3 mm	106.1 m	114.3 m
Co – A	85 ± 2 mm	93.4 mm	96.4 mm
L distance	21 mm	12.7 mm	17.9 mm

Parameter	Norms	T1	T2
Nasolabial angle	90°	106.8°	91.3°
S line U, L	0, 0 mm	3.6 mm, 1.2 mm	1.6 mm, 1.1 mm
Basic U lip thickness	15 mm	12.7 mm	16.1 mm
Upper lip strain	14 mm	15.9 mm	16.3 mm
H angle	10 ± 4°	24.3°	18.78°

Fig. 8.7 (continued)

increased overjet was reduced, deep overbite was corrected with the Class II dental malocclusion and facial appearance normalized (Fig. 8.7h–j).

8.4.2 MA with Angelalign A6

A young adolescent female, 12 years 1 month old, in permanent dentition presented with a Class II div 2 dental malocclusion and a skeletal 2 base with a normal direction of growth (Fig. 8.8a, b). Her chief concerns were her deep dental overbite and recessive lower jaw. There was mild upper and lower dental crowding with mildly constricted upper and lower dental archforms.

The Angelalign clear aligners were worn full time with a weekly change regime. The first stage

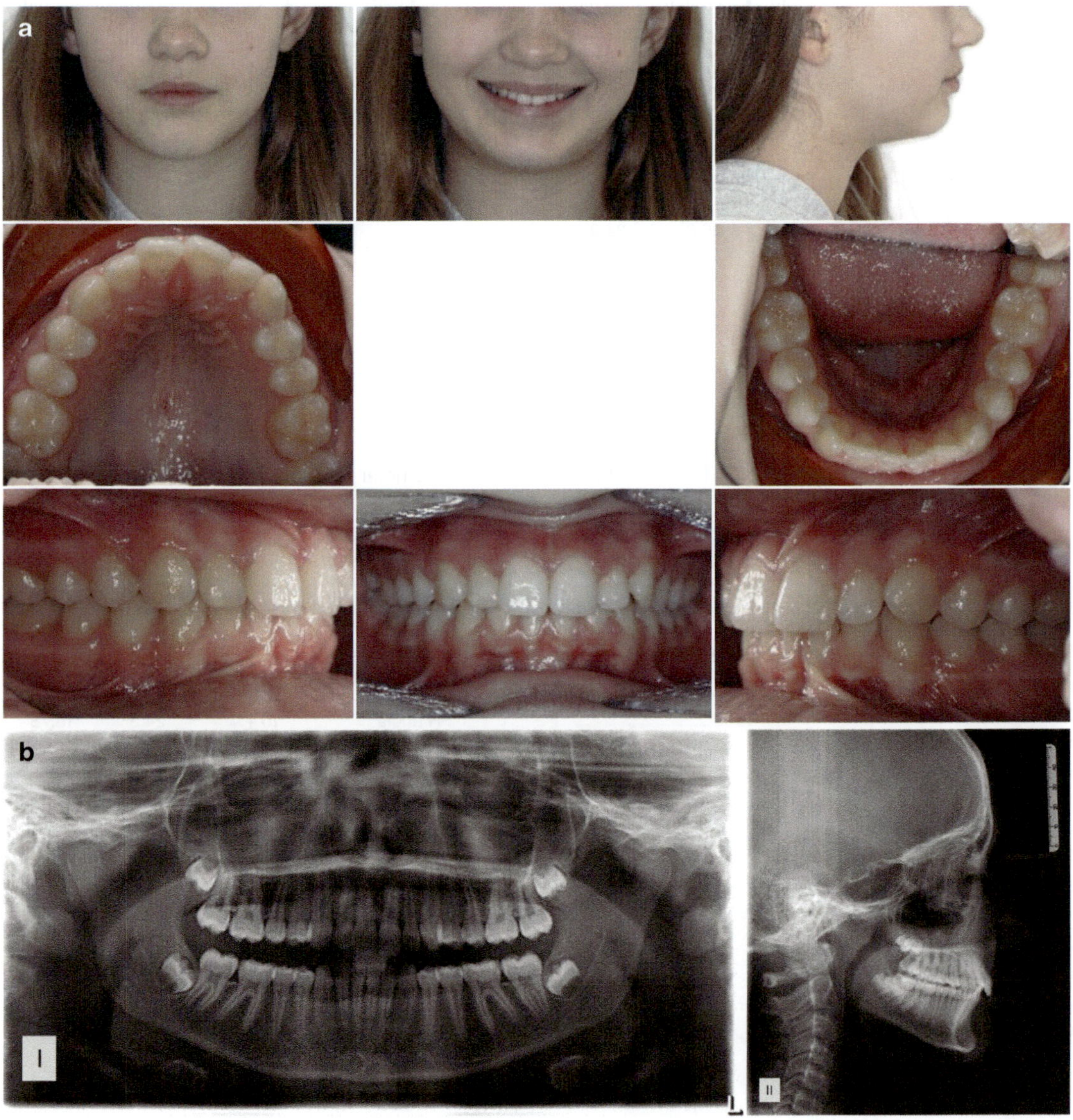

Fig. 8.8 (**a**) 12-year 1-month-old female patient: "I have a deep overbite". (**b**) Pre-treatment (I) OPG and (II) lateral cephalogram. (**c**) Images showing the completion of initial sagittal correction with an "edge-to-edge" anterior dental relationship, and a posterior open bite. (**d**) Completion of active treatment after 23 months. (**e**) Completion (I) OPG and (II) lateral cephalogram. (**f**) Comparison of (I) before and (II) after treatment with Angelalign A6 MA appliance

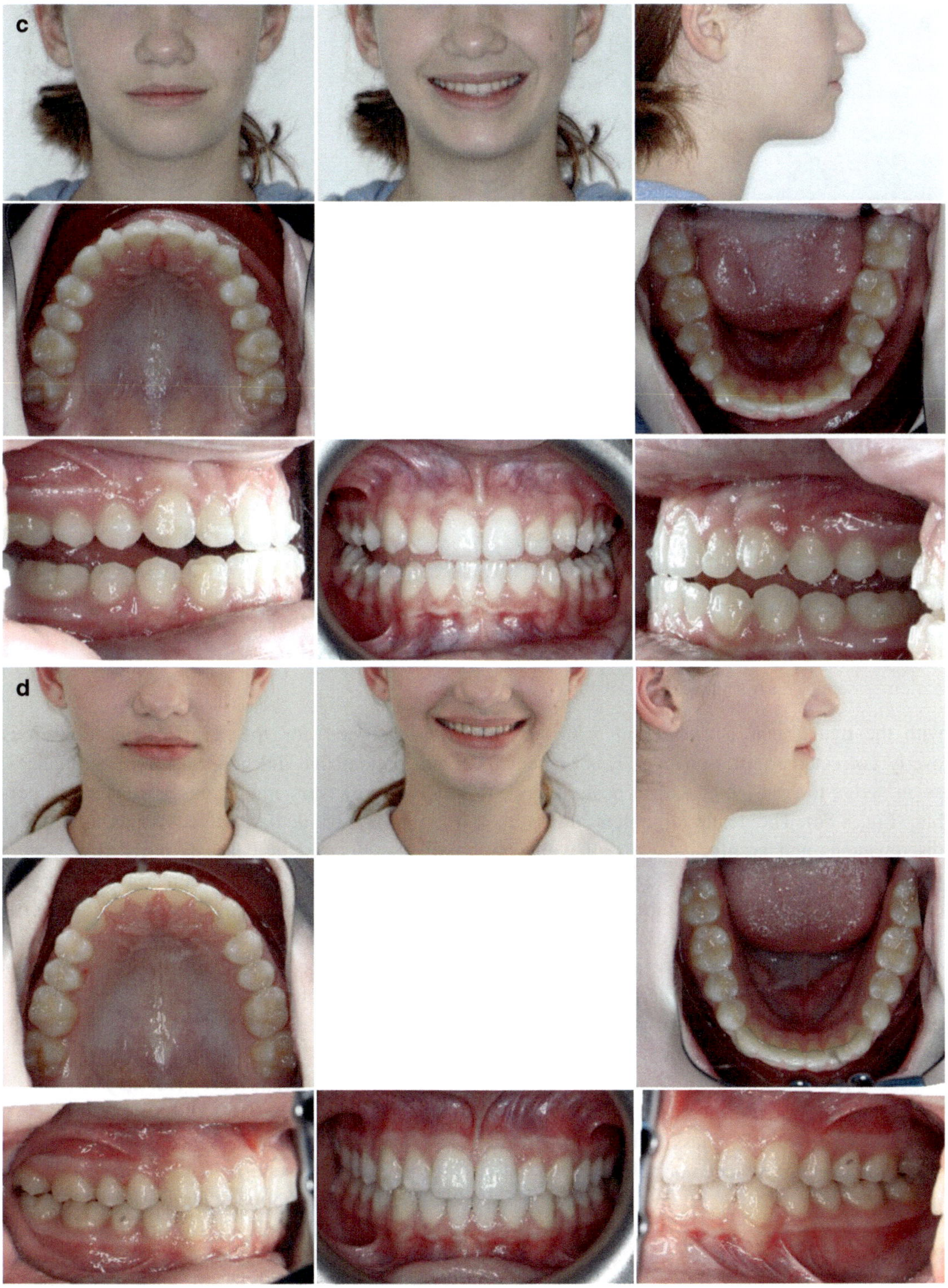

Fig. 8.8 (continued)

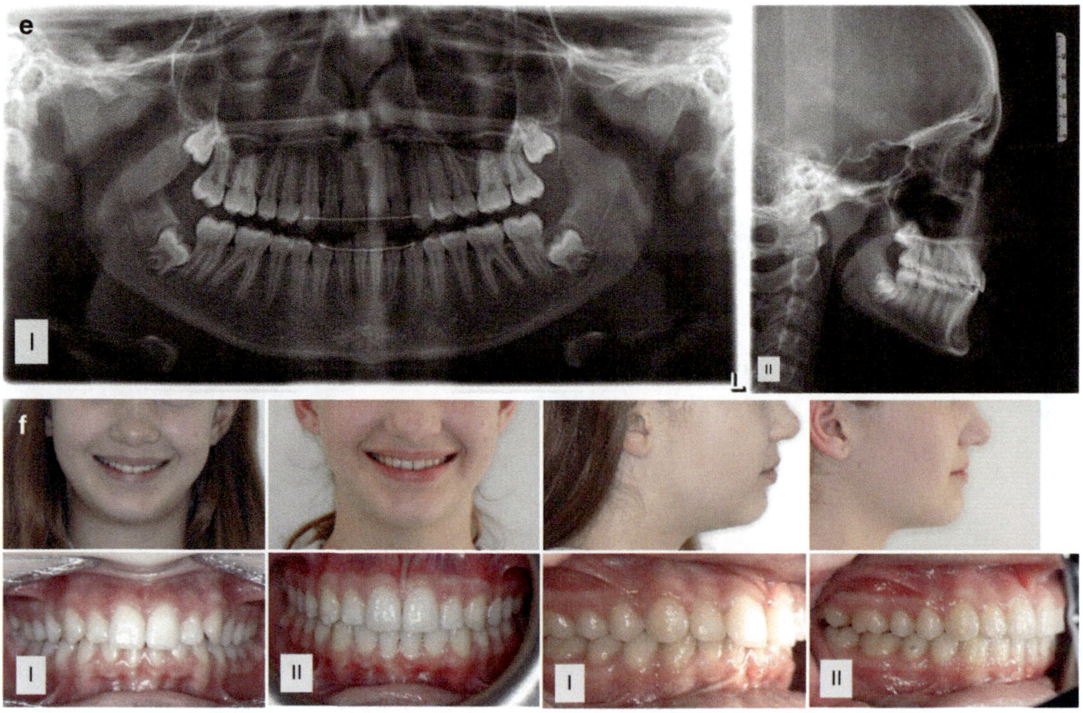

Fig. 8.8 (continued)

with the mandibular advancement achieved an overly corrected sagittal change. This presented as an "edge-to-edge" bite with a posterior open bite (Fig. 8.8c). The dental alignment, transverse discrepancies and archforms were all well corrected at this stage. The next stage followed with conventional clear aligners without the MA features. This stage concentrated on the coordination of the upper and lower arches, and to settle the bite into a good occlusion. Dental elastics may be used to help with this stage of correction where necessary. Figure 8.8d, e show the completion of the Class II correction after 23 months of active aligner treatment. The increased dental overbite was corrected, with the Class II dental malocclusion and facial appearance normalized (Fig. 8.8f).

8.5 Adolescent Class II Correction

Correction of dental malocclusions in adolescent patients has always been the bread and butter for the busy orthodontist. While clear aligners were first designed for the aesthetically conscious adult patient that did not want fixed appliances, they are now very much sought after in the correction of most dental malocclusions in younger patients. Successful Class II correction occurs readily in cases that demonstrate favourable growth potential and growth patterns. The vertical dento-alveolar growth and the biologically favourable tissue responses in younger patients enhance the treatment [13, 14].

8.5.1 Non-extraction Therapy

A 14-year 6-month-old female patient sought orthodontic intervention with concerns of her ectopically placed upper canines (Fig. 8.9a). She presented as a Class II div 1 dental malocclusion with a mild skeletal 2 base and a normal direction of growth. She had a pleasant smile, an overall convex profile with an obtuse nasal labial angle and prominent soft tissue pogonion. Although she had a full unit Class II molar relationship on the left and a half unit Class II molar relationship

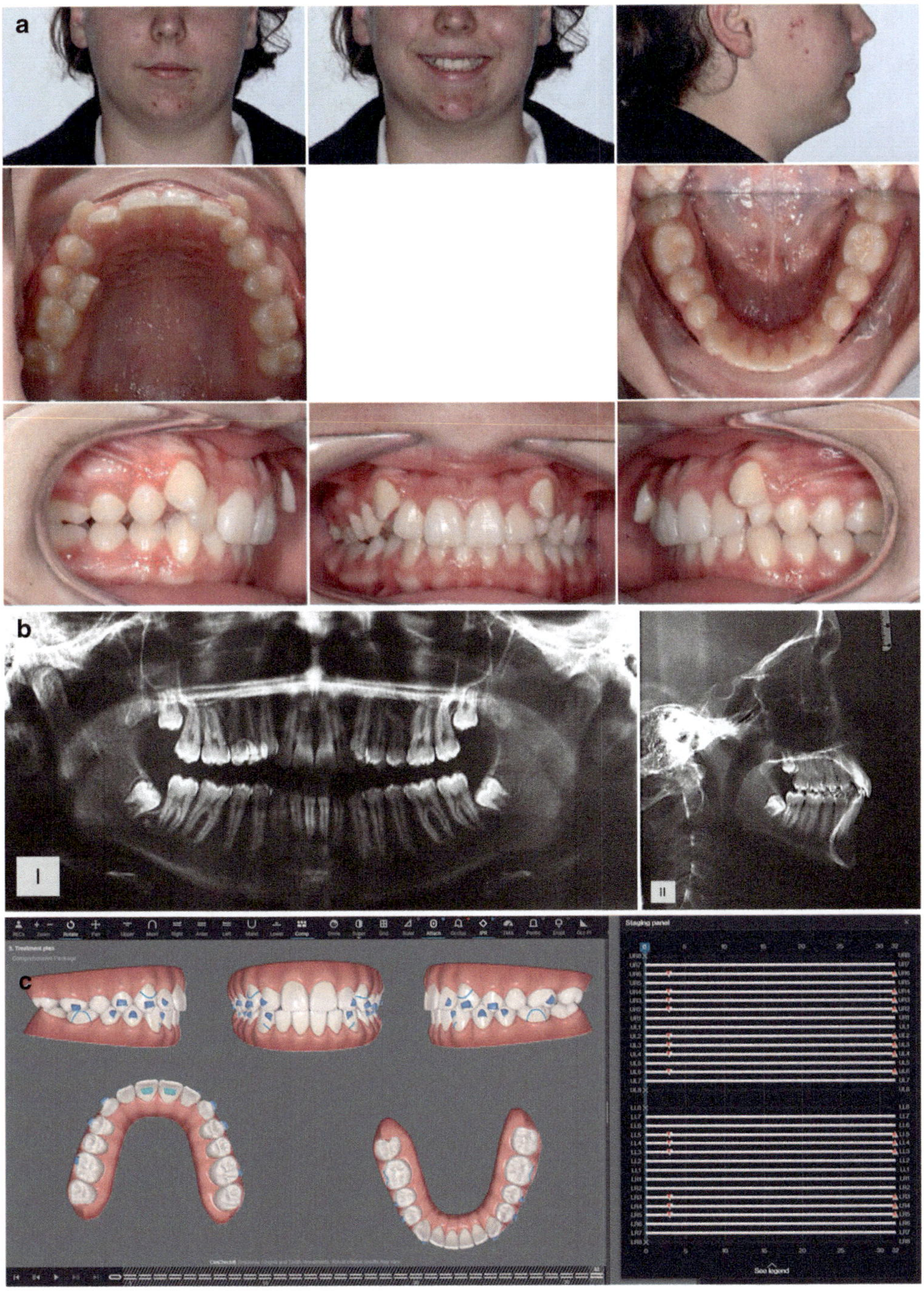

Fig. 8.9 (**a**) 14-year 6-month-old female patient sought orthodontic intervention with concerns of her ectopically placed upper canines. (**b**) Pre-treatment (I) OPG and (II) lateral cephalogram. (**c**) ClinCheck plans showing attachments, precision cuts and staging designs. (**d**) (I) Conventional Class II elastics worn from upper canines to lower first molars. (II) Triangular Class II elastics introducing a vertical vector to assist in the extrusion of the ectopic canine. (**e**) Asymmetrical elastics (stronger on the left) necessary to correct the dental midlines as treatment progressed. (**f**) Treatment progress after 31 active aligners. (**g**) Completion of active treatment after 22 months. (**h**) Completion of (I) OPG and (II) lateral cephalogram. (**i**) Intra-oral comparison of (I) before and (II) after treatment. (**j**) Extra-oral profile comparison of (I) before and (II) after treatment

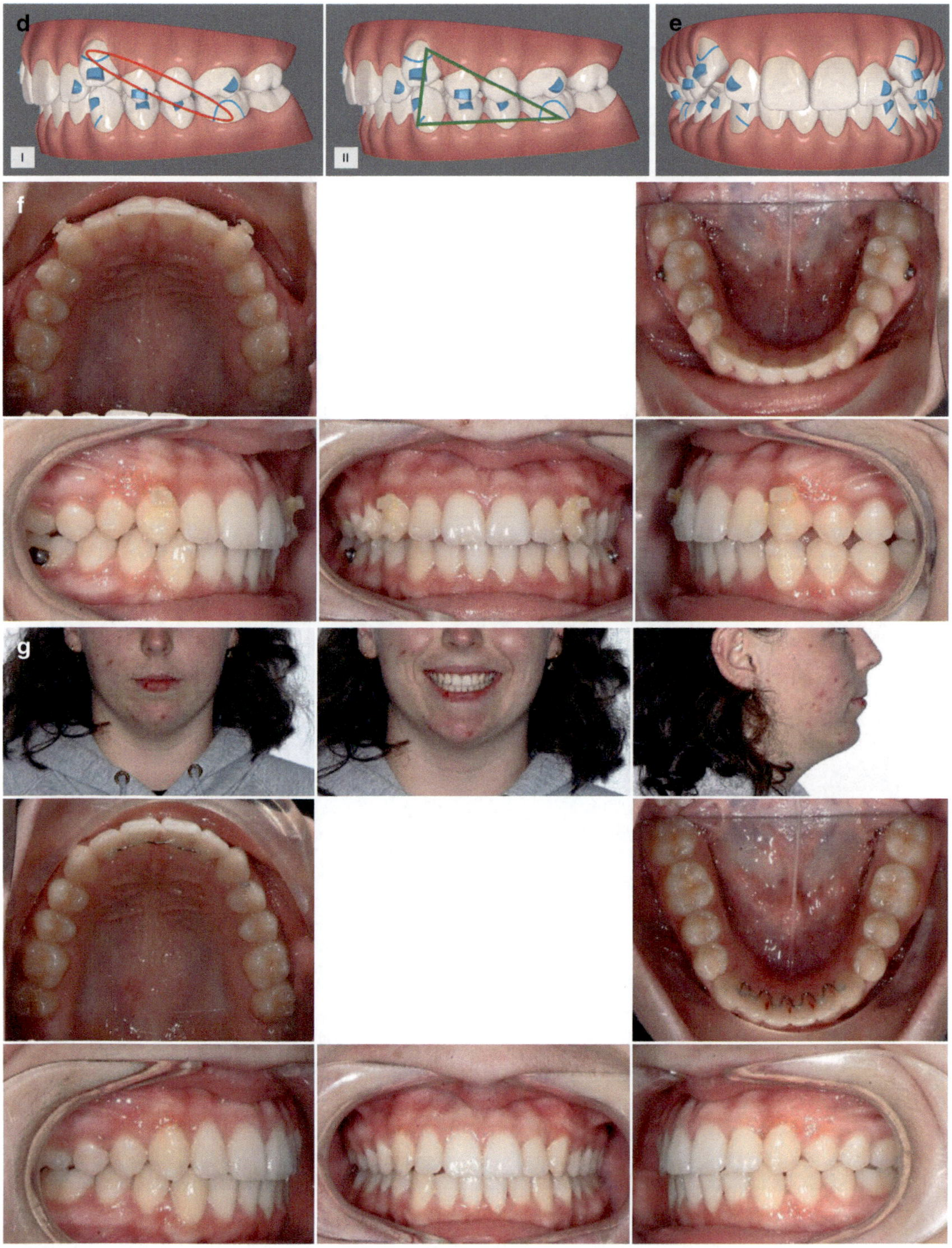

Fig. 8.9 (continued)

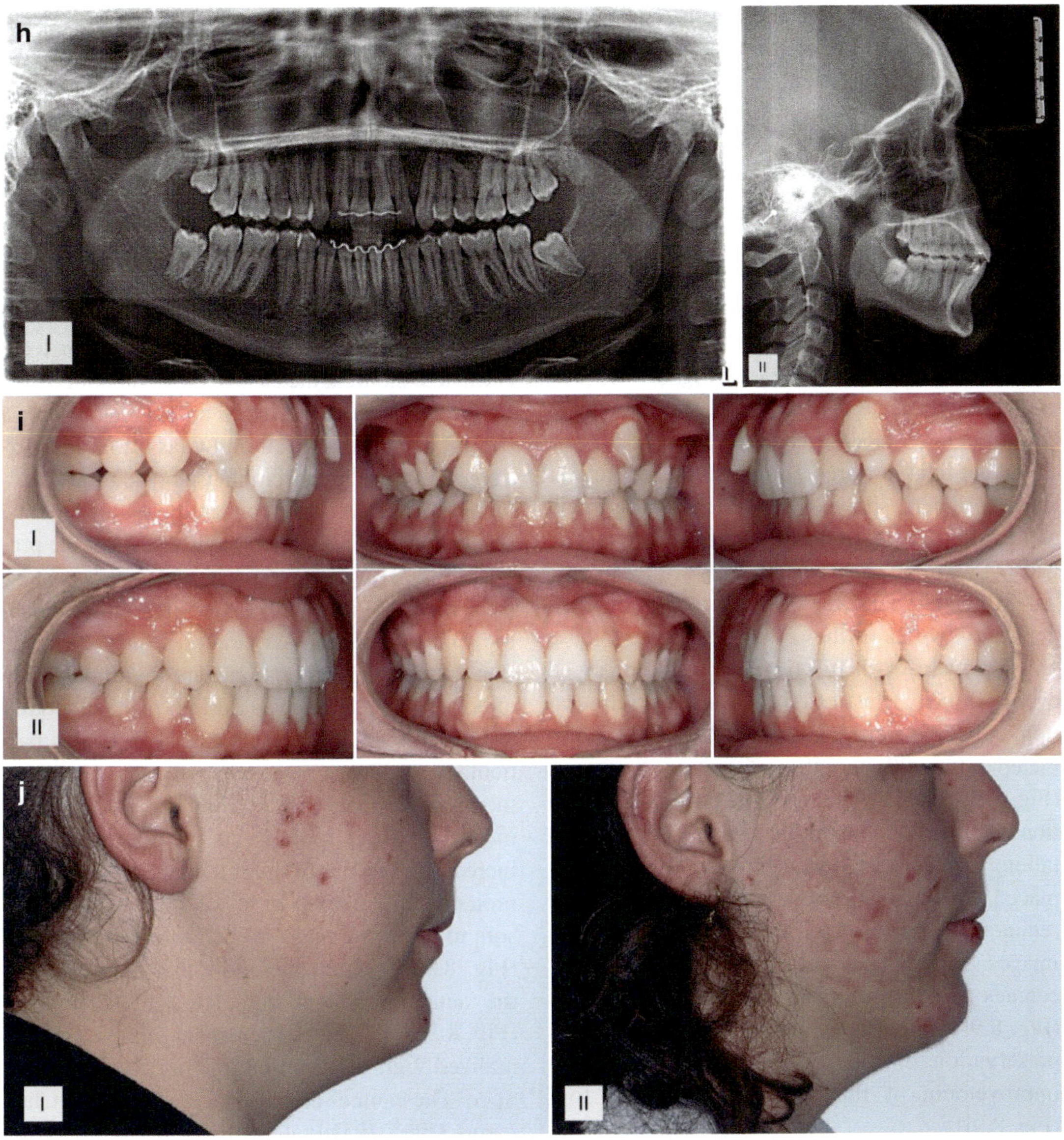

Fig. 8.9 (continued)

on the right, a non-extraction treatment plan was prescribed in order to preserve her dental profile. Even though she was 14.5 years old, her C3 cervical vertebrae showed good growth potential for our intended treatment plans (Fig. 8.9b). Once the overly retained upper right second deciduous molar and upper left deciduous canines have exfoliated, treatment with Invisalign clear aligners commenced.

The typical molar distalization plan in Class II correction utilizes a sequential staging pattern. However, in younger patients, it is possible to exploit the child's growth potential, and plan a simultaneous staging pattern (Fig. 8.9c). This allows a more efficient plan with fewer active aligners required.

The ClinCheck plans showed optimized attachments, button cut outs for elastic wear and "precision" bite ramps on the upper central incisors to support the vertical movements of the anterior teeth. The patient was instructed to change her aligners every 2 weeks, clinical Class

II elastics commenced at the fourth aligner with ¼″ 3.5 oz. strength, worn full time on both sides. The Class II elastics were changed to a triangular Class II configuration during the night and sleeping hours (Fig. 8.9d). This combination of sagittal and vertical vector of elastic forces allowed both the anterior-posterior correction, as well as the providing the guidance for the extrusion of the upper ectopic canines. At the 11th aligner, we increased the strength of the Class II elastics on the left to 3/16″ 3.5 oz. to assist with the dental midline correction (Fig. 8.9e). The elastics on the right side remained the same, with the aligners still being changed every 2 weeks. The treatment progress images taken after 31 active aligners showed good dental alignment and sagittal correction (Fig. 8.9f). The overbite and overjet were reduced significantly. Additional aligners were ordered to complete the correction with a further 21 active aligners, these aligners were worn full time daily and changed every 10 days. Elastics of the similar configuration as before were prescribed. Treatment completed after 22 months of active treatment (Fig. 8.9g, h). The images showed a full correction to Class I canine, molar and dental interdigitation. Upper and lower fixed retainers were placed with night-time wear of vacuum-formed retainers prescribed as well. The comparison images showed the correction of the ectopic canines and re-alignment of the dental midlines (Fig. 8.9i). Side profile comparison showed the preservation of the naso-labial angle and the improvement of the deep labial mental fold (Fig. 8.9j).

Simultaneous staging in growing patients is predictable and should be prescribed routinely. However, the aligners should be changed every 10–14 days. Do not rush to change the aligners as the elastics take time to achieve the sagittal correction. Monitor the sagittal correction and elastic wear very closely and in-person reviews are recommended. Often, unilateral, stronger elastics may be necessary to help correct asymmetrical cases. Consider the vector of forces required for the mechanics and plan the elastic wear and configurations accordingly.

8.5.2 Extraction Therapy

While non-extraction plans are usually indicated to preserve facial profiles, there are cases whereby dental extractions are necessary. An 11-year-old female patient presented with an upper dental protrusion. She had incompetent lips, a Class II div 1 dental malocclusion, a skeletal 1 base with mild dental crowding, a large overjet and a lower lip trap (Fig. 8.10a, b). The treatment plan was to have the upper left and right first premolar teeth extracted and treat the case to a "therapeutic Class II" occlusion finish. This is an occlusion with a Class I canine and a full unit Class II molar relationship. The ClinCheck plans showed the placement of optimized and conventional attachments, "precision cuts" and "button cut outs" for the prescription of Class II elastics and compensatory movements (Fig. 8.10c). Compensatory dental movements are necessary in cases such as extraction therapies in order to negate the tipping side effects of the appliance during planned bodily movements upon space closure [15]. In this particular case, the compensatory movements were: increased upper incisor lingual root torque, increased distal root tip of the upper canines, increased mesial root tip of the upper second premolars and increased intrusion of the lower incisors to allow an anterior open bite were planned (Fig. 8.10d). After one additional aligner order, the active treatment completed in 21 months (Fig. 8.10e, f). The overjet and overbite were normalized with the levelling of the lower curve of Spee. The canines and molars completed in Class I and Class II dental relationships respectively showed good buccal inter-digitation. The lip competency was improved and the OPG radiograph showed good root parallelism.

Aligner therapy in young patients that require extractions has been demonstrated to be a powerful alternative to traditional fixed appliances. With thorough understanding of the patient's biological response to aligner movement, and designing compensatory movements to overcome the shortfall of the aligners in controlling bodily translational movements, it is possible to achieve excellent results.

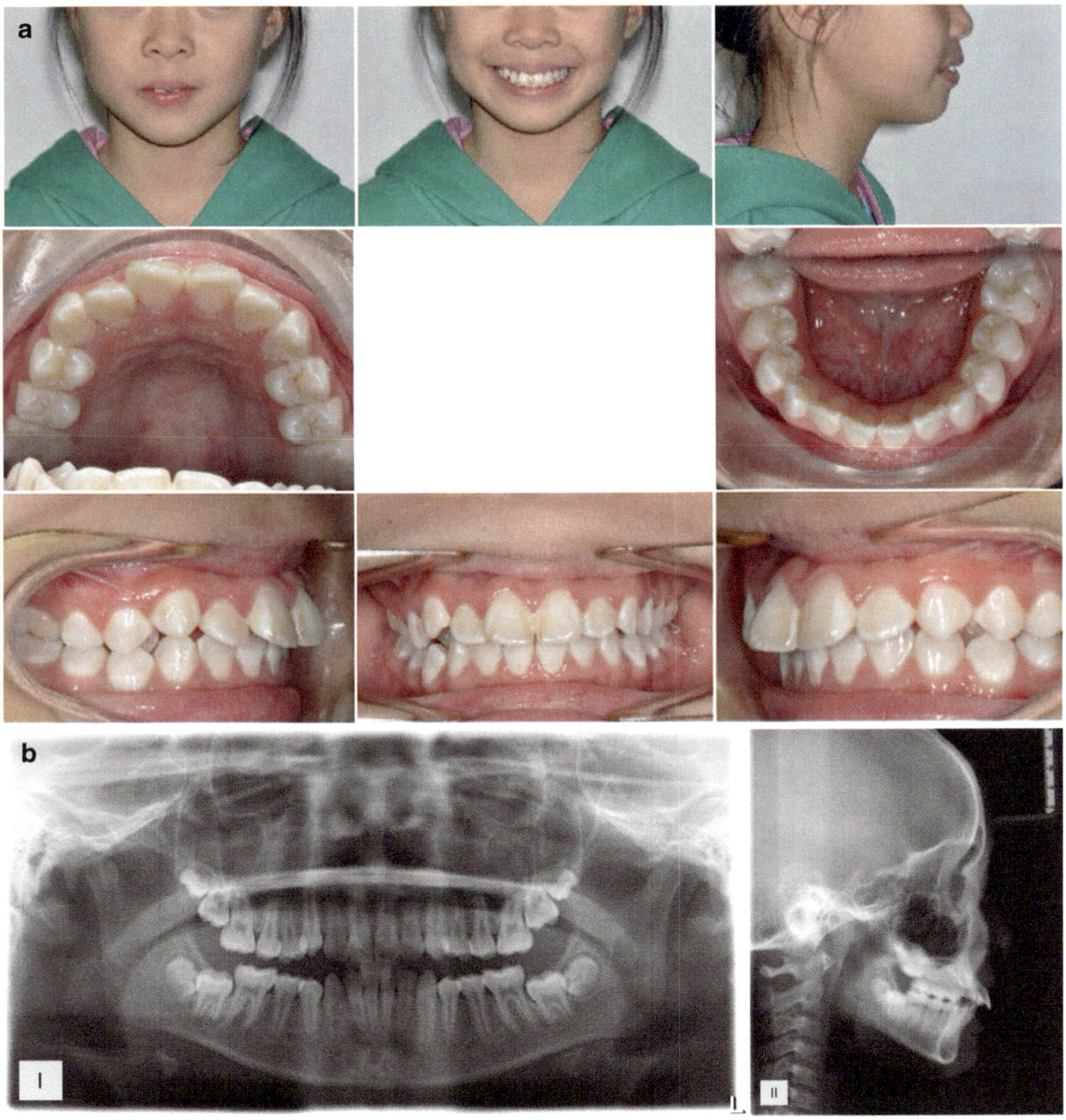

Fig. 8.10 (**a**) 11-year-old female patient presented with an upper dental protrusion and incompetent lips. (**b**) Pre-treatment (I) OPG and (II) lateral cephalogram. (**c**) ClinCheck plans showing attachments, precision cuts and elastic wear designs. (**d**) ClinCheck plans showing compensatory movements. (**e**) Completion of active treatment after 21 months. (**f**) Completion (I) OPG and (II) lateral cephalogram

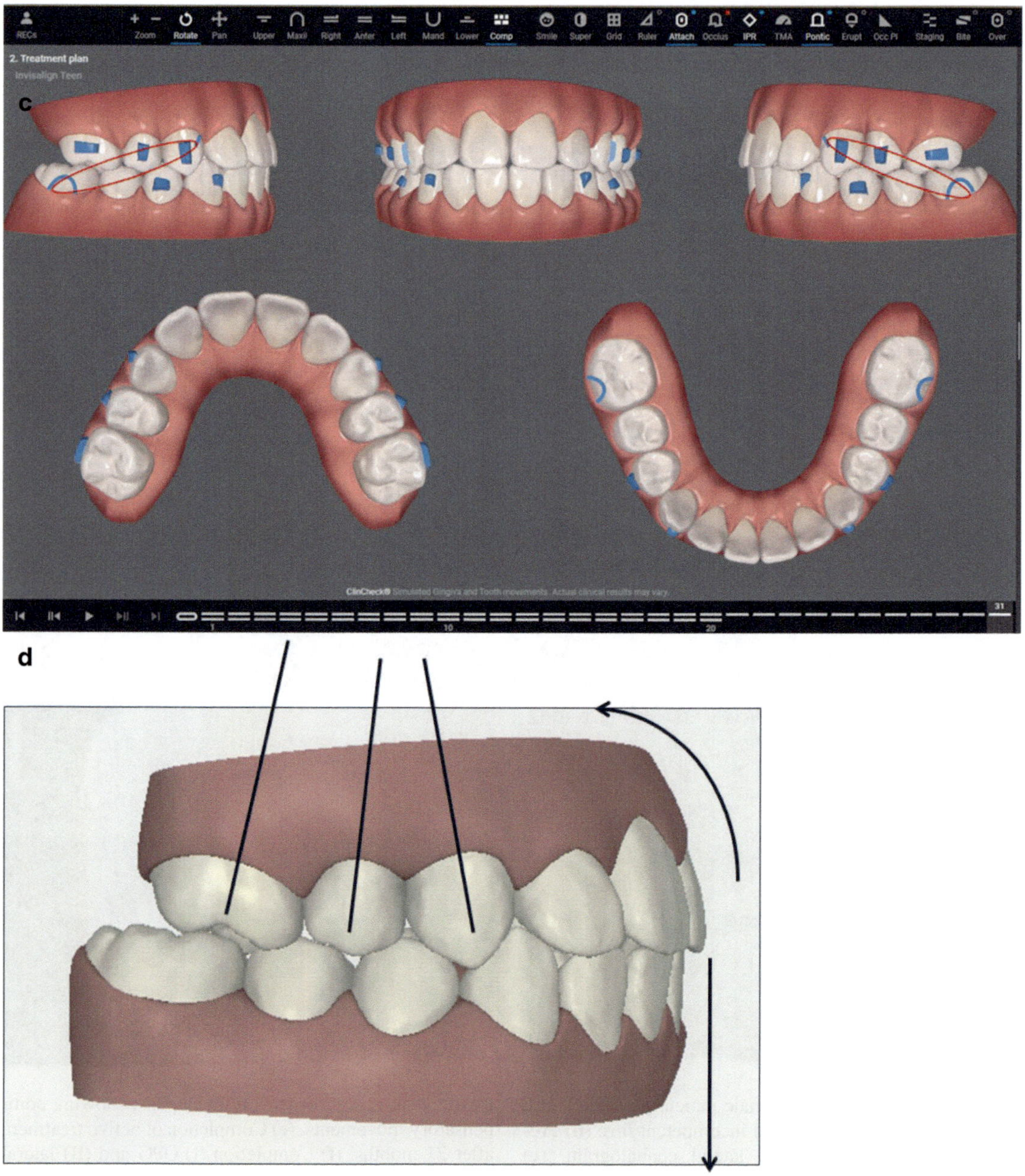

Fig. 8.10 (continued)

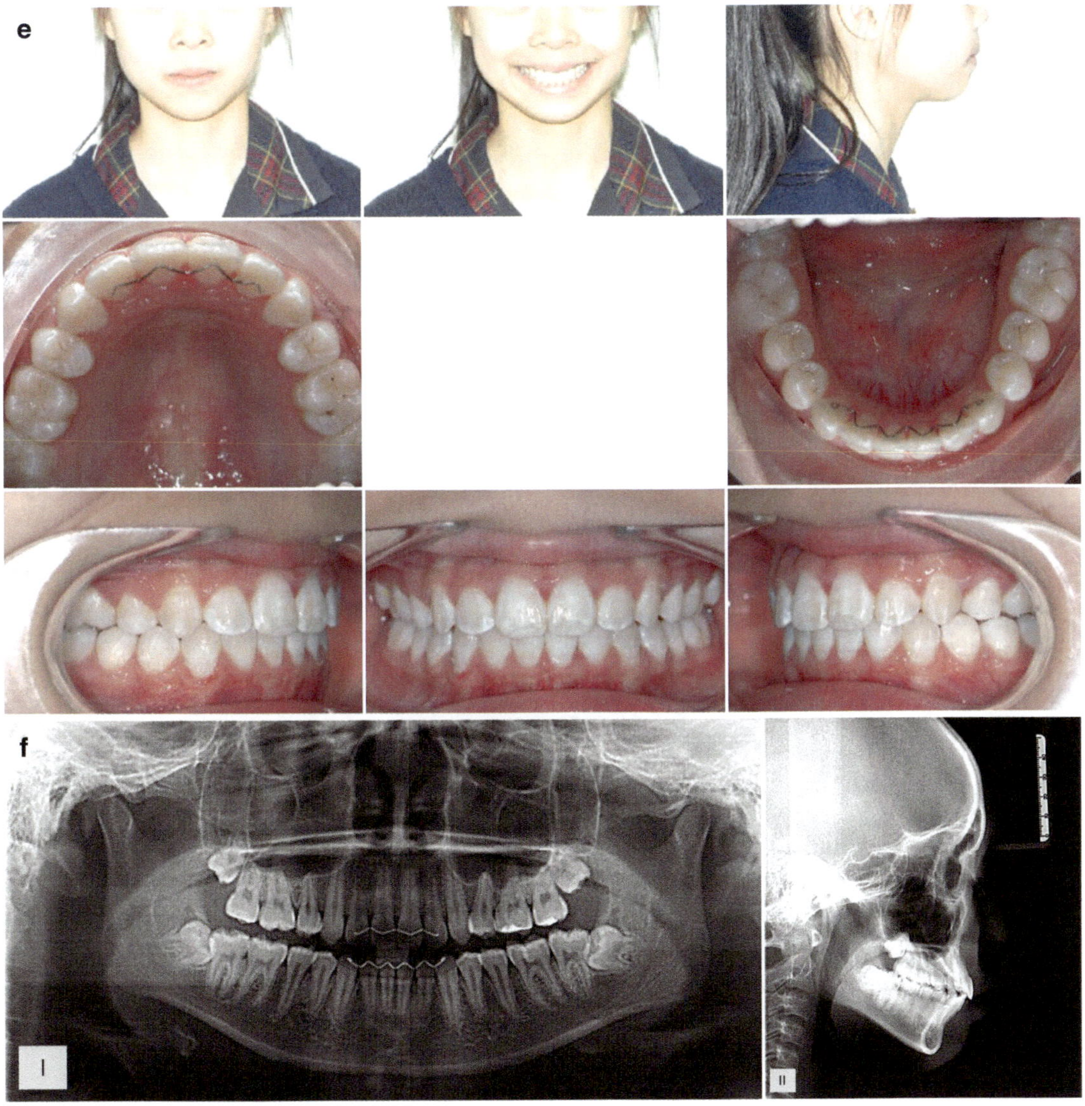

Fig. 8.10 (continued)

8.6 Adult Class II Correction

Class II correction in adults is planned differently primarily due to the lack of their vertical dento-alveolar growth. Non-surgical sagittal correction is mostly achieved with either upper molar distalization or with dental extractions.

8.6.1 Non-extraction Therapy

A female adult patient with upper dental protrusion sought a non-extraction treatment therapy with clear aligners. She presented as a Class II division 1 dental malocclusion on a mild skeletal 2 base with normal to horizontal direction of growth (Fig. 8.11a, b). There was an increased

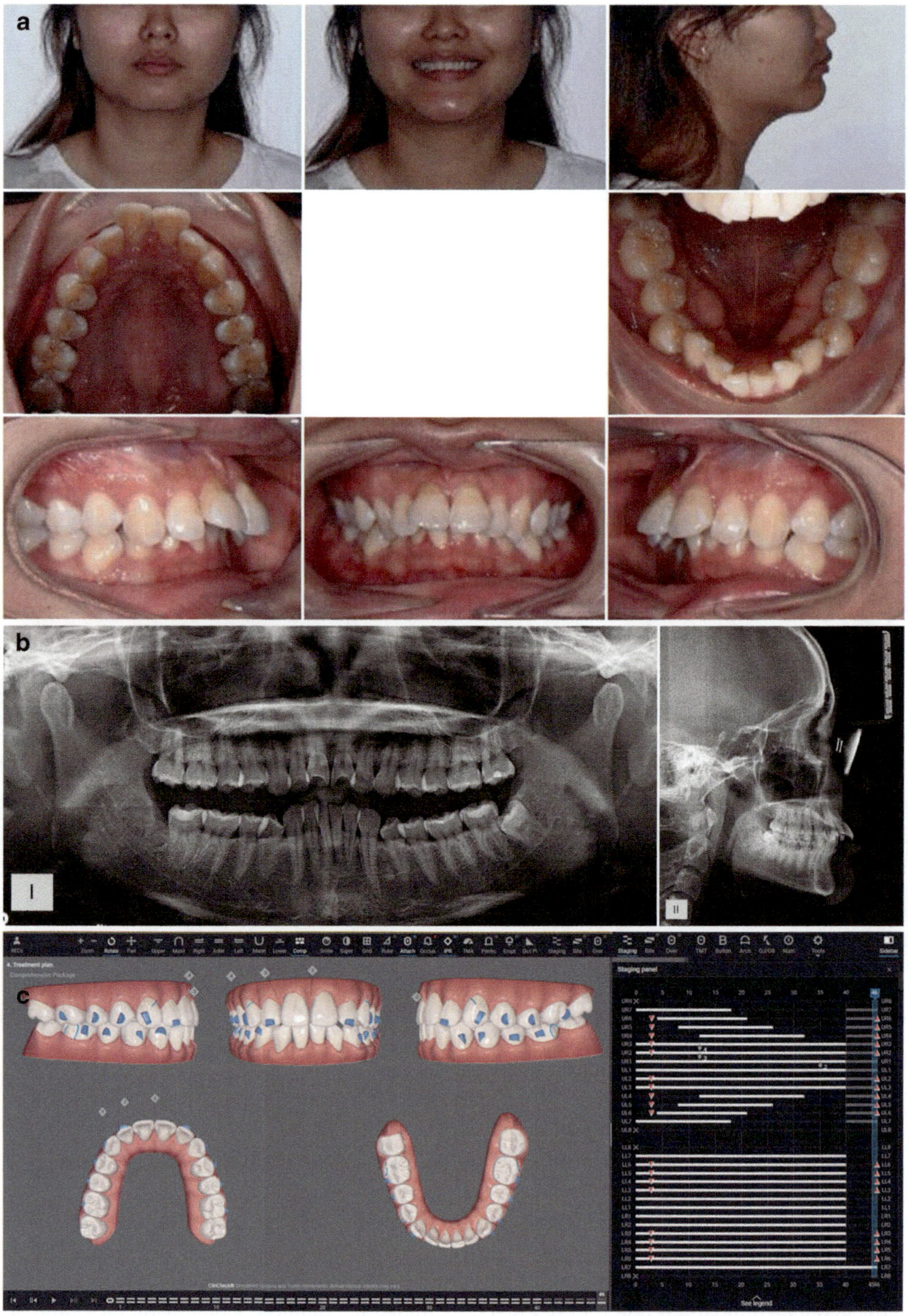

Fig. 8.11 (**a**) Adult female patient with upper dental protrusion sought a non-extraction treatment therapy with clear aligners. (**b**) Pre-treatment (I) OPG and (II) lateral cephalogram. (**c**) ClinCheck plans showing attachments, precision cuts and staging designs. (**d**) Completion of active treatment after 18 months. (**e**) Completion (I) OPG and (II) lateral cephalogram. (**f**) Progress of treatment from (I) initial, (II) additional aligner order to (III) completion (**g**) Extra-oral profile comparison of (I) before and (II) after treatment

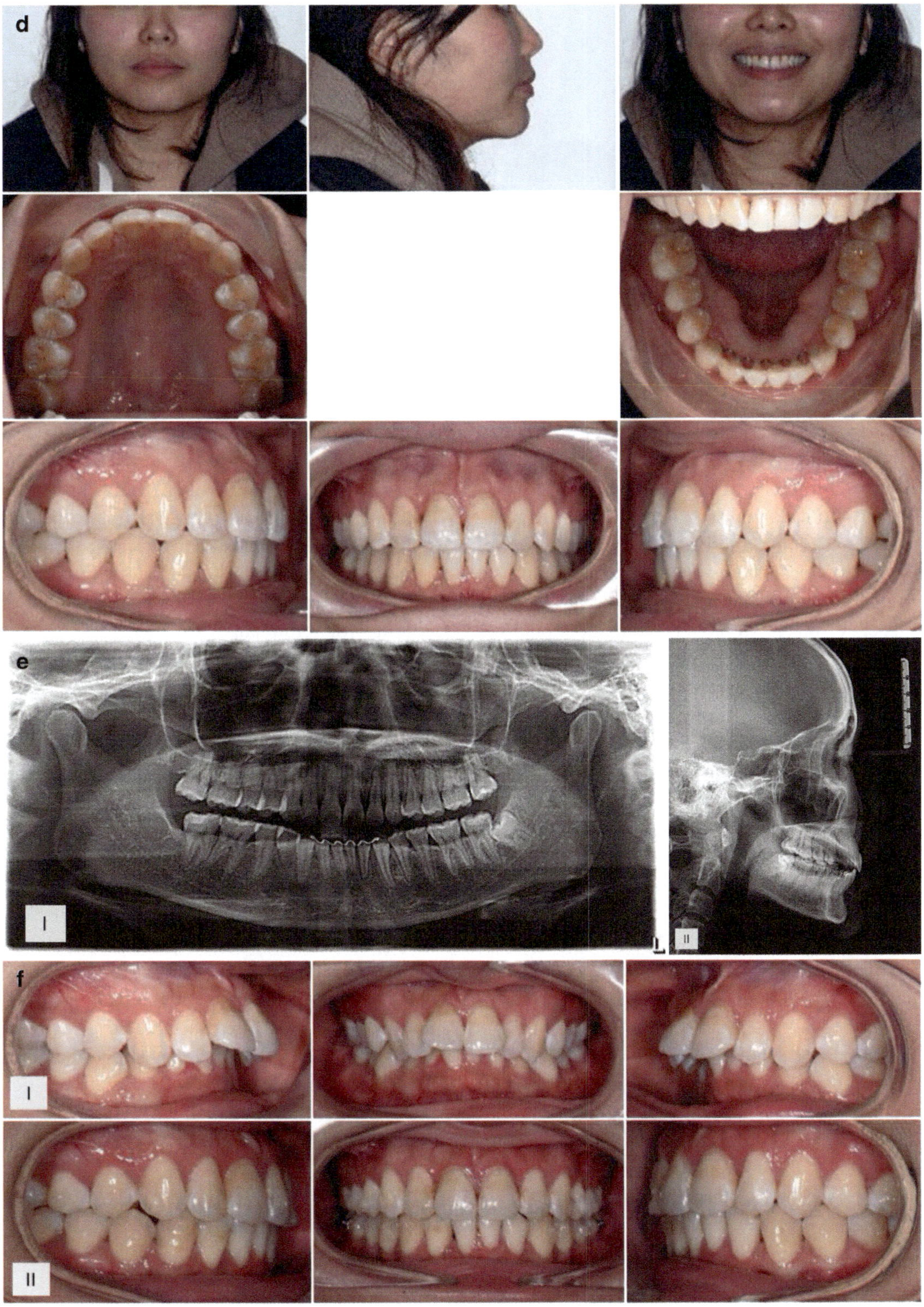

Fig. 8.11 (continued)

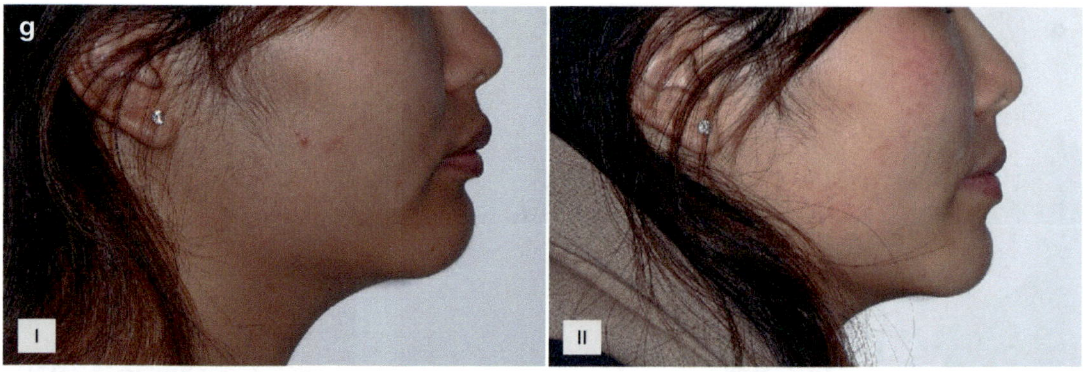

Fig. 8.11 (continued)

dental overjet, a deep overbite with a deep lower curve of Spee, moderate upper and lower dental crowding with rather constricted upper and lower dental archforms.

Sequential staging with upper molar distalization is a common approach to the correction of Class II malocclusions. However, the default set up is often drawn out with upwards of 60 active aligners or more. Moreover, while the molar distalization is occurring, the default set up often does not allow any upper anterior movements. Hence, the patient's chief concerns of misaligned upper front teeth are usually not addressed until the second half of the active treatment. These shortfalls can be managed by re-staging the ClinCheck plans.

(i) During the modification process of the ClinCheck plans, request for an early upper anterior aesthetic start while the upper molars are distalizing. This shows up as an "arrowhead" staging pattern instead of the conventional "v" shape pattern (Fig. 8.11c). This initial upper anterior alignment occurring in concurrent with the upper molar distalization addresses the patient's misalignment concerns early.

(ii) The usual default in sequential molar distalization distalizes the second molar over 8 stages, before the first molar distalizes a further 8 stages. This is then followed by the second premolar and first premolar distalizing 8 stages each respectively. This distalization pattern stretches out the total number of active aligners and may be unrealistically long for clinicians. During modification, request to start the distalization of the second molar from stage 1, the first molars commences distalization from stage 4, the second premolar from stage 8 and so on. This less truncated sequential staging will condense the total number of active aligners to improve both the patient and clinician's experience.

However, with these modifications, early anchorage demand and control needs to be addressed. The use of Class II elastics is paramount in Class II corrections. Start elastic wear as early as stage 4, or immediately after the attachments, buttons and "precision cuts" are placed. The ClinCheck plan in this case showed the placement of attachments and commencement of Class II elastics from stage 4 (Fig. 8.11c). Aligners were changed 2 weekly initially and only with good treatment response and compliance observed, from stage 15 onwards, they were changed every 10 days. The initial strength of Class II elastics used were ¼" 3.5 oz. As treatment progressed, they were increased to 3/16″ 3.5 oz. (from stage 9). The final occlusion shows the complete resolution of the increased overjet, deep overbite and deep lower curve of Spee (Fig. 8.11d, e). Figure 8.11f shows the treatment progress to completion. There was improvement of the facial profile with the slight increase of the lower facial height and shallowing of the deep labial mental fold (Fig. 8.11g). Active treatment was completed in 18 months.

8.6.2 Extraction Therapy

An adult female patient presented with a Class II dental subdivision malocclusion with a skeletal 1 base and normal direction of growth (Fig. 8.12a, b). She had a bimaxillary protrusive profile with incompetent lips. There were moderate degrees of upper and mild degrees of lower dental crowding, upper and lower dental protrusion with a constricted upper dental arch form. There was also a lingual crossbite on the left terminal molars. The canine and molar relationships were Class II ½ unit and Class I on the right and left respectively. The patient's oral hygiene was not good and she was sent away for a few months of careful dental debridement and oral hygiene care before commencement of her orthodontic treatment.

The extraction of four premolars was indicated. On the right, the Class II ½ unit side, teeth #14 and #45, while on the left, the Class I side, teeth #24 and #34 were extracted. The ClinCheck plans showed a simultaneous staging pattern, the indicated teeth may be extracted right at the beginning of the treatment or within the first 2–4 aligners depending on clinical preferences. Conventional attachments and "precision cuts" were placed at stage 4 (Fig. 8.12c). Compensatory dental movements are necessary in cases such as extraction therapies in order to negate the tipping side effects of the appliance during planned bodily movements upon space closure [13]. In this particular case, increased upper incisor lingual root torque, increased distal root tip of the upper canines, increased mesial root tip of the distal abutment premolars and molars from the extraction spaces and increased intrusion of the lower incisors to allow an anterior open bite were planned (Fig. 8.12d). The aligners were worn full time with a 2-weekly change regime. Class II elastics were worn from precision hooks on the upper canines to bonded buttons on the lower first molars commenced from stage 4 as well. The initial elastics used were ¼″ 3.5 oz. this was further increased to 3/16″ 3.5 oz. after approximately 6 months (stage 12). The biological response and patient compliance was exemplary and at approximately 12 months into treatment (stage 27) the aligners were changed every 10 days. There were 44 active aligners in the first stage of treatment (Fig. 8.12e), followed by an additional aligner order of 13 more aligners (10 days change). Treatment was completed in 23 months with good bilateral Class I interdigitation, normalized overjet and overbite with good facial profile and lip changes (Fig. 8.12f, g). Upper and lower fixed retainers were placed to be worn concurrently with night-time vacuum-formed retainers.

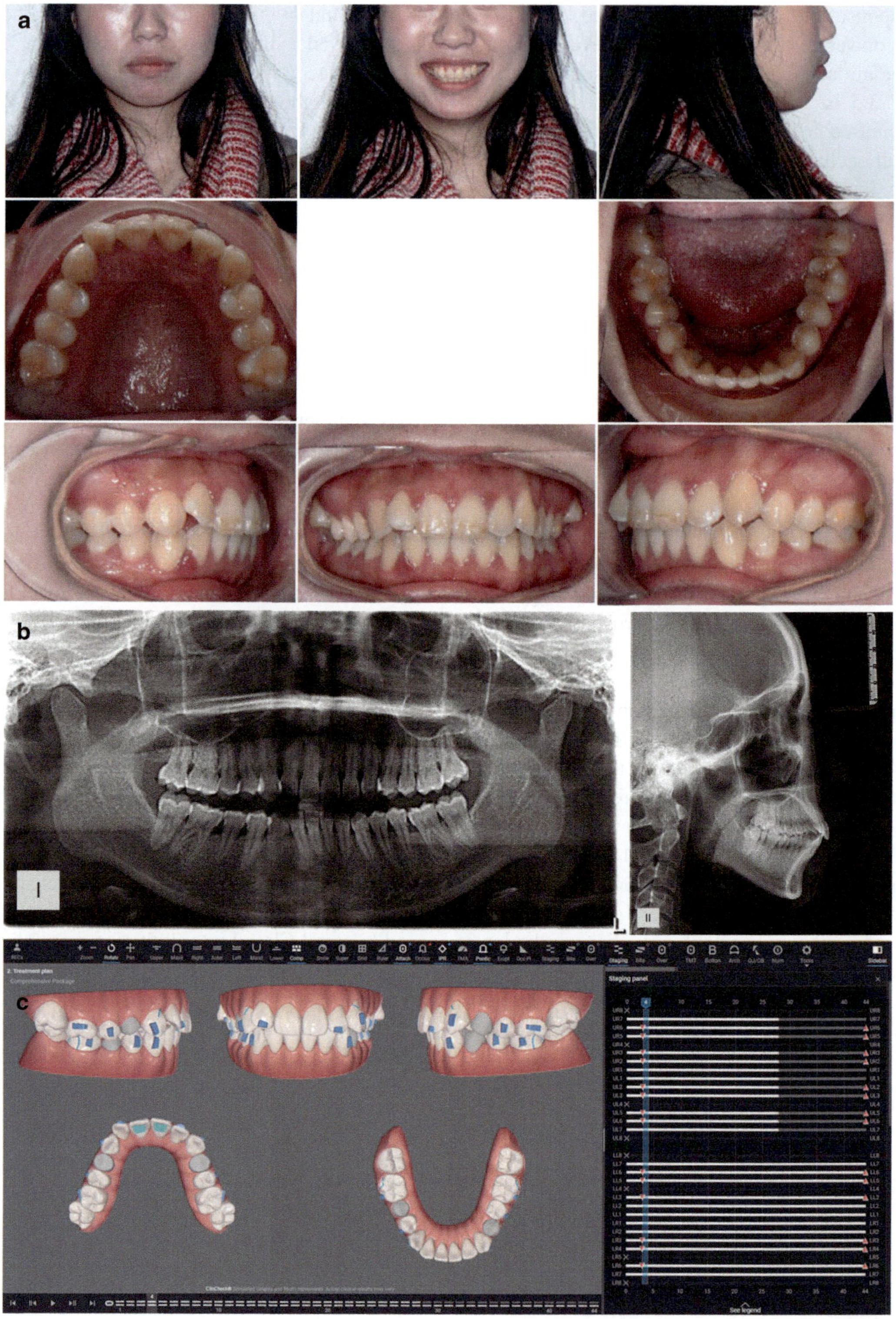

Fig. 8.12 (**a**) Adult female patient with dental crowding and protrusion. (**b**) Pre-treatment (I) OPG and (II) lateral cephalogram. (**c**) ClinCheck plans showing attachments, precision cuts and staging designs. (**d**) ClinCheck plans showing compensatory movements. (**e**) Treatment progress after 44 active aligners. (**f**) Completion of active treatment after 23 months. (**g**) Completion (I) OPG and (II) lateral cephalogram

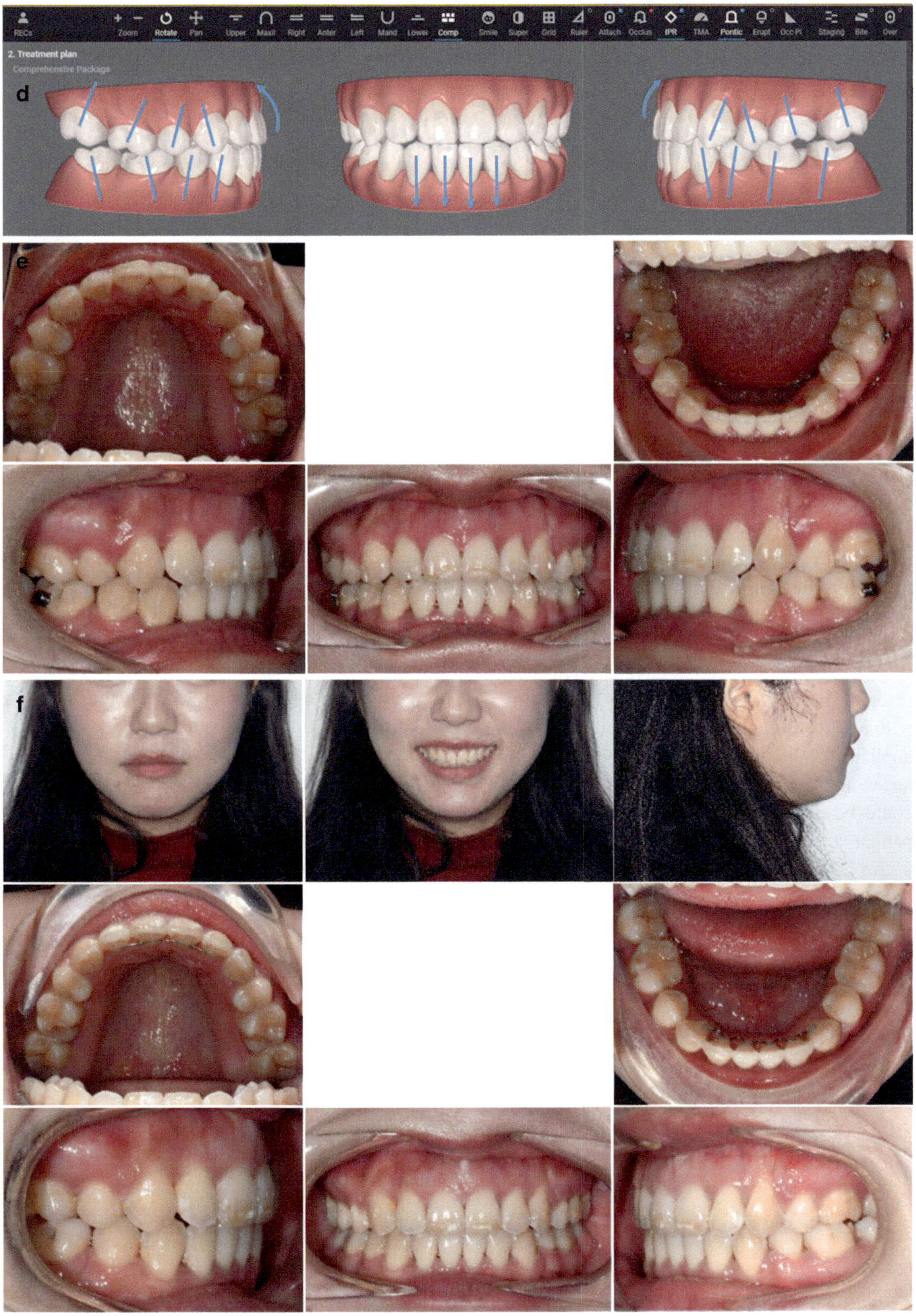

Fig. 8.12 (continued)

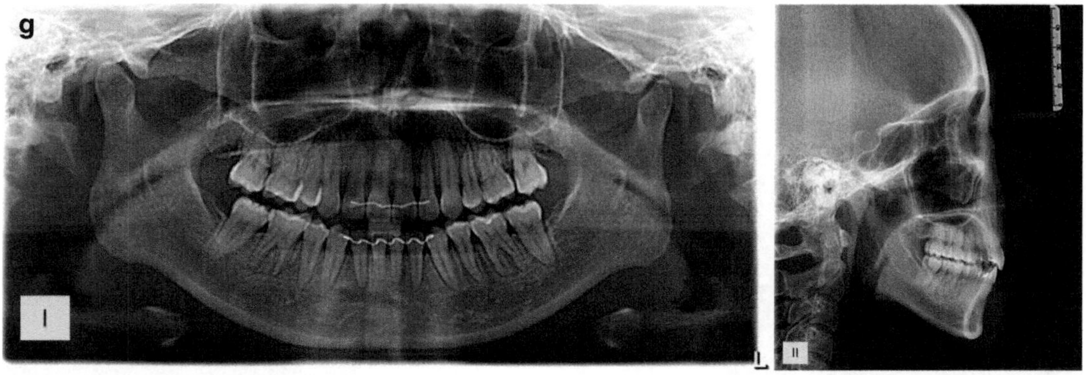

Fig. 8.12 (continued)

8.7 Surgery

Conventionally, orthognathic surgery planned in conjunction with traditional orthodontics required fixed appliances to help with the fixation of the surgical splints during surgery and stabilization after surgery. However, there are advantages for patients undergoing orthognathic surgery without the need to have fixed appliances placed. The digital planning could be seamless, with no transition and re-adaptation to a different appliance. Without the presence of fixed appliances and surgical wire fixations, oral hygiene could be much better managed. This promotes patient comfort and optimizes wound healing.

An adult male patient presented with a deep dental overbite and a recessive chin (Fig. 8.13a, b). He was concerned with his retrognathic mandible and would like to seek orthodontic treatment incorporating orthognathic surgery. There was a deep dental overbite, retroclined upper incisors, rather constricted archforms with mild to moderate upper and lower dental crowding. The lower dental midline was deviated to the right. Decompensation pre-surgical orthodontics was performed with clear aligners for approximately 14 months (Fig. 8.13c). Once the arches were ready for surgery, buttons were bonded on the upper and lower, left and right canines and first molars with corresponding "precision button cut-outs" placed in the aligners (Fig. 8.13d). The orthognathic surgical movements performed were maxillary posterior impaction, asymmetrical mandibular BSSO advancement, and an advancement genioplasty. Without the need to have fixed appliances placed during the orthognathic surgical procedure, oral hygiene was immaculately maintained (Fig. 8.13e). Once the patient had regained full jaw movements, additional aligners were ordered to detail and complete the treatment. The completed images showed a balanced and harmonious facial change. The deep dental overbite, dental crowding, deviated midlines, recessive mandible and chin were normalized (Fig. 8.13f–h). Fixed and night-time removable retainers were prescribed to retain the orthodontic correction.

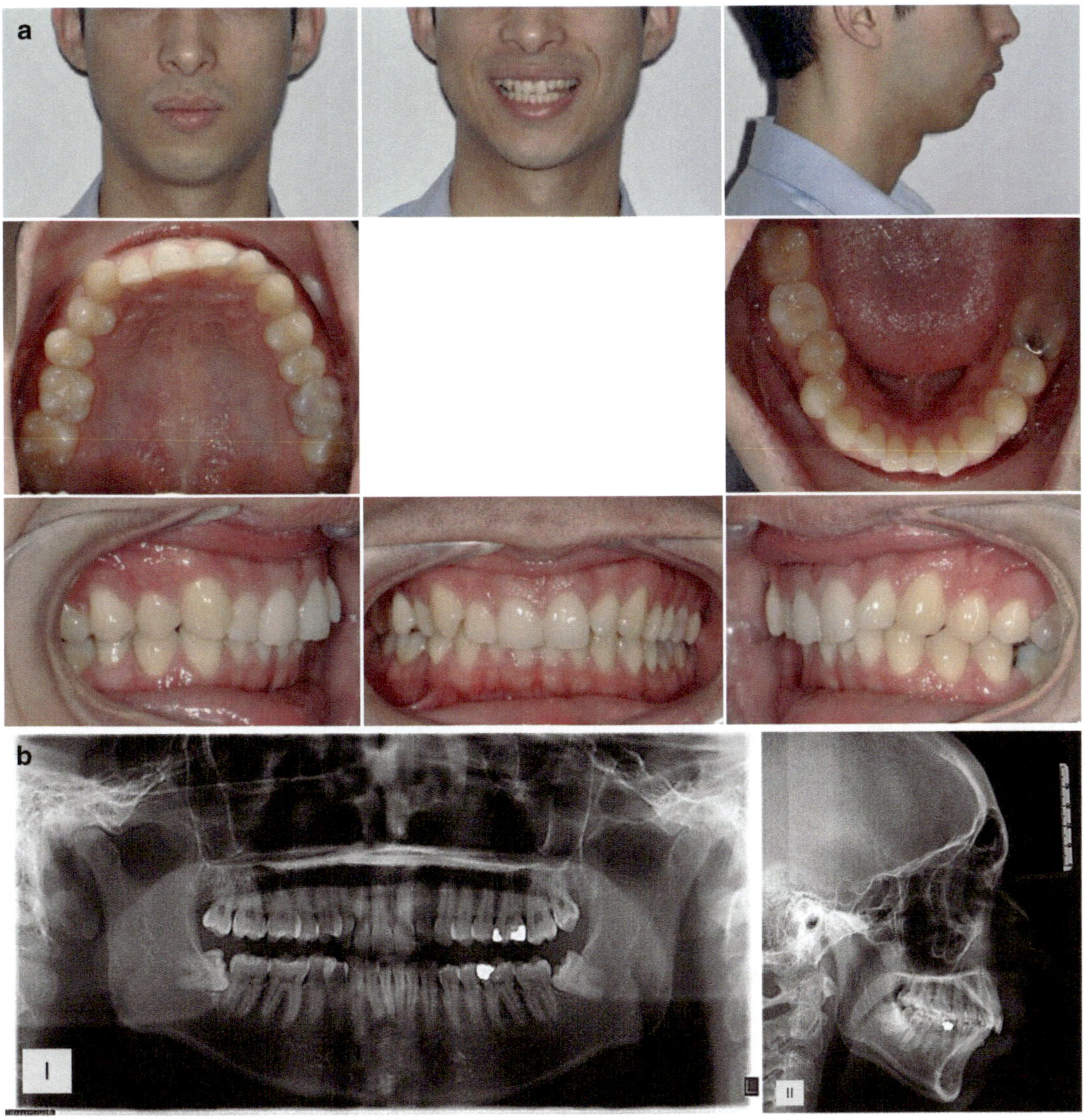

Fig. 8.13 (**a**) Adult male patient with a deep dental overbite and a recessive chin. (**b**) Pre-treatment (I) OPG and (II) lateral cephalogram. (**c**) ClinCheck plans showing attachments and precision cut designs. (**d**) Treatment progress after 14 months. The pre-surgical movements are complete. (**e**) (I) Extra and (II) intra-oral photos at 3 weeks post orthognathic surgery. (**f**) Post-surgery (I) OPG and (II) lateral cephalogram. (**g**) Completion of active treatment. (**h**) Extra-oral profile and lateral cephalogram comparison of (I) before and (II) after treatment

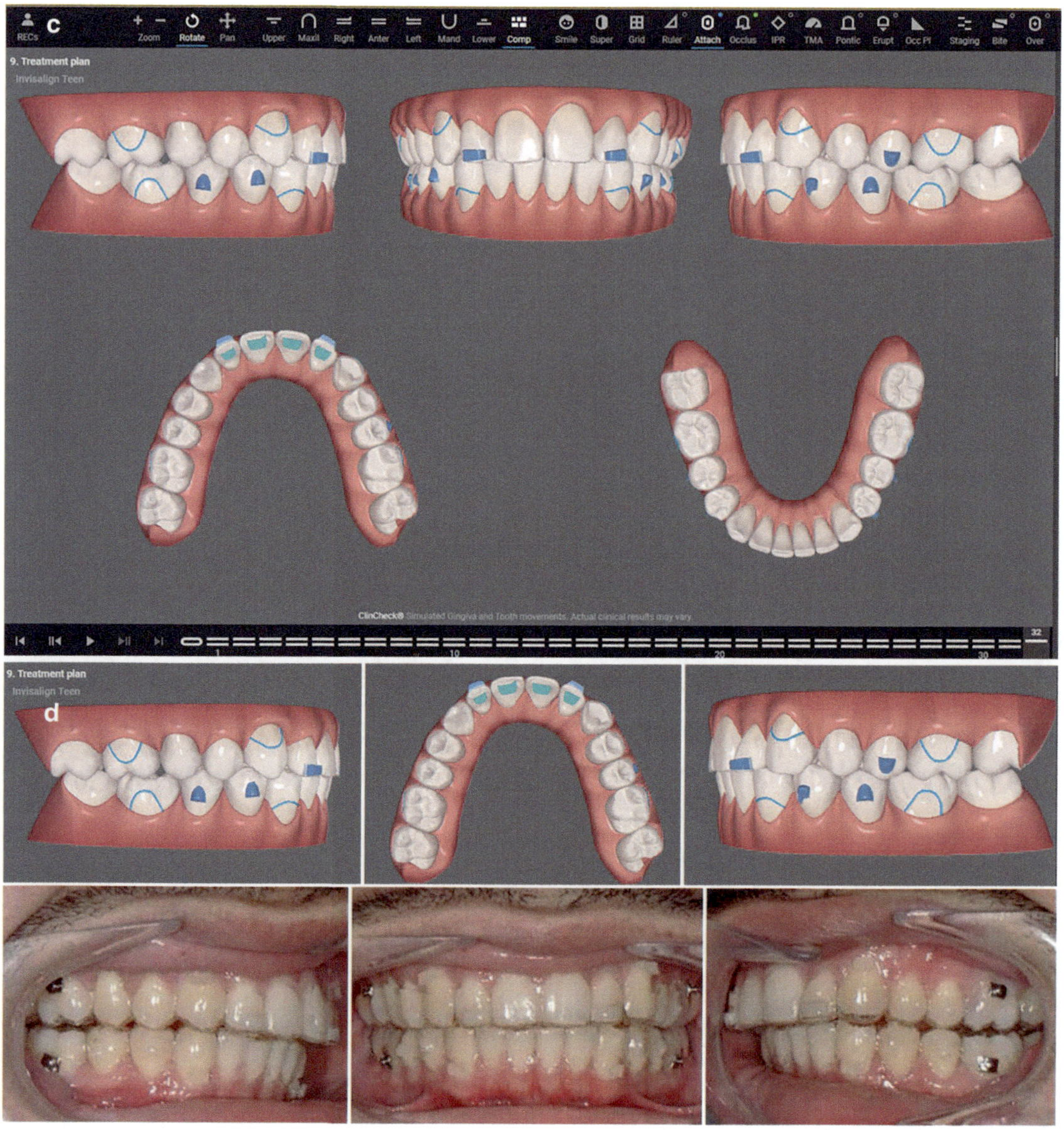

Fig. 8.13 (continued)

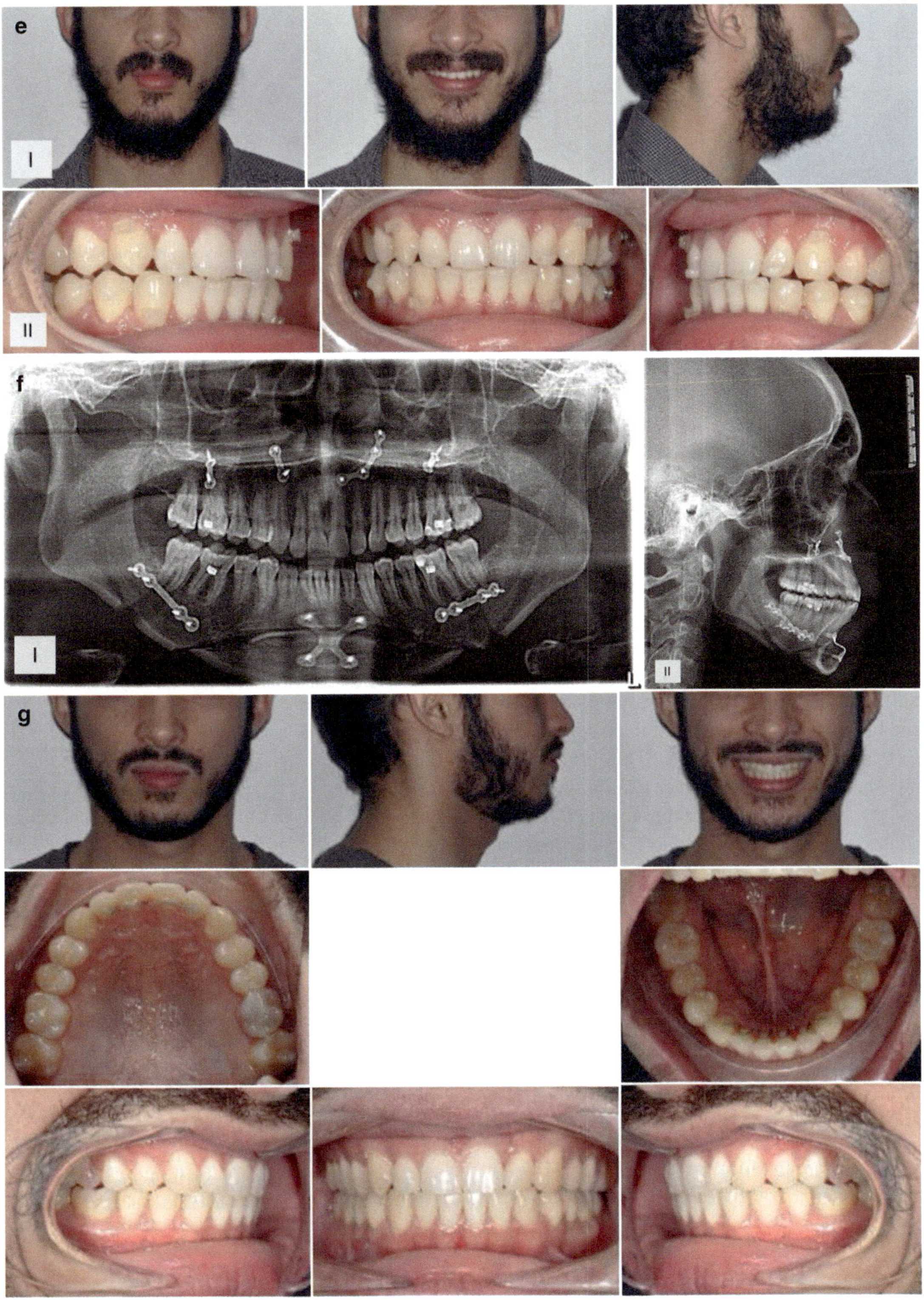

Fig. 8.13 (continued)

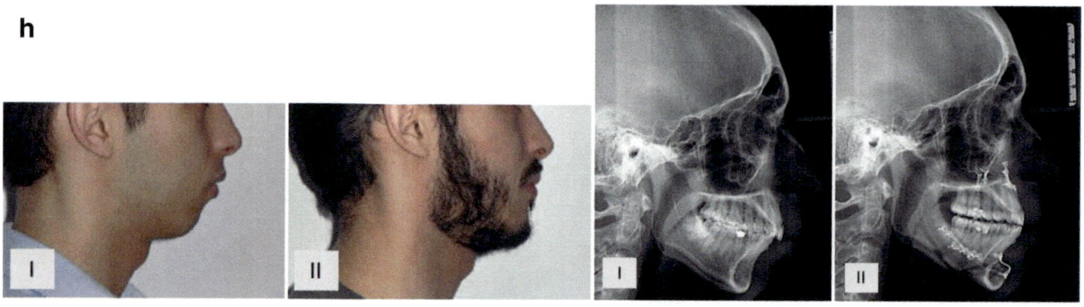

Fig. 8.13 (continued)

8.8 Conclusions

A Class II malocclusion has a variety of different aetiologies and may present with different morphologies. The skeletal and dental influences, coupled with maxillary and/or mandibular contributions and age-related treatment responses, further complicate treatment plans and their executions.

Using clear aligners to treat complex comprehensive orthodontic cases is still relatively new. Shifting the mindset and applying knowledge and biomechanics learnt from fixed appliances to clear aligners requires time. This brief chapter introduces what clear aligner can do with dental and skeletal Class II correction under different contexts and conditions. Incorporating the clinician's knowledge, embracing digital technology in orthodontics and with cooperative subjects, treatment with clear aligners in complex comprehensive Class II cases can eventuate with excellent results.

References

1. Harris EF. Effects of patient age and sex on treatment: correction of class II malocclusion with the Begg technique. Angle Orthod. 2001;71(6):433–41.
2. Brodie A. On the growth of the jaws and the eruption of the teeth. Angle Orthod. 1942;12:109–23.
3. Mellion ZJ, Behrents RG, Johnston LE Jr. The pattern of facial skeletal growth and its relationship to various common indexes of maturation. Am J Orthod Dentofacial Orthop. 2013;143:845–54.
4. Perinetti G, Contardo L. Reliability of growth indicators and efficiency of functional reatment for skeletal class II malocclusion: current evidence and controversies. Biomed Res Int. 2017;1367691
5. Tulloch JFC, Lenz BE, Phillips C. Surgical versus orthodontic correction for class II patients: age and severity in treatment planning and treatment outcome. Semin Orthod. 1999;5(4):231–40.
6. Linder-Aronson S, Woodside DG, Daigle DJ. A longitudinal study of the growth in length of the maxilla in boys between ages 6-20 years. Trans Eur Orthod Soc. 1975:169–79.
7. Baccetti T, Lorenzo F, Toth LR, McNamara JA Jr. Treatment timing for twin-block therapy. Am J Orthod Dentofacial Orthop. 2000;118(2):159–70.
8. Dugoni SA, Lee J. Early mixed dentition treatment: post-retention evaluation of stability and relapse. Angle Orthod. 1995;65:311–9.
9. Janson G, Barros SEC, Simão TM, Freitas MR. Relevant variables of class II malocclusion treatment. Rev Dental Press Ortod Ortop Facia. 2009;14:149–57.
10. Tadic N, Woods M. Contemporary class II orthodontic and orthopaedic treatment: a review. Aust Dent J. 2007;52:168–74.
11. Hassel B, Farman AG. Skeletal maturation evaluation using cervical vertebrae. Am J Orthod Dentofacial Orthop. 1995;107:58–66.
12. Hagg U, Rabie AB, Bendeus M, Wong RWK, Wey MC, Du X, Peng J. Condylar growth and mandibular positioning with stepwise vs maximum advancement. Am J Orthod Dentofacial Orthop. 2008;134:525–36.
13. King GJ, Keeling SD, Hocevar RA, Wheeler TT. The timing for class II malocclusions in children: a literature review. Angle Orthod. 1990;60(2):87–97.
14. Tulloch JFC, Phillips C, Koch G, Proffit WR. The effect of early intervention on skeletal pattern in class II malocclusion: a randomized clinical trial. Am J Orthod Dentofacial Orthop. 1997;111:391–400.
15. Chan E, Darendliler MA. The invisalign appliance today: a thinking person's orthodontic appliance. Semin Orthod. 2017;23:12–64.

Class II Division 2 Malocclusion

9

Zamri Radzi, Siti Adibah Othman, and Mang Chek Wey

9.1 Introduction

Class II division 2 malocclusions are described as having excessive lingual inclination of the maxillary central incisors, often overlapped on the labial by the maxillary lateral incisors and accompanied by a deep overbite and minimal overjet. Class II division 2 malocclusion is reported to be present in about 10% of children in the UK. Its prevalence is between 5% and 12% in other European populations with slightly less in the USA, which is between 3% and 4%.

In cases with extreme overbite, the lower incisor edges may contact the soft tissues of the palate. In a few Class II division 2 cases, the mandibular labial gingival tissues may be also traumatized by the lingually inclined maxillary incisors, particularly in the absence of an overjet.

A Class II division 2 incisor relationship is defined by the British Standards classification as being present when the lower incisor edges occlude posterior to the cingulum plateau of the upper incisors and where the upper central incisors are retroclined. The overjet is usually minimal but may be increased [1].

Z. Radzi · S. A. Othman · M. C. Wey (✉)
Faculty of Dentistry, Department of Paediatric Dentistry and Orthodontics, Universiti Malaya, Kuala Lumpur, Malaysia
e-mail: zamrir@um.edu.my; sitiadibah@um.edu.my; weymc@um.edu.my

9.2 Aetiology

The aetiological basis of Class II division 2 malocclusion can be considered in terms of the skeletal pattern, dentoalveolar and soft tissue features.

9.2.1 Skeletal Pattern and Facial Growth

Growth of the skeletal craniofacial complex involves an increase in the absolute size of the various bones as well as changes in their position and form. Class II division 2 malocclusion is commonly associated with a Class II skeletal pattern; however, it may also occur in association with a Class I or even a Class III skeletal base. The vertical dimension is also important, and typically is reduced. When comparing Class II division 2 and Class I and Class II division 1 individuals, the posterior cranial base is often larger in Class II division 2 cases. The low gonial angle giving rise to a square facial profile is commonly due to the forward rotational pattern of the mandible.

The presence of a strong hereditary component is apparent from an examination of families of individuals who tend to have similar facial features. A study on identical twins demonstrated 100% concordance for Class II division 2 malocclusion, indicating a strong genetic influence,

M. T. Cobourne (ed.), *Orthodontic Management of Class II Malocclusion*,
https://doi.org/10.1007/978-3-031-57530-3_9

autosomal dominant with incomplete penetrance or polygenic model in the development of Class II division 2 deep-bite malocclusions.

9.2.2 Dentoalveolar

The upper anterior dentition is thought to play an important role in the development of Class II division 2 malocclusion. A study on the upper incisors of Class II division 2 subjects showed that retroclination starts prior to emergence, continued during emergence, and then for several years thereafter [2]. The more upright position of the upper incisors among division 2 subjects allows the mandible to over rotate. There is a negative relationship between upper incisor angulation and lip height, with greater coverage associated with greater incisor retroclination. Patients with Class II division 2 malocclusion have higher lower lip line, with resting lip pressures greater in the incisal areas and less in the cervical areas which be a causal factor in determining the axial position of the incisors. In addition, a retroclination of the upper incisors is frequently associated with an abnormal crown-root angle.

9.2.3 Soft Tissues

The influence of the soft tissues in Class II division 2 malocclusions is usually secondary to discrepancy in the skeletal pattern. If the lower facial height is reduced, the lower lip line will effectively be higher relative to the crown of the upper incisors. A special lip morphology and behaviour as well as a high resting lower lip line will tend to retrocline the upper incisors giving the appearance of marked labio-mental groove beneath the lower lip. It has also been suggested that the lips act as a local genetic factor in Class II division 2 malocclusion and that maxillary incisor retroclination results from excessive non-physiological pressure between the lips and teeth. The activity shown in perioral electromyography indicated that the local epigenetic factors had an important role in the development of imbalanced vertical relationship between the lips and the maxillary anterior dentoalveolar structures.

Class II division 2 also features high masseteric muscle forces where fibre-type properties are very closely associated with variations in vertical growth of the face. Biting forces with strong musculature have been reported to be higher in Class II division 2 patients with reduced lower facial height. The presence of strong masticatory muscle pattern in Class II division 2 cases could have been explained by the genetically determined muscular and neuromuscular system.

9.3 Features

9.3.1 Extraoral

Due to an anterior or anticlockwise growth rotation of the mandible, a patient with Class II division 2 malocclusion may present with a straight or convex lateral profile (Fig. 9.1). The chin may even appear pronounced with greater mandibular rotation, and this may present as a mildly concave lateral profile. At the same time, with the upward mandibular growth rotation pattern, the patient may present with a decreased or almost average vertical facial proportion [3]. All these extraoral features combined with a flat mandibular plane fit into a brachycephalic facial pattern. Along with an acute angle of the mandible, this may result in a more 'squarish' shape of the face (Fig. 9.1). The forward mandibular growth rotation may also cause an over-closed soft tissue appearance, with reduced lip thickness and deep labiomental fold. The lips may appear retrusive relative to a prominent chin from an anteriorly rotated mandible. Should the lower lip get trapped behind the palatal surface of the upper lateral incisors, the subsequently proclined lateral incisors may cause lip incompetence at rest.

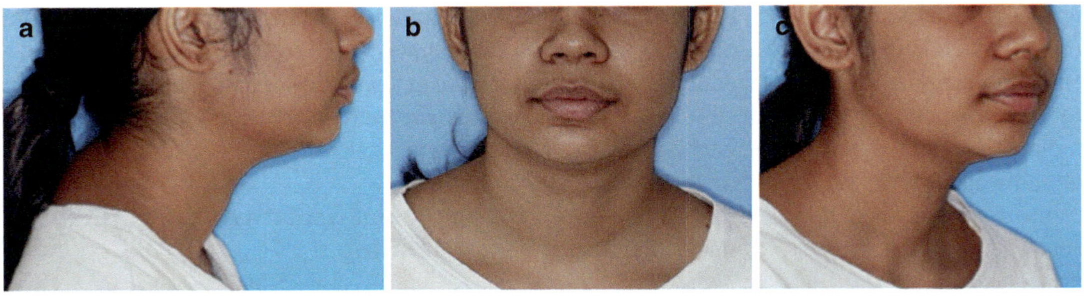

Fig. 9.1 (**a**) Convex lateral facial profile with decreased gonial angle, flat mandibular plane, and prominent labiomental fold; (**b**) Squarish brachycephalic face shape; (**c**) Decreased gonial angle, flat mandibular plane and prominent labiomental fold. *(Pictures courtesy of Dr Pang Yee Rui)*

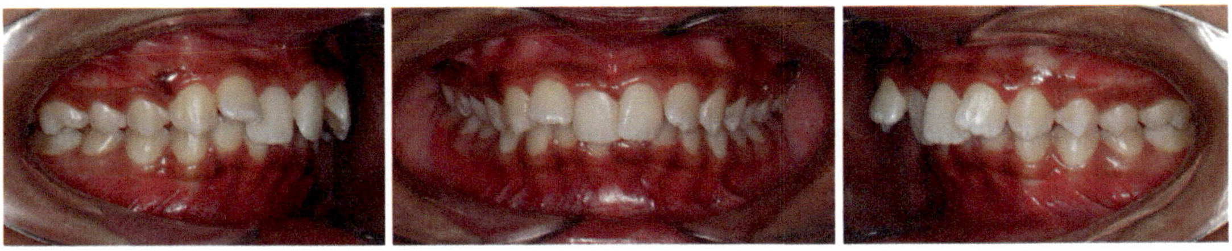

Fig. 9.2 Retroclined upper central incisors, proclined upper lateral incisors, increased overbite, Class II canine and molar relationships. (*Pictures courtesy of Dr Pang Yee Rui)*

9.3.2 Intraoral

In the permanent dentition, the lower incisor edges occlude posterior to the cingulum plateau of the upper incisors [1]. The overjet may be reduced, average or increased, depending on the severity of the sagittal skeletal discrepancy combined with retroclination of incisors.

The upper labial segment is often retroclined, especially the central incisors (Fig. 9.2). Along with the upward mandibular rotation, the lower lip level may cover the labial surface of the upper incisors [3], exerting a palatally directed force on the labial incisor surface during function. The lateral incisors, however, may be proclined due to their more superior position, above the level of the lower lip. If the lower lip gets trapped behind the palatal surface of the upper lateral incisors, this will then exert a labially directed pushing force on the lateral incisors, resulting in their proclination. As for the lower incisors, the lower labial segment rotates upwards and backwards with the anticlockwise rotation of the mandible, to appear retroclined.

The overbite is usually increased [4] with over-eruption of the anterior segments, resulting from a lack of occlusal stop on the palatal surface of the retroclined upper incisors. This may present with increased gingival show and gummy smile, and increased curve of Spee in the lower arch. There may be attrition of palatal surfaces of upper incisors, resulting in the loss of the cingulum shape and decreased labio-palatal crown width. A severely increased overbite can result in traumatic palatal gingival stripping of the upper incisors and labial gingival stripping of the lower incisors.

Bimaxillary retroclination of both upper and lower labial segments will result in various degrees of upper arch and lower arch crowding. The interincisal angle is also increased [3, 4], and this may present as flattened anterior segments resulting in a squarish arch shape, with broader transverse dimensions and frequent scissors bite in the premolar region.

In the posterior region, the molars are usually in Class II relationships, with the mesiobuccal cusps of the upper first molars occluding anterior to the mesiobuccal groove of the lower first molars (Fig. 9.2). Similarly, the canines are usually in Class II relationships, with the upper canines' cusp tip occluding anterior to the embrasure between the lower canines and first premolars.

9.3.3 Lateral Cephalometric Analysis

The lateral cephalometric values are usually in tandem with the extraoral and intraoral features and reflect the anterior rotational growth pattern of the mandible. The Class II maxillary-mandibular skeletal relationship presents as an increased ANB angle of more than the population norm, although sometimes this may be mild or average as compared to the population norm. The Class II skeletal pattern can be contributed by either a prognathic maxilla indicated by an increased SNA, or a retrognathic mandible indicated by a decreased SNB or a combination of both. A short mandibular length is common, with an anteriorly angled condylar head, and a flat lower border. The inferior alveolar canal may be curved downwards. The lips may be retrusive if measured from an E-line comprising an anteriorly positioned soft tissue Pogonion.

The cephalometric values for reduced vertical proportions such as a decreased Frankfort-Mandibular Plane Angle (FMPA) or Maxillary-Mandibular Plane Angle (MMPA) and decreased lower facial height proportion may be presented [5]. This decrease in angular measurements reflects the decrease in the anterior facial height relative to the posterior facial height in keeping with the anticlockwise rotation of the mandible.

The upper incisor angle traced from the retroclined incisors would be decreased but purposeful tracing of the proclined lateral incisors would result in an increased upper incisor angle. With upward rotation of the mandible, this would result in lower labial segment retroclination and a decrease in lower incisor angle. Interincisal angle is usually increased.

9.4 Facial Growth and Treatment Timing

Genetically predetermined facial growth expresses itself fully during the pubertal growth spurt. Growth of the mandible is in an anticlockwise growth rotation, with a resulting deep overbite and reduced vertical facial height. Treatment involving enhanced eruption of the posterior teeth is more successful during growth because the dentoalveolar vertical development could enhance vertical eruption of the posterior teeth in deep overbite correction, contributing to a stable treatment outcome. For a more severe mandibular retrusion, or vertical skeletal discrepancies, growth modification with a functional appliance, such as to enhance mandibular growth, is best just before, or at the peak of pubertal growth spurt. Should the sagittal or vertical discrepancy be too severe in a non-growing patient, surgery may be a better option than camouflage, but cessation of growth is a requirement.

9.5 Interceptive Treatment

9.5.1 Correction of the Deep Traumatic Overbite

Deep overbite is a common classic feature for a Class II division 2 malocclusion. Normally the deep overbite is traumatic and needs urgent intervention. In a growing patient it can be corrected by using an upper removable appliance incorporated in an anterior bite plane, which will free the occlusion posteriorly. This then induces over-eruption of the lower posterior teeth, levelling the curve of Spee and eventually decreases the overbite.

Retroclined upper incisors are also one of the classic features for a Class II division 2 malocclusion. An expansion screw or z-springs can be added to the upper removable appliance to procline the upper incisors to their normal inclination. At least 3-points of retention are needed for this mechanic. For example, if an anterior expansion screw is used, retention can be placed anteriorly (Southend clasp on both upper central incisors) and posteriorly (Adams clasp on both upper first molars) (Fig. 9.3).

9.5.2 Correction of the Buccal Segment

The buccal segment is normally in a Class II relationship, in a Class II division 2 malocclusion. The correction of it can be aided in growing patients by using an extraoral traction. A straight pull headgear can be used to distalize the upper buccal segments. A cervical pull headgear can be utilized too, taking the advantage of correcting the deep overbite as well. It acts by extruding the posterior teeth and the wedge effect will reduce the deep overbite.

9.5.3 Growth Modification

The aims for growth modification in a growing patient are to correct the overjet, overbite, buccal segment relationships, as well as the antero-posterior and transverse relationships. The Class II division 2 incisor relationship first needs to be converted to a Class II division 1 incisor relationship. A modified Twin Block appliance can be utilized. Anteriorly an expansion screw can be incorporated to procline or to convert the upper incisors to a Class II division 1 malocclusion (Figs. 9.4 and 9.5).

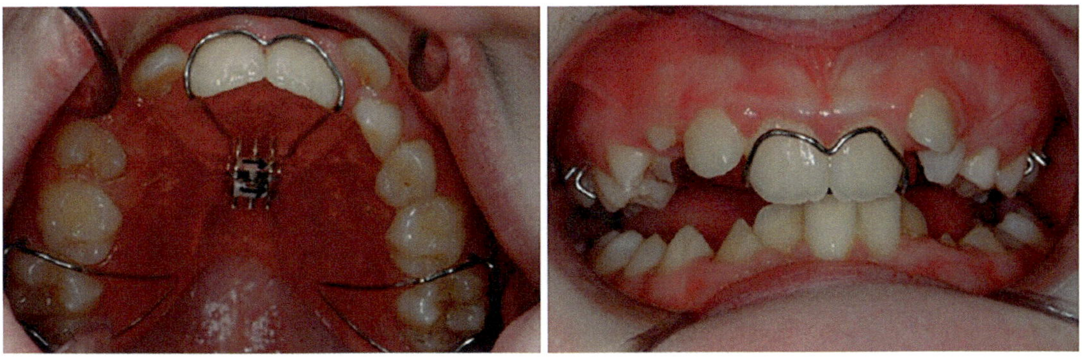

Fig. 9.3 Overbite reduction. An upper removable appliance with anterior bite plane together with an anterior expansion screw. Retention is through a Southend clasp on the upper central incisors and Adams clasp on both the upper first molars

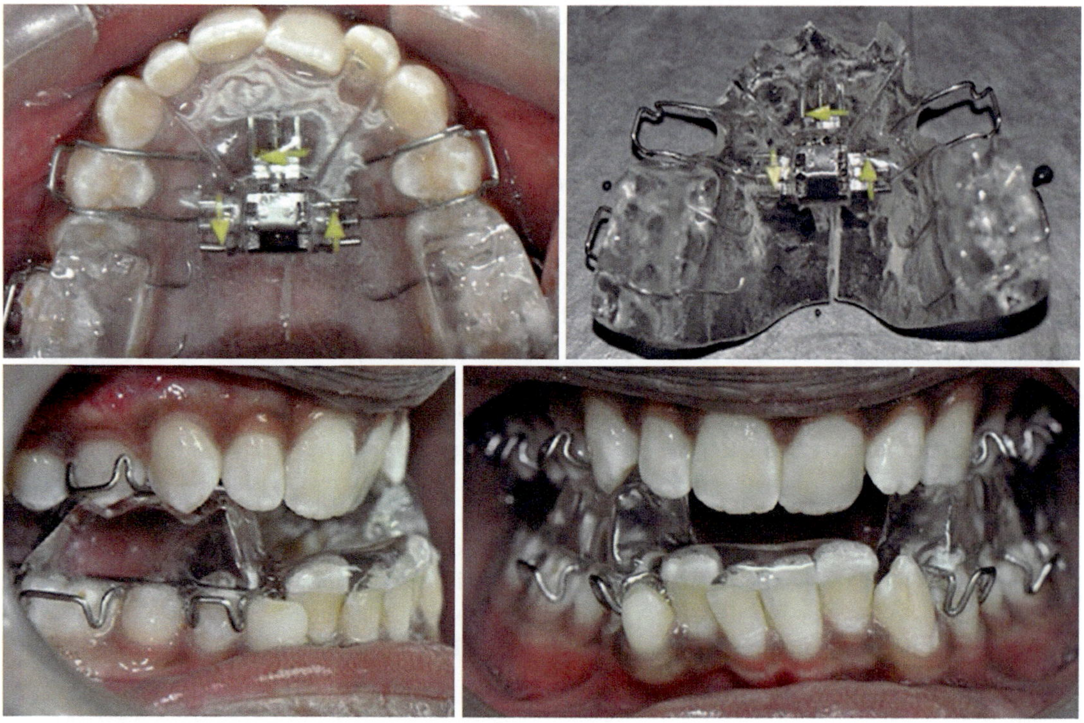

Fig. 9.4 Modified Twin Block appliance for the correction of a class II division 2 discrepancy. The upper anterior screw is to procline the retrocline upper incisors to achieve normal inclination

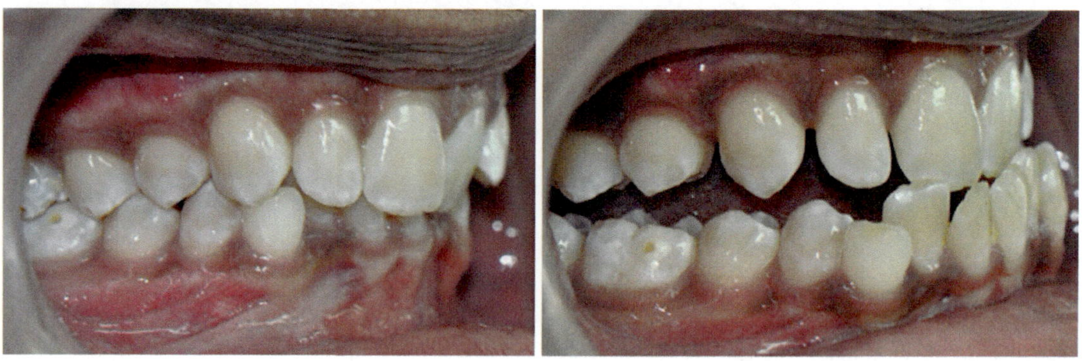

Fig. 9.5 Changes in the case shown in Fig. 9.4 before and after treatment with a modified Twin Block appliance

9.6 Orthodontic Camouflage

9.6.1 Indication

In a mild to moderate skeletal Class II discrepancy, the camouflage treatment option using a comprehensive orthodontic fixed appliance can be attempted in the permanent dentition. This is also indicated in any situation contra-indicating surgical treatment.

9.6.2 Deep Overbite

The common difficulty in fixed orthodontic treatment of Class II division 2 is the correction of the increased overbite. Extrusion of the posterior teeth with orthodontic fixed appliance can flatten the curve of Spee and help with overbite reduction. This is more stable with the presence of vertical dentoalveolar growth in growing patients [3, 6]. By rotating the mandible downwards and backwards, this can increase the vertical proportion, increase the FMPA and MMPA and improve the short face appearance with prominent chin. Extrusion of posterior teeth can be achieved by sequential archwire progression, banding of second molars, reverse curve of Spee arch wires, intrusion loops bent on upper archwire, employing anterior bite plane and anterior bite turbos.

The anterior bite plane can be incorporated into a removable acrylic splint with retentive Plint clasp to be worn over buccal molar tubes and ball-ended clasps to be fitted over a concurrent fixed orthodontic appliance. The working bite for the splint should register the required thickness of the bite plane depending on the amount of overbite that is intended to be reduced. There is tendency for favourable lower incisor proclination with use of anterior bite plane. In reduced overjet deep bite patients, this appliance can also disengage the anterior segment to allow bonding brackets on the lower labial segment and prevent dislodgement of lower anterior brackets during function (Fig. 9.6).

Another form of anterior bite plane can be a modification of the Nance appliance with the acrylic disc placed further anteriorly over the incisal edges of the lower labial segment in occlusion. There is however risk of trauma of the acrylic disc to the palatal tissues, and hygiene difficulties with long-term use of fixed anterior bite plane. Therefore, short-term use is advocated, and removal of the fixed anterior bite plane must precede retraction of the upper labial segment in extraction cases.

Proclination of incisors within biological boundaries similarly will also reduce the overbite [3], especially when aligning crowded arches without extraction of teeth. Lower incisor proclination helps to flatten the increased curve of Spee, which can change the arch shape from squarish to a more ovoid shape. Considering the risk of gingival recession, care should be taken to ensure good oral hygiene and proclination may be contraindicated in patients with thin gingival biotypes [7].

With an excessively increased overbite, more anterior teeth intrusion may be required [8] in addition to posterior extrusion in decreased vertical facial proportions or without posterior extrusion with average vertical proportions. This can be achieved with various intrusion techniques

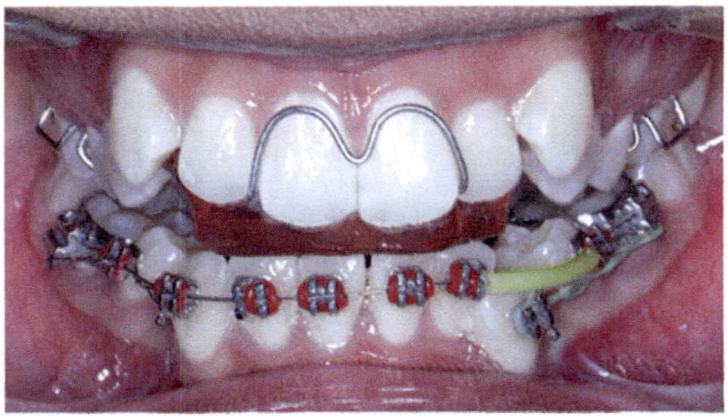

Fig. 9.6 Upper removable appliance with flat anterior bite plane to disengage the anterior segment and allow the bonding of brackets to the lower arch

ranging from the 2 × 4 Mulligan bypass arch, Rickett's utility arch, and segmented arch mechanics [9] such as Burstone's technique, to temporary anchorage devices.

9.6.3 Decision for Extraction

Extraction of teeth can complicate overbite reduction as the overbite will tend to deepen during space closure, which is undesirable in many Class II division 2 malocclusions with an increased pre-treatment overbite. The more anterior the extraction, the more the overbite will tend to deepen. Therefore, the choice of extraction needs careful consideration and space closure requires careful overbite control to avoid bite deepening.

Planning for extractions depends on anchorage requirements and the anchorage mechanics planned. Should the crowding be too severe, extractions may be necessary. Depending on the required soft tissue changes [10], extraction of second premolars can result in some amount of incisor proclination and this can contribute to overbite reduction. Should incisor proclination not be conducive to the lip profile, extraction of the upper first premolars may be required (Fig. 9.7). Just as in any Class II malocclusions, the extraction pattern in the lower arch may sometimes involve lower second premolars; however, extraction of first premolars is hardly indicated in Class II division 2 malocclusions, as residual space closure by retroclining the lower labial segment can complicate bite opening.

By incorporating any form of anchorage reinforcement, or anchorage-preserving mechanics such as frictionless space closure, extraction pattern may change or can even be avoided. Using various methods to distalize upper buccal segments such as temporary anchorage device or cervical pull headgear, which can also increase vertical facial proportions, can also influence the need and pattern of extraction.

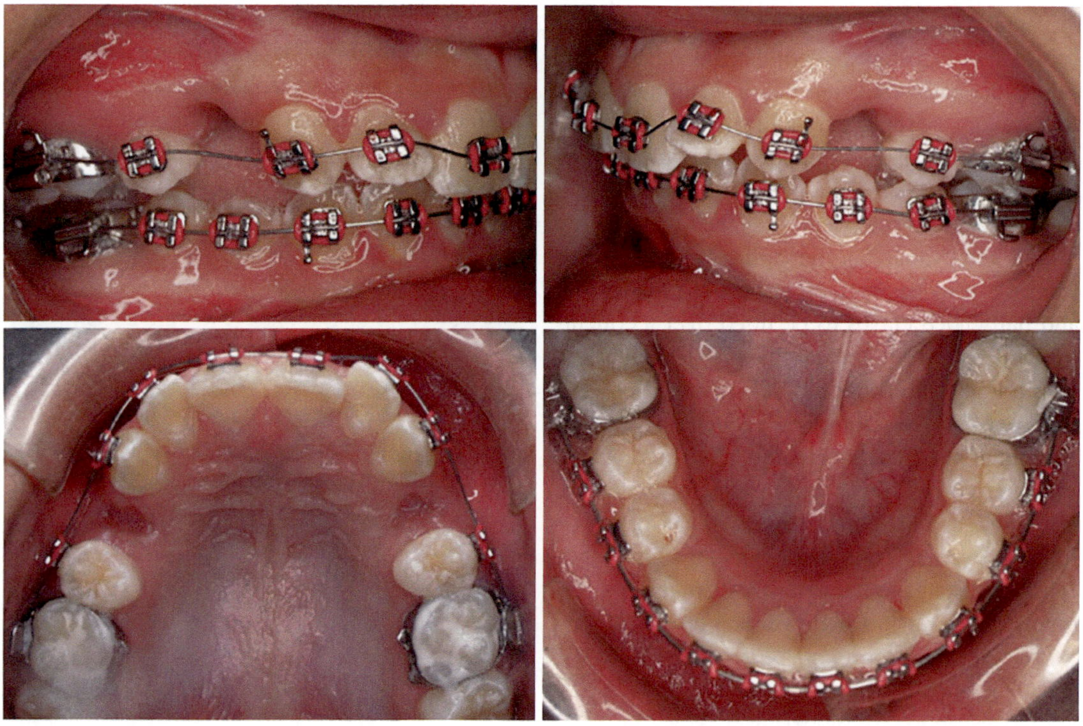

Fig. 9.7 Extraction of upper first premolars and non-extraction in the lower arch

9.6.4 Alignment of the Anterior Segments

Early engagement of resilient NiTi archwires can proline incisors, especially if retroclined central incisors are engaged to proclined lateral incisors and in a crowded non-extraction treatment option. This is desired when incisors are retroclined, overbite is deep and lip profile is flat. Proclining the upper and lower incisors can reduce interincisal angle, resulting in a more stable edge-centroid relationship [11].

When extractions are required, however, engaging anterior labial segments will result in initial proclination followed by retraction in subsequent extraction space closure. This is a form of round tripping that carries the risk of root resorption. This can be avoided by delaying engaging and aligning of retroclined incisors until space is available from retraction of canine into extraction spaces. After completion of space closure, increasing upper labial segment inclination can be achieved by palatal root torque. This would maintain lip profile should this be the desired treatment aim. Due to the acute incisor crown-root angle, increasing upper labial segment inclination by employing palatal root torque techniques may require a longer alignment duration using light force to carefully avoid root resorption, especially when palatal alveolar bone is thinner than normal.

9.6.5 Transverse Discrepancy

Lingually tilted lower dentition or omega-shaped lower arch with constriction at premolars region contributing to scissors bite can be expanded with normal archwire sequence to increase lower transverse dimension and torque lower posterior crowns buccally. Employing use of cross elastics and expansion appliances such as a lower quad-helix together with bite disengagement can be considered for severely constricted lower arches.

Proclination of upper labial segment together with constriction of upper posterior teeth and carefully finishing by coordinating upper and lower arch can address scissors bite commonly presented in Class II division 2 malocclusions.

9.7 Orthognathic Surgery

When the case is too severe for orthodontic treatment alone, an orthognathic surgery approach in a non-growing patient is warranted. The treatment objectives include establishing a functional occlusion aiming to achieve normal overbite/overjet and transverse relationship; providing a stable result in normalizing the facial balance and proportions in three dimensions and providing long-term stability.

Typically, a patient with severe Class II division 2 presents with mandibular retrognathia, prognathic maxilla, reduced lower face height, reduced gonial angle, and reduced MMPA, anterior deep bite, and an excessive curve of Spee in the lower arch.

The treatment planning and execution are conducted in a collaborative manner in the form of a multidisciplinary team (MDT) to ensure a successful outcome can be obtained when managing patients undergoing orthognathic treatment. Orthodontics plays an integral part in preparing the patient for orthognathic surgery involving three distinct stages which are pre-surgical orthodontics, surgery and post-surgical orthodontics. It is crucial to plan this treatment in all three planes of space: anteroposterior, vertical and transverse. Pre-surgical orthodontics typically involves relief of crowding and alignment, decompensation and arch coordination.

One of the key differences in presurgical orthodontics for Class II division 2 as compared to other malocclusions is how the curve of Spee is corrected. In a case with deep overbite and a reduced face height, curve of Spee is maintained during pre-surgical orthodontics as extrusion of the molars can easily be accomplished during the post-surgical orthodontic phase. During the pre-surgical orthodontics, a three-point landing is created. When the mandible is advanced, the face height is increased leaving tooth contact between the incisors and molars with a deep curve of Spee observed immediately after surgery. This curve of Spee can later be corrected post-surgery by extruding the premolar teeth. In a case with a combination of deep curve of Spee and some degree of lower incisor crowding, extraction of teeth is sometimes needed for space creation to level the arch and to align the teeth. Care must be taken to avoid the stretching of the muscles of the pterygomandibular sling which can lead to post-orthognathic surgery instability and relapse.

9.8 Stability and Retention

9.8.1 Stability

The correction of the overbite with a good reduction of the inter-incisor angle is important for stability in a Class II division 2 malocclusion. For maximal chances of stability, the upper root centroid should be at least 2 mm behind the lower incisor edge and the inter-incisor angle is reduced as much as possible toward 125° [12]. Intrusion and palatal root torquing of the upper incisors are needed to decrease and normalize the interincisal angle. Proclination of the lower labial segment after intrusion of the upper labial segment has been suggested as treatment that will be stable as the lower incisors would take up positions previously occupied by the uppers [3, 13].

9.8.2 Retention

The standard approach of retention in a Class II division 2 malocclusion is bonding a fixed lingual retainer behind the lower right canine to left canine. This is to ensure a stable antero-posterior and transverse position of the lower labial segment. The upper arch often requires little or no retention unless the upper laterals were rotated mesiolingually. The upper incisors will be supported automatically by a properly positioned lower labial segment once overbite and inter-incisor angle are corrected [13].

As relapse is unpredictable, it is recommended that long-term retention is maintained. A normal night-time wear retention regime can be followed. In a growing patient, an upper anterior bite plane can be incorporated into the Hawley retainer to maintain the corrected deep overbite.

References

1. British Standards Institute. Glossary of dental terms (BS 4492). London: BSI; 1983.
2. Leighton BC. Some observations on vertical development and the dentition. Proc R Soc Med. 1968;61:1273–7.
3. Mills JRE. The problem of overbite in class II, division 2 malocclusion. Br J Orthod. 1973;1:34–48.
4. Al-Khateeb EA, Al-Khateeb SN. Anteroposterior and vertical components of class II division 1 and division 2 malocclusion. Angle Orthod. 2009;79:859–66.
5. Brezniak N, Arad A, Heller M, Dinbar A, Dinte A, Wasserstein A. Pathognomonic cephalometric characteristics of angle class II division 2 malocclusion. Angle Orthod. 2002;72:251–7.
6. Ng J, Major PW, Heo G, Flores-Mir C. True incisor intrusion attained during orthodontic treatment: a systematic review and meta-analysis. Am J Orthod Dentofacial Orthop. 2005;128:212–9.
7. Melsen B, Allais D. Factors of importance for the development of dehiscences during labial movement of mandibular incisors: a retrospective study of adult orthodontic patients. Am J Orthod Dentofacial Orthop. 2005;127:552–61.
8. Lapatki BG, Mager AS, Schulte-Moenting J, Jonas IE. The importance of the level of the lip line and resting lip pressure in class II, division 2 malocclusion. J Dent Res. 2002;81:323–8.
9. Stellzig A, Basdra EK, Kube C, Komposch G. Extraction therapy in patients with class II/2 malocclusion. J Orofac Orthop. 1999;60:39–52.
10. Selwyn-Barnett BJ. Rationale of treatment for class II division 2 malocclusion. Br J Orthod. 1991;18:173–81.
11. Houston WJB. Incisor edge-centroid relationships and overbite depth. Eur J Orthod. 1989;11:139–43.
12. Selwyn-Barnett BJ. Class II division 2 malocclusion: a method of planning and treatment. Br J Orthod. 1996;23:29–36.
13. Mills JRE. The stability of the lower labial segment. A cephalometric survey. Dent Pract Dent Rec. 1968;18:293–306.

10 Orthodontic-Surgical Management of Class II Malocclusion

Farhad B. Naini and Mehmet Manisali

10.1 Introduction

The purpose of this chapter is to describe the role of the orthodontist and surgeon team in the clinical management of patients with moderate to severe Class II malocclusions of predominantly skeletal aetiology requiring orthognathic surgical correction.

10.2 Classification and Terminology

The term 'Class II,' originally introduced by Edward Angle to classify sagittal dental-occlusal relationships, is now widely used to describe a variety of attributes of the bimaxillary complex. A Class II skeletal pattern refers to mandibular retrusion *relative* to the maxilla in the sagittal plane. Class II may also refer to the incisor relationship (separated into divisions 1 and 2), the buccal segment relationships, or the overall malocclusion. The term is also sometimes used to describe the facial soft tissue morphology.

In relation to the skeletal pattern, a Class II relationship may be due to sagittal maxillary excess (prominence of the maxilla due to a forward position, referred to as prognathism, or infrequently, an excessive size, referred to as macrognathia). More commonly, a Class II skeletal relationship is due to sagittal mandibular deficiency. This may be due to posterior positioning of the mandible in relation to the craniofacial complex, known as mandibular retrognathia or retrognathism, reduced size of the mandible, known as micrognathia, or both.

Vertical overgrowth of the entire maxilla, known as vertical maxillary excess, or overgrowth of the posterior maxilla and maxillary dentoalveolus, described as posterior vertical maxillary excess, can lead to a posterior (backward or clockwise) rotation of the mandible, which will exacerbate a Class II malocclusion and appearance by moving the chin downwards and backwards.

A Class II facial appearance may also be exacerbated by sagittal or combined sagittal and vertical osseous chin deficiency.

F. B. Naini (✉)
Department of Orthodontics, Maxillofacial Unit, Kingston Hospital NHS Foundation Trust, and The Gillies Unit, Queen Mary's Hospital, King's College Hospital NHS Foundation Trust, London, UK
e-mail: Farhad.Naini@kcl.ac.uk

M. Manisali
Maxillofacial Unit, St George's University Hospital NHS Foundation Trust, London, UK
e-mail: Mehmet.Manisali1@nhs.net

M. T. Cobourne (ed.), *Orthodontic Management of Class II Malocclusion*,
https://doi.org/10.1007/978-3-031-57530-3_10

10.3 Clinical Evaluation

Clinical evaluation should begin with the frontal facial examination, and go on to assess the face from different viewpoints and using various diagnostic records. Comprehensive clinical diagnosis is beyond the scope of this chapter and has been described elsewhere [1, 2], but the most pertinent information related to the Class II patient is summarized below. The patient should be in their natural head position (NHP), though the clinician may need to make minor manual adjustments to the patient's head position, as patients may have developed a compensatory head posture, or more commonly, may habitually posture the mandible forward, in order to minimize the aesthetic impact of a mandibular deficiency.

The aesthetic parameters described below serve as useful guidelines for clinical evaluation. A useful starting point is the evaluation of the vertical facial thirds, which may be undertaken in frontal or profile view. This proportional canon, known as the vertical facial trisection (Vitruvian trisection), was described by the Roman architect Vitruvius and popularized by Leonardo da Vinci [1]. The face may be vertically divided into thirds (Fig. 10.1):

- Upper facial third: trichion (hairline) to soft tissue glabella.
- Middle facial third: soft tissue glabella to subnasale.
- Lower facial third: subnasale to soft tissue menton. The lower facial third may be slightly greater than the middle third in males.

The lower facial third may be further subdivided. Leonardo da Vinci described the upper lip as forming the upper third and the lower lip and chin forming the lower two-thirds. Albrecht Dürer subdivided the lower anterior face height into quarters, with the upper lip height ¼ of lower facial height. Subsequent attractiveness research has found that Leonardo's proportion appears to be the ideal, though a range of variability exists from the upper lip being anything from ½ to ¼ of lower anterior face height (LAFH) [3, 4].

Vertical chin height should be assessed whilst considering the vertical facial proportions.

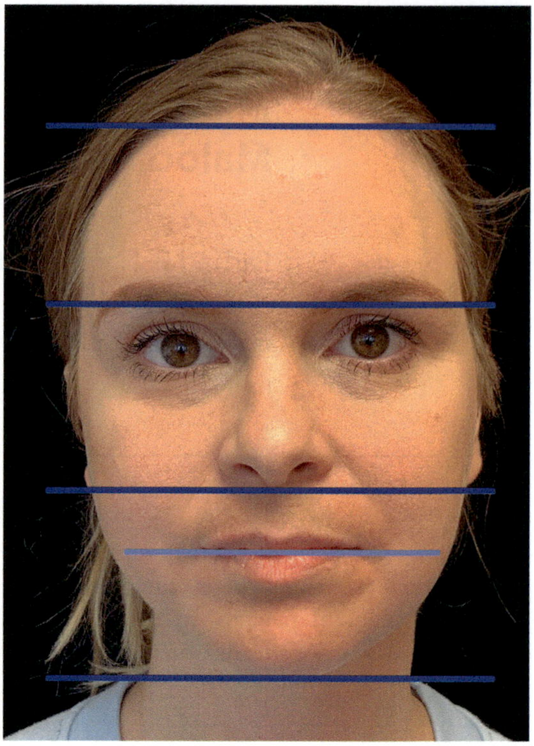

Fig. 10.1 Vertical facial trisection. The upper facial third is from trichion (hairline) to soft tissue glabella (the most prominent midline point of the forehead between the brow ridges). Midface height is from soft tissue glabella to subnasale (the deepest midline point where the base of the nasal columella meets the upper lip). Lower face height is from subnasale to soft tissue menton (the most inferior midline point of the soft tissue chin). The upper lip height is approximately one-third of lower face height

Sagittal correction of mandibular position often alters the appearance of the mentolabial fold region and lower facial height proportions, as the mandible may be moved forward and downward (see later), potentially improving the chin height to face height proportion. Therefore, in such cases, vertical reduction or augmentation genioplasty may be undertaken, simultaneously or as a secondary procedure if necessary.

The sagittal position of the maxilla may be evaluated in profile view using a true vertical line (TrV or facial vertical) from soft tissue nasion, soft tissue glabella or a point midway between the two (perpendicular to the true horizontal line), with the patient in NHP (Fig. 10.2). Subnasale and soft tissue A-point should be approximately on this line.

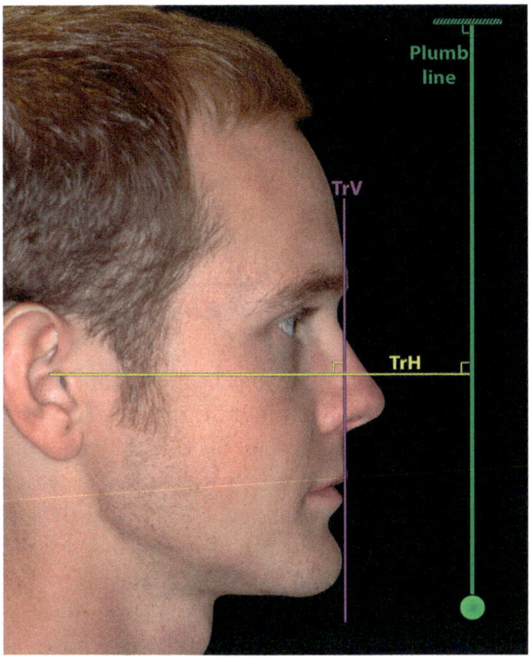

Fig. 10.2 A patient in natural head position (NHP), demonstrating the true facial vertical (TrV) and true horizontal (TrH) lines used to evaluate facial aesthetics. The true vertical may be taken as a line parallel to a plumb line hanging from the ceiling. The true horizontal will be at right angles to this. In some patients the Frankfort plane may be parallel to the true horizontal; however, the inclination of the Frankfort plane is subject to individual variability. (From: Naini FB. *Facial Aesthetics: Concepts and Clinical Diagnosis*. Oxford: Wiley-Blackwell, 2011. Reprinted with permission)

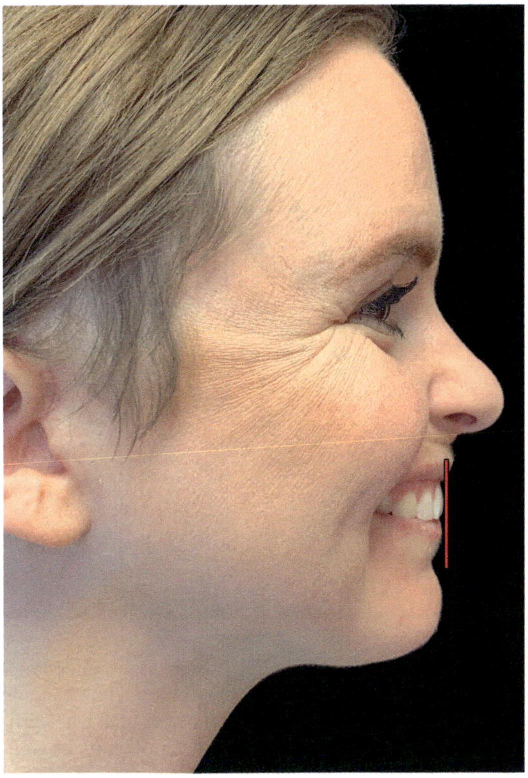

Fig. 10.3 The labial face tangent. The most accurate measurement of maxillary incisor *crown* inclination, from an aesthetic viewpoint, is that of a tangent to the labial face of the maxillary central incisor crown, with the patient in natural head position. This tangent should be approximately parallel to the true vertical plane and thereby approximately perpendicular to the true horizontal plane

Maxillary incisor inclination should be evaluated in profile smiling view. A tangent to the labial face of the maxillary central incisor crown should be approximately parallel to a true facial vertical line (TrV) (Fig. 10.3) [5].

Maxillary incisor position in the sagittal plane should be approximately level with a true vertical line dropped from soft tissue nasion, glabella or a point between the two, depending on the morphology of the glabellar-nasal region, and considering ethnic variation. Cephalometrically, the maxillary incisors should be approximately 4 mm anterior to the nasion-perpendicular (which is very similar to their proposed position in relation to the true vertical line dropped from soft tissue nasion).

The sagittal chin position may be evaluated using a true vertical line as described above. Soft tissue pogonion should be approximately 0 ± 2 mm to this line. If the patient has normal sagittal projection of the midface, subnasale (rather than soft tissue nasion) may be used to drop a TrV line, perpendicular to the true horizontal line (TrH), with the patient in NHP. This analysis is useful for planning treatment in mandibular retrognathia or retrogenia, where the maxillary position is correct. The sagittal prominence of the soft tissue chin ideally should not be further ahead than the lower lip. An angular relationship relating the prominence of the chin to the lower lip may be useful (Fig. 10.4) [6].

It is important to assess the soft tissue thickness anterior to the bony chin (which may be observed on the lateral cephalometric radiograph, and palpated clinically), as an over-pro-

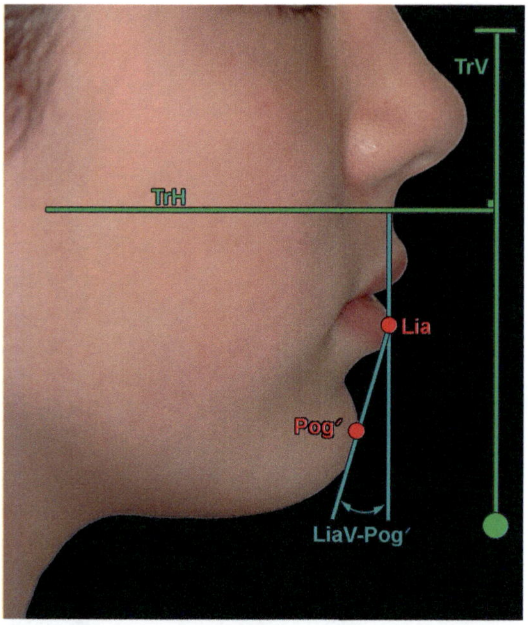

Fig. 10.4 The lower lip-chin prominence (LiaV-Pog′) angle. In front of the patient there is a plumb line hanging from the ceiling, which acts as an extra-cranial true vertical line (TrV). Perpendicular to the TrV may be constructed the true horizontal line (TrH). A line parallel to the TrV, and perpendicular to the TrH, may be constructed through the Lia point (labrale inferius anterioris, which is the most anterior/prominent midline point of the lower lip, with the lips in repose, teeth lightly in occlusion and the subject in natural head position), which may be referred to as the Lia-Vertical line, or "LiaV." This is effectively a true vertical line through the most prominent point on the lower lip. From Lia point, a second line is constructed to soft tissue pogonion (Pog′). The angle formed between the LiaV line and the Lia-Pog′ line may be termed the LiaV-Pog′ angle, i.e. the lower lip-chin prominence angle. The advantage of an angular relationship is that it is unaffected by magnification if being measured on a photographic or radiographic image. The "ideal" angular relationship appears to be 0°, i.e. with the chin on the LiaV, or just behind it. Chin retrusion or prominence up to an angle of 15° retrusion to 5° prominence is deemed acceptable. Angular deviations outside this range are likely to be deemed unattractive, with a desire for surgical correction from most observers

jection of the chin may be entirely due to the soft tissue thickness. The submental length (soft tissue menton to C-point, which is the junction of submental plane and vertical plane of the anterior aspect of the neck) is on average approximately 50 mm, with a proportional value of approximately 80% of lower anterior face height. The submental-cervical angle describes the contour of the transition from the submental plane to the anterior aspect of the neck, with an average value of 110° (range 100–135°). Mandibular and/or chin advancement surgery tends to improve the submental-cervical contour by stretching the submental-cervical soft tissues.

10.4 Cephalometric Analysis

Cephalometric analysis may be used as an adjunct to the clinical evaluation of the patient. Two useful methods of analysing sagittal skeletal relationships are the nasion perpendicular, which provides linear measurements, and a group of angular measurements which relate the maxilla (SNA angle), mandible (SNB angle) and chin (SND angle; SN-Pog angle) to the anterior cranial base (sella-nasion or SN plane). An extension of the latter is the ANB angle, which relates the maxilla to the mandible.

Nasion perpendicular (McNamara) (Fig. 10.5): With the patient's head oriented in NHP, the most direct method to determine the sagittal position of the maxilla and mandible is to measure the horizontal linear distance to the nasion perpendicular (N-perpendicular), a vertical line perpendicular to the true horizontal, dropped from bony nasion. McNamara's original data was based on the Frankfort plane rather than the true horizontal plane. Points anterior to N-perpendicular are assigned a positive value, and posterior a negative value. In white Caucasian patients [7]:

- Maxillary point A is on or slightly ahead of nasion perpendicular (0 to +1 mm).
- Mandibular point B is 2–3 mm behind nasion perpendicular.
- A-B difference (horizontal distance between points A and B when both are projected onto the true horizontal) is approximately 4 mm.
- Hard tissue pogonion (the most anterior point on the bony chin) is:
  - −4 to 0 mm behind N-perpendicular (in adult women).
  - −2 to +5 mm to N-perpendicular (in adult men).

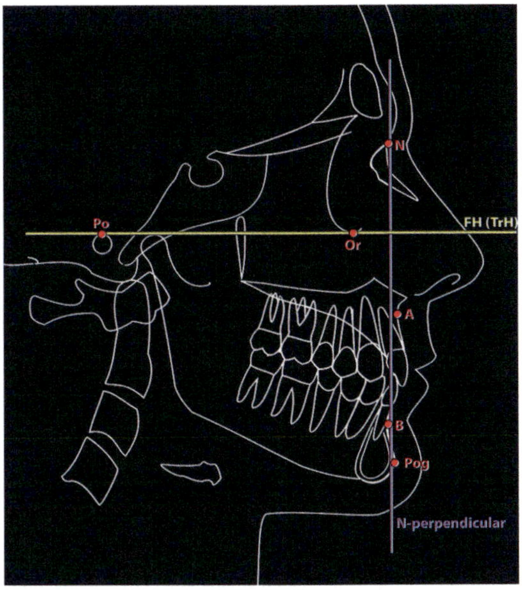

Fig. 10.5 The nasion perpendicular is a vertical line perpendicular to the Frankfort (FH) plane, or ideally the true horizontal plane (TrH), dropped from bony nasion (N). A, Skeletal A-point; B, skeletal B-point; Or, orbitale; Po, porion; Pog, pogonion. (From Naini FB. Facial Aesthetics: Concepts and Clinical Diagnosis. Oxford: Wiley-Blackwell; 2011. Reprinted with permission)

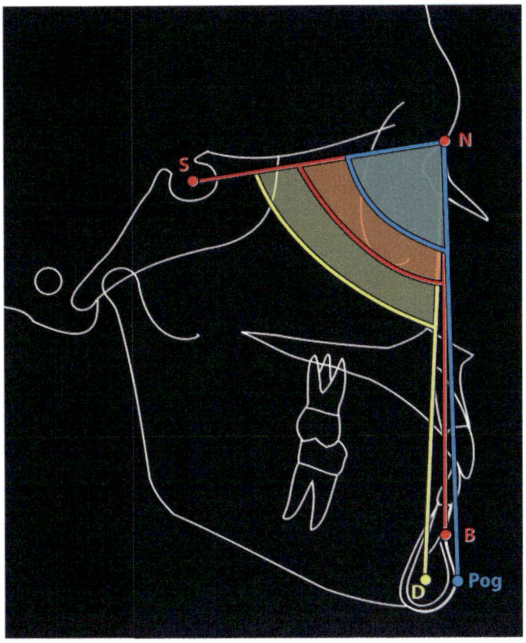

Fig. 10.6 The SNB, SND and SN-Pog angles provide an indication of the sagittal position of the mandibular apical base, mandible, and chin, respectively, in relation to the anterior cranial base and in relation to each other. (From: Naini FB. Facial Aesthetics: Concepts and Clinical Diagnosis. Oxford: Wiley-Blackwell, 2011; reprinted with permission)

SNA angle (82 ± 3°): Relates the sagittal position of the maxillary apical base (A-point) to the anterior cranial base (SN). The SNA angle provides an *indication* of the sagittal position of the maxilla relative to the anterior cranial base.

SNB angle (79 ± 3°): Relates the sagittal position of the mandibular apical base (B-point) to the anterior cranial base (SN). The SNB angle provides an *indication* of the sagittal position of the mandible relative to the anterior cranial base (Fig. 10.6).

It should be noted that A-point and B-point are alveolar points and do not necessarily represent the true position of the skeletal bases, though they tend to provide a useful indication of the relative sagittal position of the maxilla and mandible. Additionally, the inclination of the SN plane is variable, therefore these analyses may only be employed if the SN plane has a normal inclination of 6–7° relative to the true horizontal, and sella and nasion are in normal sagittal and vertical positions.

SND angle (76–77°): Point 'D' is the centre of the body of the symphysis (bony chin) and is estimated visually. The SND angle provides an assessment of the *sagittal position of the mandibular skeletal base* in relation to the anterior cranial base (see Fig. 10.6).

SN-Pog angle (80 ± 3°): This angle is formed between the most anterior point on the bony chin (pogonion) and the SN plane. It is important to compare the value of SNB to SN-Pog. In patients with a prominent chin but mandibular dentoalveolar (apical base) retrusion, the facial profile may be acceptable even though the dentoalveolar relationship is unfavourable. This relationship is common in Class II division 2 type malocclusions. If SN-Pog is smaller than SNB, the patient is likely to have an excessively recessive bony chin in the sagittal plane (see Fig. 10.6).

ANB angle (3 ± 1°): The ANB angle represents the difference between the SNA and SNB angles, providing an indication of the sagittal discrepancy between the maxillary and mandibular apical bases (Fig. 10.7). The ANB angle is positive if point A lies anterior to NB. If NA and NB coincide, the ANB angle is zero. If point A lies posterior to NB, ANB will be negative. The skeletal pattern is described as:

- Class I: the ANB angle is in the range 2–4°.
- Class II: if ANB angle greater than 4°.
- Class III: if ANB angle less than 2°.

When assessing sagittal skeletal pattern using the angle ANB, it should be borne in mind that variations in the position of nasion will affect the ANB angle. Additionally, the sagittal skeletal and dental-occlusal relationships do not always match due to dentoalveolar compensation, e.g. a significant sagittal skeletal Class II may have a relatively small incisor overjet if the mandibular incisors are excessively proclined.

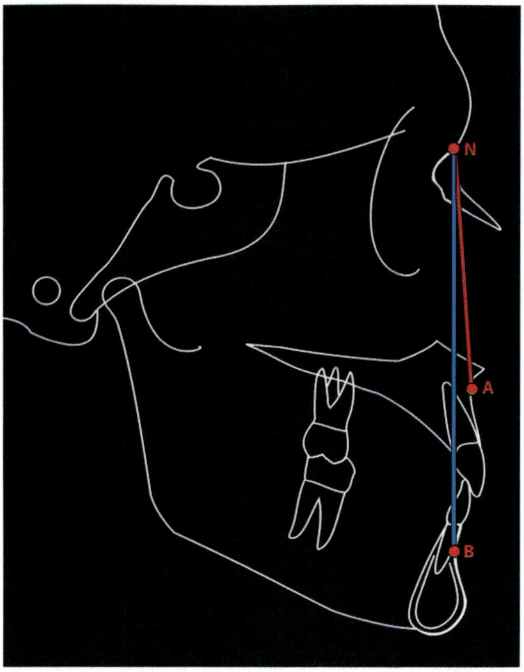

Fig. 10.7 The ANB angle represents the difference between the SNA and SNB angles, providing an indication of the sagittal discrepancy between the maxillary and mandibular apical bases. (From: Naini FB. Facial Aesthetics: Concepts and Clinical Diagnosis. Oxford: Wiley-Blackwell, 2011; reprinted with permission)

10.5 Treatment Planning

A logical treatment plan will follow from a thorough and accurate clinical diagnosis [8]. At the initial joint orthognathic clinic, a preliminary treatment plan is provided to the patient. This is sometimes referred to as a 'plan in principle,' which is usually a general discussion of the type of surgery required, e.g. bimaxillary vs. single jaw, with or without genioplasty, and any potential adjunctive procedures that may be required. It is also explained that the final treatment plan may alter following the orthodontic preparation.

The final treatment plan is reached at the presurgical joint clinic, following preparatory orthodontic treatment. Once the region(s) at fault have been identified, the next step may be termed vectorial analysis, in which the direction and approximate magnitude of movement of each jaw is determined [8]. This process is based predominantly on clinical observation of the patient, and is thereby qualitative in nature. It is not, however, entirely subjective; the reason is that most trained clinicians are likely to obtain similar findings. After accurate preoperative diagnosis, vectorial analysis is the most important stage of the treatment planning process.

Having decided the direction and approximate magnitude of the skeletal movements required, the exact movements are confirmed using orthognathic prediction planning. The different methods of prediction planning have been described elsewhere [8]. For the purposes of this chapter, the modern technique of three-dimensional virtual surgical planning (3D-VSP) will be described [9].

A cone beam computed tomography (CBCT) scan is acquired. Due to the limited spatial resolution of CBCT, the upper dentition, lower dentition and bite registration are directly or indirectly scanned. The CBCT and dental scan are subsequently aligned, in preparation for the multidisciplinary 3D-VSP meeting, which should include the treating surgeon, orthodontist and 3D-VSP engineer. Virtual osteotomies may be made, based on the plan (Fig. 10.8), with virtual adjustments made to the osteotomies based on potential a

b

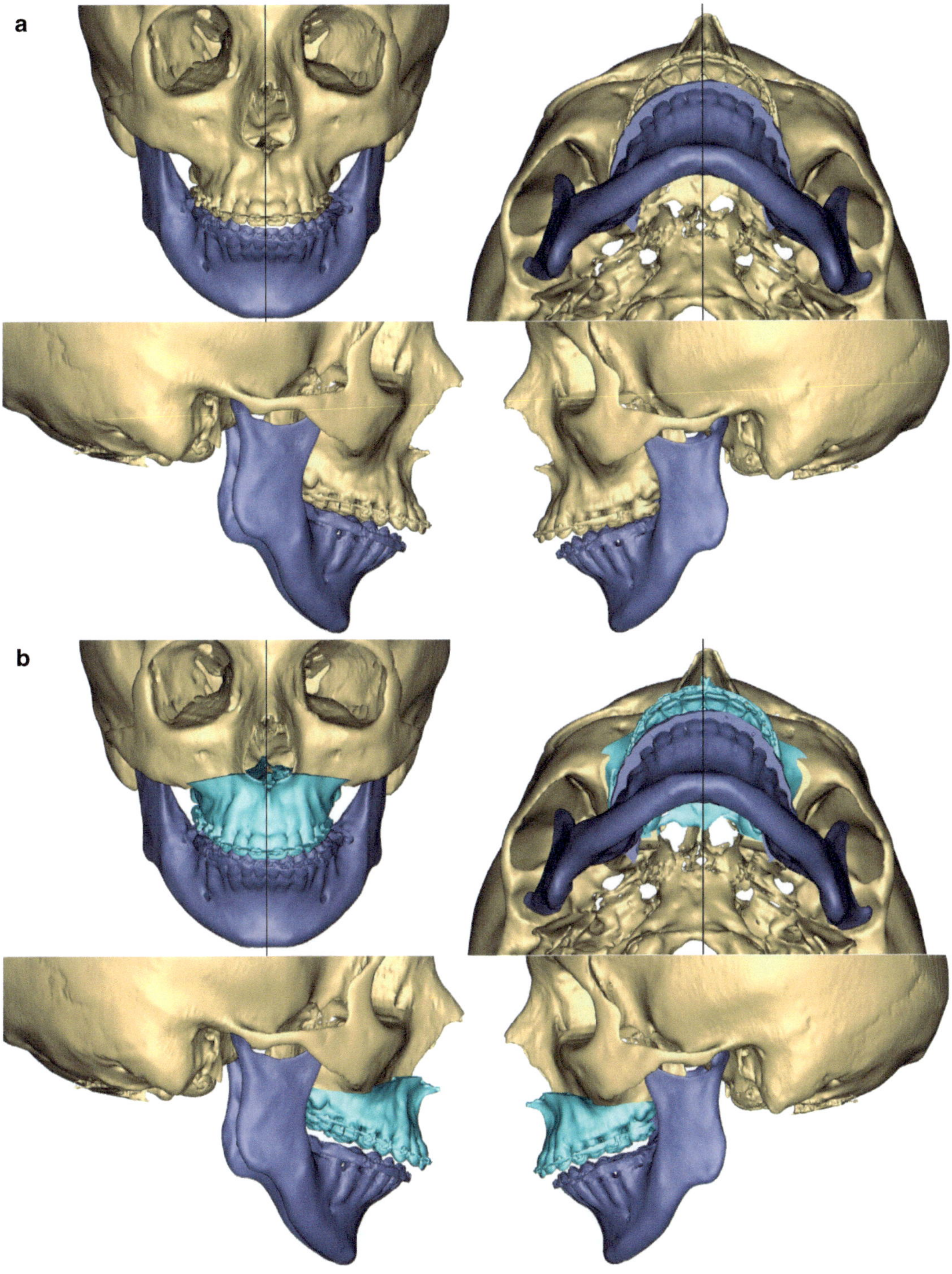

Fig. 10.8 (**a**) Class II patient with mandibular retrognathia, a skeletal anterior open bite and retrogenia, planned using 3D-VSP. (**b**) Differential posterior impaction of the maxilla (shown in light blue). (**c**) Forward autorotation and advancement of the mandible (shown in yellow). (**d**) Advancement osseous genioplasty (shown in dark blue)

c

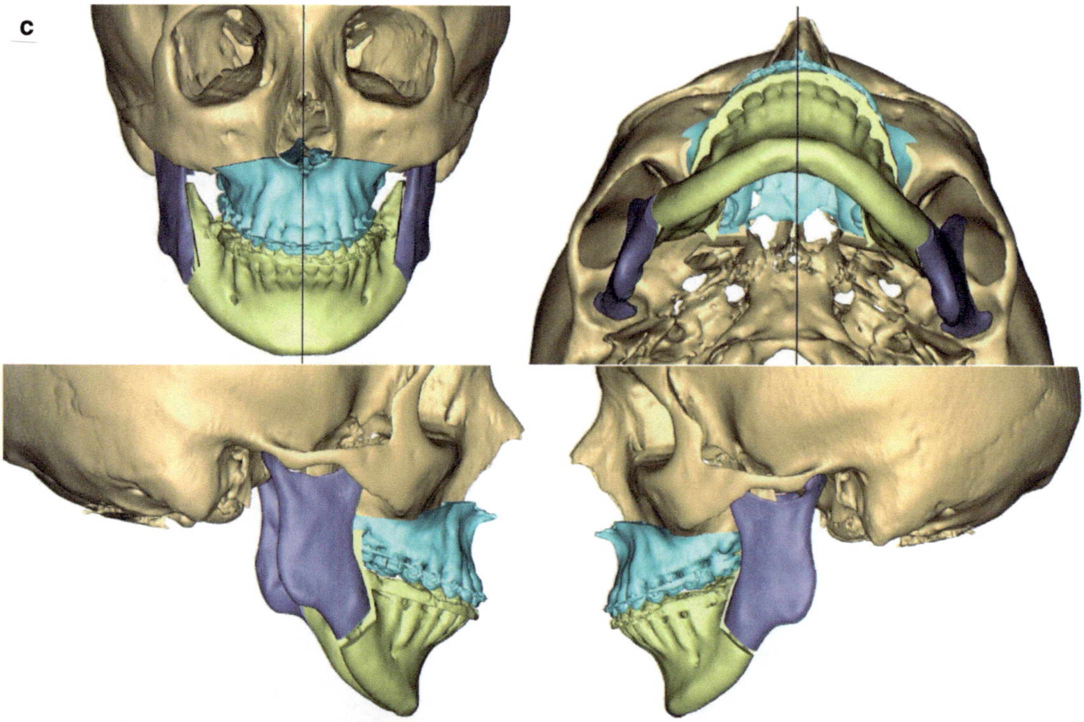

d

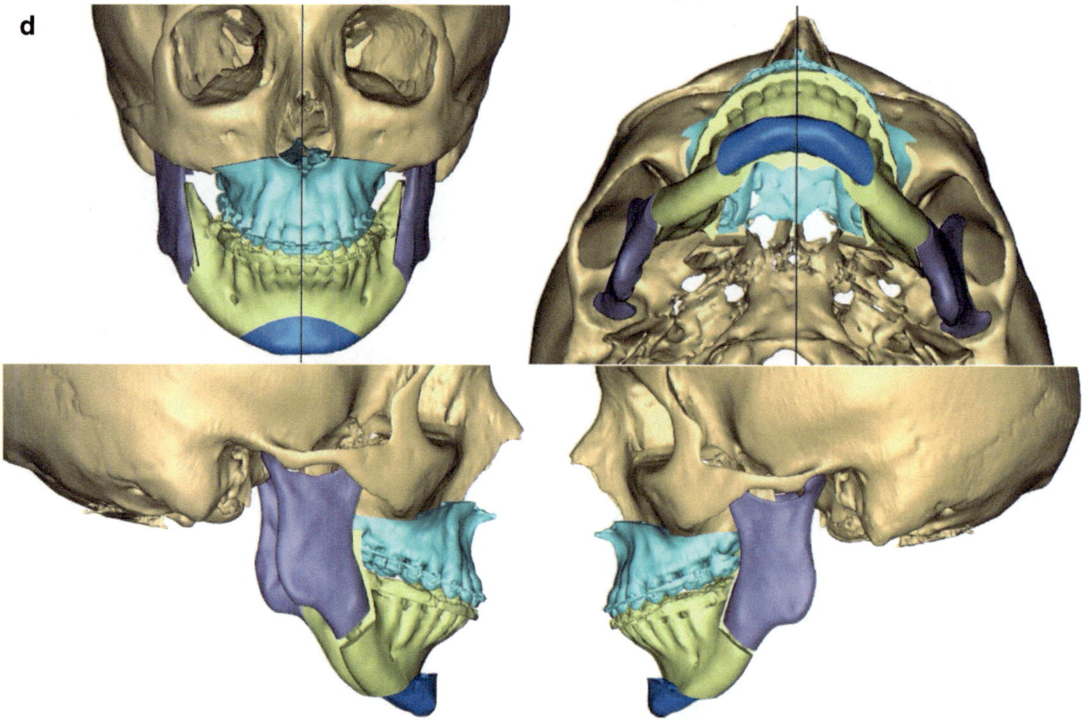

Fig. 10.8 (continued)

occlusal collisions or bony interference collisions, which may be clearly visualized from different directions (Fig. 10.9).

Le Fort I, bilateral sagittal split osteotomy (BSSO) and osseous genioplasty cutting guides (Figs. 10.10 and 10.11) and plates (Fig. 10.12) are constructed in preparation for surgery. When determining the locations of plate screw holes, root positions in the alveolar bone, the mandibular nerve, the maxillary

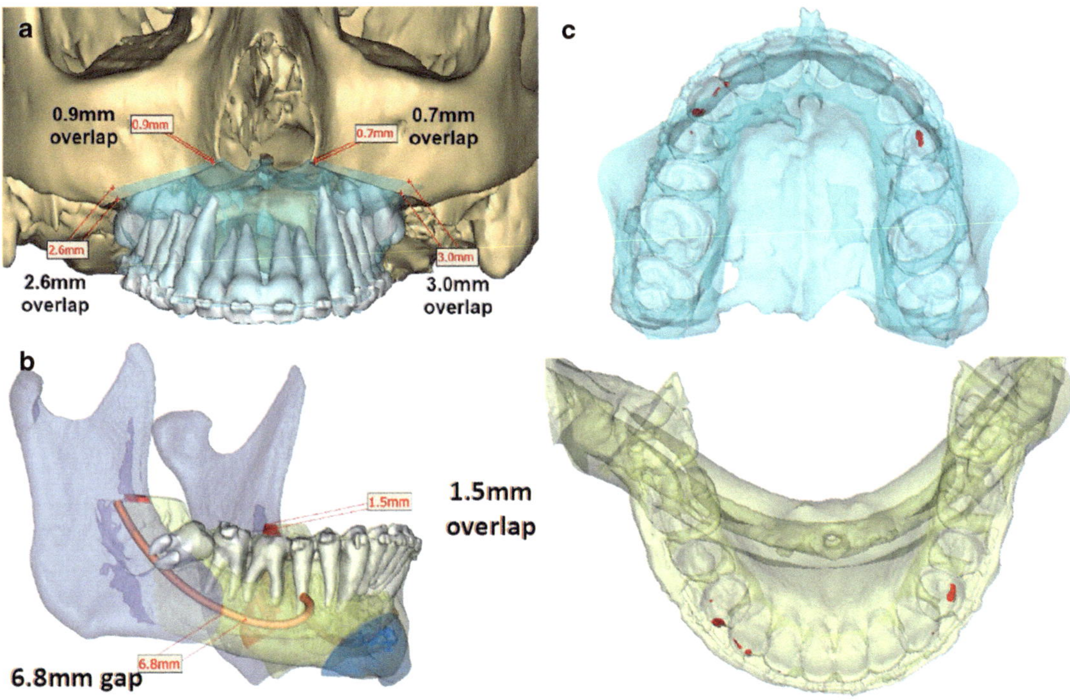

Fig. 10.9 (**a**) Overview of the planned maxillary movement, showing root positions and areas of bony overlap. (**b**) Overview of the planned mandibular movement, showing the position of the mandibular nerve and tooth roots. (**c**) Dental-occlusal interferences are shown with red dots

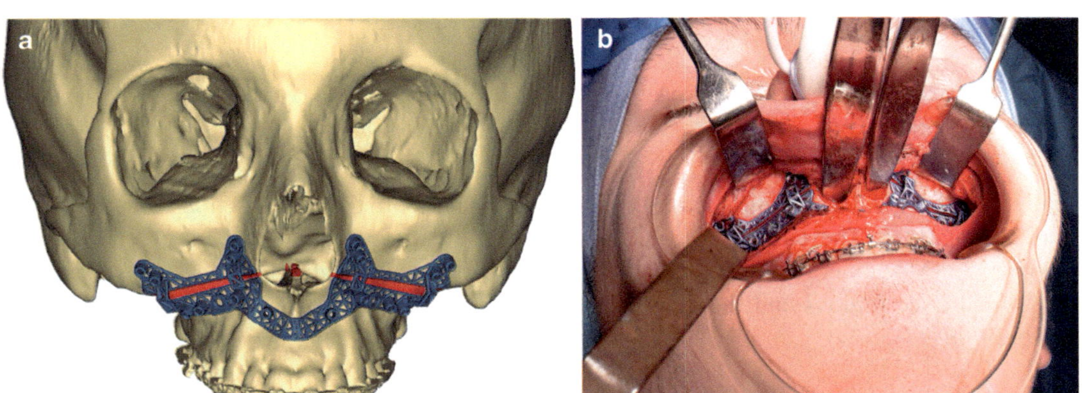

Fig. 10.10 (**a**) Maxillary cutting guides. (**b**) Intraoperative view of the maxillary cutting guides in preparation for a Le Fort I osteotomy

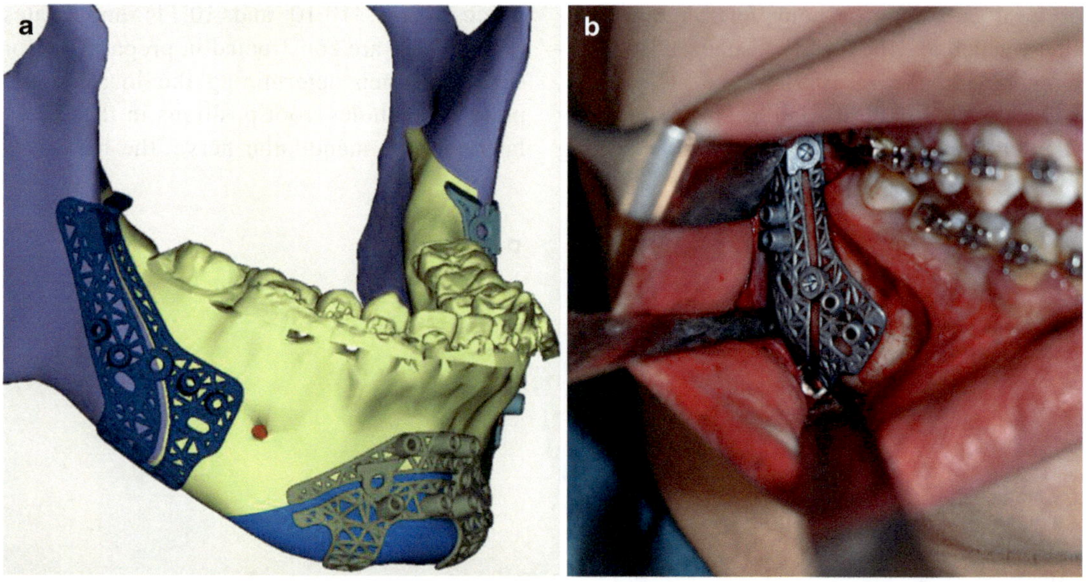

Fig. 10.11 (**a**) Mandibular sagittal split osteotomy and osseous genioplasty cutting guides. (**b**) Mandibular sagittal split osteotomy cutting guide in preparation for the osteotomy

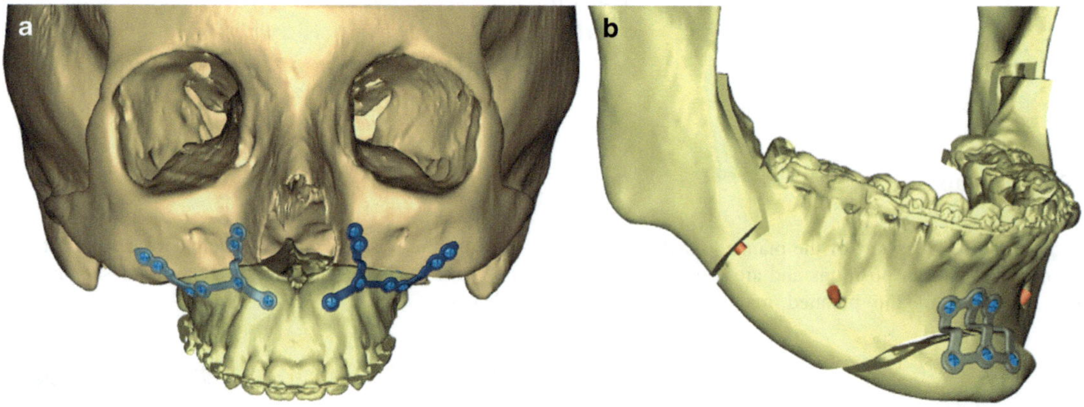

Fig. 10.12 (**a**) Maxillary plates. (**b**) Genioplasty plate. All the required plates will be three-dimensionally printed in preparation for the surgery

sinus, and the quality and thickness of bone can be visualized. The cutting guides can be designed with pilot hole locators aligned to best-suited bone regions and the drilling vectors built in.

Facial soft tissue predictions can be undertaken but their reliability is still questionable, as they are based on algorithms, whereas facial soft tissue responses to surgery are variable (Fig. 10.13).

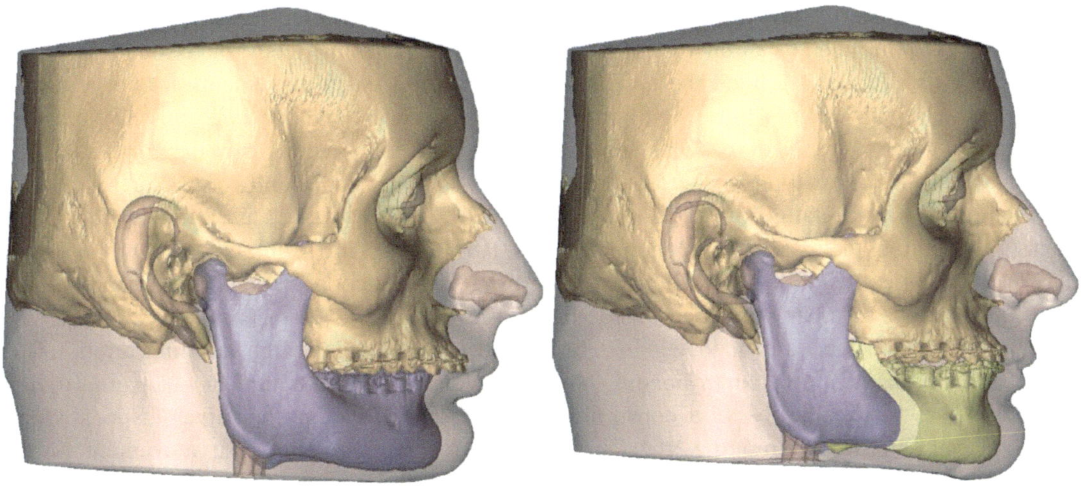

Fig. 10.13 Facial soft tissue predictions can be undertaken but their reliability is still questionable

10.6 Orthodontic Preparation

The overall purpose of preoperative orthodontic treatment is to place the teeth into the correct position for their respective jaw, so that on repositioning the jaws, the surgeon may attain the desired skeletal movements *and* obtain the best possible dental occlusion. *The preparatory orthodontic tooth movements should be determined in relation to the proposed surgical movements of the jaws*. The intended tooth movements may be described in relation to the six objectives of preparatory preoperative orthodontic treatment [10]:

- Alignment.
- Levelling.
- Decompensation.
- Incisor inclination preparation.
- Arch coordination.
- Elimination of occlusal interferences.

There is a seventh objective if segmental surgery is required:

- Creating interdental space for osteotomy cuts.

These objectives of orthodontic preparation are not always achieved in the same order. For example, decompensation may occur prior to arch levelling, or maxillary arch expansion to coordinate the arches may be required at the beginning of treatment. In certain circumstances, some of these phases occur together. They are described separately below for descriptive clarity.

Alignment: Alignment is usually, though not always, the first step in preoperative orthodontics (arch expansion is sometimes undertaken prior to alignment). Some arch levelling also begins at the same time as alignment, i.e. when the initial archwire is engaged into the brackets the teeth will begin to level. However, for the purpose of clarity, levelling will be described separately in the next section. The purpose of alignment is to correctly angulate ('tip') the crowns of the teeth into the correct position for their respective jaw and to correct tooth rotations.

Time taken to accurately position the brackets is never wasted. The brackets must be bonded into the correct position for each tooth. Minor variations in bracket positioning may be required in some patients. In orthognathic patients, the coordination of the maxillary and mandibular labial segments, i.e. the canine-to-canine region, is paramount. Often, interference may occur between the tip of the mandibular canine and the mesio-palatal aspect of the maxillary canine, which prevents the intercuspation of the teeth. Therefore, it is advisable to bond the maxillary canine bracket approximately ½ to ¾ of a millimetre mesial to the long axis of the tooth, leading to slight mesio-labial rotation of the tooth, and better ultimate interdigitation of the labial segment [10]. Bonding the maxillary second molars may lead to their extrusion, which will become a major interference in attempting arch coordination. If they must be bonded/banded, e.g. to derotate, then care should be taken to bonding the brackets somewhat occlusally. If a convertible tube is placed onto the first molar, vertical steps can be added to an archwire to also minimize extrusion of the second molar.

For archwire selection, a thin, round archwire is ideal for initial alignment, producing little binding and friction, and permitting relatively free tipping of the tooth crowns. The forces should be as light as possible, whilst permitting tooth movement. Nickel-titanium alloy (NiTi) is the initial aligning archwire material of choice, having both shape memory (i.e. it returns to its original form following plastic deformation, e.g. being ligated to a malpositioned tooth) and superelasticity (i.e. a flat 'superelastic' plateau in the middle of the force-deflection curve, allowing appreciable distortion of the wire in order to engage brackets on considerably displaced teeth whilst maintaining acceptable force levels) [11].

Typical sequencing of archwires for an orthognathic patient is variable, depending on the desired goals of treatment. Assuming a 0.022 × 0.028-in. bracket slot, the preliminary archwire is usually a round 0.014-in., followed by a 0.016-in. NiTi or 0.018-in. copper NiTi after one to two visits of religation. If sliding mechanics are required, e.g. to correct a dental midline shift, a working archwire of 0.018-in. stainless steel may be used, though a working wire should always be ligated into the brackets for at least a month, allowing levelling of the bracket slots, prior to any sliding mechanics being undertaken. This helps to make the archwire passive and thereby avoids binding of the brackets onto the archwire. The 0.018-in. stainless steel archwire is also very useful for correcting the inclination of incisor teeth, as the teeth rotate round the transverse axis. If such movements are not required, then an interim 0.019 × 0.025-in. NiTi archwire is used to help prepare for the ligation of the 0.019 × 0.025-in. stainless steel archwires, on which surgery is usually carried out. 0.019 × 0.025-in. stainless steel archwires are also useful for coordinating the dental arches and for levelling.

Levelling: Dental arch levelling refers to the stage of orthodontic treatment which aims to flatten (or almost flatten) the curve of Spee, by permitting the relative vertical movement of the teeth in each arch to bring their marginal ridges to lie approximately in the same horizontal plane. A relatively flat (i.e. 'level') curve of Spee is one of the prerequisites to a normal dental occlusion.

In the Class II orthognathic patient, levelling may be undertaken preoperatively or postoperatively, depending on the requirements of the respective case:

- Preoperatively—In patients with an average or increased lower anterior face height (LAFH) most or all the levelling may be undertaken prior to surgery.
- Postoperatively—In patients with a reduced LAFH some or most of the levelling is undertaken following surgery, e.g. a three-point or tripod landing (interarch tooth contact at the incisors and terminal molars only) is used to increase the LAFH and reduce the incisor overbite (Fig. 10.14) (see below).

The decision on how to level the maxillary arch is predominantly based on the final desired position of the maxillary incisors in relation to the upper lip and face. Once the desired postoperative position of the maxillary incisors has been planned, the decision on how to level the mandibular arch depends on the planned postoperative position of the mandibular incisors in relation to the maxillary incisors and the effect of this position on the LAFH. If no increase in LAFH is desired, the mandibular arch is levelled preoperatively by incisor intrusion. However, if an

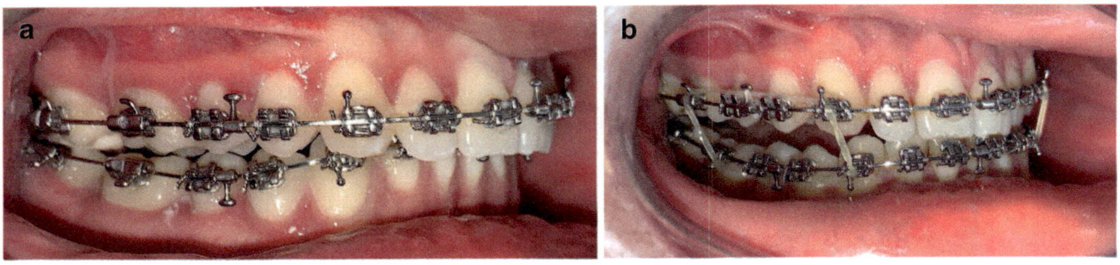

Fig. 10.14 (**a**) Preoperative dental occlusion in a Class II patient with mandibular retrognathia and reduced lower anterior face height (LAFH), prepared for a mandibular advancement to a three-point landing. (**b**) Postoperative dental occlusion following mandibular advancement to a three-point landing. With a flexible lower archwire in place, bilateral box elastics may be used to close the lateral open bites

increase in LAFH is desired, the mandibular arch curve of Spee is either partially levelled if only a small increase in LAFH is desired, the curve is maintained if already present at the required depth, or the curve is accentuated if a significant increase in LAFH is desired, i.e. the degree of preoperative levelling depends on how much of an increase in LAFH is desired. As the mandible is advanced, the degree of anterior-inferior movement of the mandibular incisors will determine the increase in LAFH (Fig. 10.15).

There is a space requirement for orthodontic levelling, with approximately 1 mm of space required to level a 3 mm depth curve of Spee [6].

Decompensation: The discrepancy between the jaws in all three planes of space has an indirect yet considerable influence on the dental occlusal relationship as a result of dentoalveolar compensation. Dentoalveolar compensation describes the variations in the positions of the teeth, in the sagittal, vertical and transverse dimensions, that may compensate for variations in the skeletal pattern, i.e. it is nature's way of trying to get the teeth to meet when the jaws are growing away from one another. In the normal situation, the erupting maxillary and mandibular teeth are guided towards each other by the surrounding soft tissue envelope of the tongue, lips and cheeks; hence, they erupt into a position of soft tissue equilibrium between the opposing forces of the tongue and lips/cheeks. Therefore, in the presence of sagittal or transverse skeletal discrepancies, alterations in the inclination of the teeth may compensate for the skeletal discrepancy. In such cases, the occlusal discrepancy will appear less severe than the underlying skeletal discrepancy. For example, in a patient with a severe Class II skeletal pattern, the dentoalveolar compensation may involve proclination of the mandibular incisors. This compensatory mechanism may be unsuccessful either because the skeletal discrepancy is too severe or because the soft tissue pattern is unfavourable. For example, in a Class II skeletal discrepancy, if the soft tissues are unfavourable and the lower lip is unable to control the labial aspect of the maxillary incisors and instead falls behind them it will lead to their proclination and thereby magnify rather than compensate for the skeletal discrepancy.

In the vertical plane, the incisors will tend to overerupt to compensate for increasing lower anterior face height, unless a forward tongue position prevents their overeruption. If the face height is dramatically increased, the incisors may not be able to fully compensate and an anterior open bite (AOB) will ensue.

Orthodontic preparation for orthognathic surgery requires orthodontic decompensation of the dental arches in all three planes of space, i.e. the process of removing the dentoalveolar compensations that may be present in the sagittal, transverse and vertical planes, and re-establishing the correct position of the teeth with regard to their own skeletal base thereby permitting adequate surgical correction of skeletal discrepancies. An important objective of preparatory orthodontics

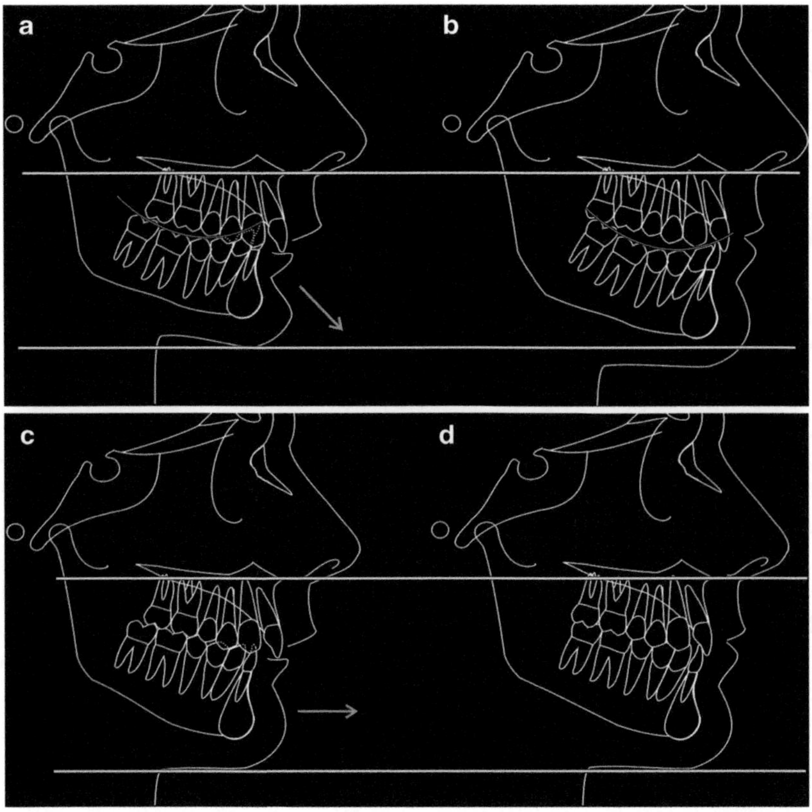

Fig. 10.15 (**a**) Maintaining or accentuating an increased curve of Spee before mandibular advancement. (**b**) Mandibular advancement to a three-point landing (incisors and terminal molars) occurs by a downward and forward vector of movement of the mandibular incisors. This will increase the lower anterior face height (LAFH) and unfurl the mentolabial fold, improving the soft tissue contour of the lower face. The lateral open bites are closed orthodontically by extrusion of the mid-arch mandibular dentition (i.e., postoperative levelling of the curve of Spee). (**c**) If the LAFH does not need to be increased, the mandibular dental arch is levelled in the preoperative orthodontic preparatory phase (i.e., preoperative levelling of the curve of Spee). (**d**) As such, mandibular advancement does not lead to any significant change in the LAFH. (From Naini FB, Gill DS, eds. Orthognathic Surgery: Principles, Planning and Practice. Oxford: Wiley-Blackwell; 2017. Reprinted with permission)

in a Class II patient is to remove the dental compensations and to make the dental-occlusal discrepancy match the skeletal discrepancy, which will allow correction of the dental occlusion with the skeletal repositioning.

There may be a 'worsening' effect on the dental occlusion and facial appearance in this stage of preoperative orthodontics. Just as dentoalveolar compensation tends to mask the extent of the underlying skeletal discrepancy, orthodontic decompensation unmasks the true extent of the underlying skeletal discrepancy. For example, in a patient with a Class II skeletal discrepancy and proclined/compensated mandibular incisors, often mandibular first premolars are extracted, and the space is used to retrocline the mandibular incisors towards their ideal inclination for their skeletal base. There may be a significant increase in the incisor overjet. Dental-occlusal function may also deteriorate during this stage of treatment. As such, it is extremely important that patients are made aware of this issue prior to embarking on treatment, and as part of informed consent.

Class III interarch elastics may be required in order to help mandibular incisor retroclination.

This is the opposite to their use in Class II orthodontic camouflage mechanics.

Dental extractions, when required, will be to permit the maximum extent of decompensation achievable, and thereby allow the desired extent of surgical movement of the jaws. In preparation for orthognathic surgery dental extraction patterns are usually the opposite of those used in conventional orthodontics.

If maxillary surgery is not required, maxillary dental midline deviation correction may well require dental extractions to create space. This usually involves extraction of the first premolar on the side to which the dental midline is to be moved. However, all things being equal, it is better to avoid extractions in the maxillary arch only, as there is a tendency to narrowing of the arch width, making arch coordination more difficult. This is particularly true in a Class II patient with a narrow maxilla relative to the mandible. All extraction patterns should be planned after undertaking a comprehensive space analysis [12, 13].

Incisor inclination preparation: The orthodontic treatment required to prepare the maxillary and mandibular incisor inclinations for surgery often occurs as part of incisor decompensation (see above). However, preoperative incisor inclination changes are not always, by definition, strictly speaking decompensation. For example, Class II patients with mandibular retrognathia often develop a lower lip trap, i.e. the lower lip gets caught behind the maxillary incisors, and leads to their proclination. This is not a compensatory proclination, but the inclination of the maxillary incisors needs to be corrected prior to mandibular advancement surgery.

Incisor inclination preparation for orthognathic surgery depends on whether surgery is being planned for a jaw, and whether that surgery involves rotation of the jaw round the transverse axis (also referred to as a change in pitch). If surgery is not being planned, then the incisor inclination for that jaw should be corrected prior to surgery, e.g. proclined maxillary incisors should be corrected preoperatively when only mandibular advancement surgery is being planned. If surgery is being planned for either jaw that will only entail sagittal bodily translation of the jaw, or if only vertical maxillary movement is required, then the incisor inclination for that jaw should again be corrected prior to surgery. However, if either jaw is being planned for surgery that will involve the rotation of the jaw round the transverse axis, such as differential posterior impaction of the maxilla, or autorotation of the mandible, which thereby alters the relative inclination of the incisors, then the incisor inclination should be prepared preoperatively to take into account the change in incisor inclination that will occur as part of the surgical repositioning of the respective jaw [8, 10].

Arch Coordination: Dental arch coordination refers to the aspects of orthodontic treatment which ensure that the maxillary and mandibular dental arches will fit well together in occlusion, with maxillary and mandibular arch forms that correspond to one another, and with normal incisor, canine and buccal segment overjet. Of all the parameters that must be dealt with in orthodontic preparation, the coordination of the maxillary arch with the mandibular arch is often the most important, commonly the most challenging, and usually the most likely to cause problems at the time of surgery and in the postoperative phase of treatment.

Ideally, the dental arches should be as well-coordinated as possible prior to surgery. However, in some patients, if the occlusion is so well-interdigitated as to make expansion difficult, particularly in low angle patients, glass ionomer cement blocks may be placed on the occlusal surface of the maxillary first molars to disclude the arches and permit easier expansion. Conversely, some of the posterior buccal segment expansion (perhaps 3–4 mm, i.e. no more than 2 mm per side) may be completed postoperatively. However, the coordination of the canine-to-canine region of the maxilla to that of the mandible is the single most important preparatory requirement of preoperative orthodontics [2]. Good preoperative coordination of this region is mandatory.

Judging the arch width of the opposing jaws for arch coordination is best accomplished by hand articulating the dental study models, which will demonstrate the requirement for arch expan-

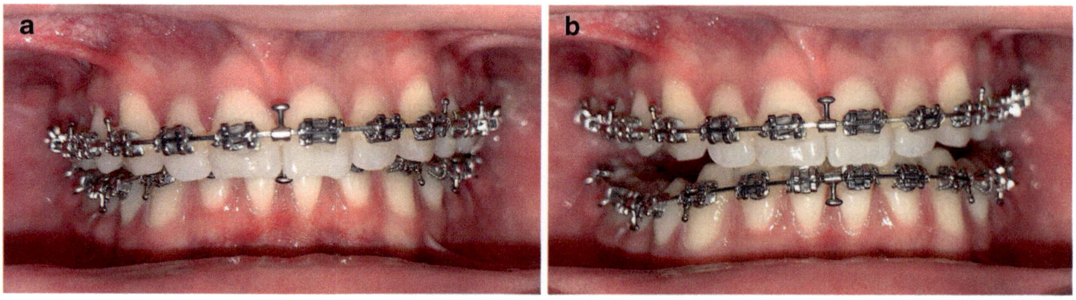

Fig. 10.16 (**a**) Preoperative Class II patient, with reduced or average lower anterior face height, in occlusion. (**b**) Posturing the mandible into a Class I incisor relationship allows comparison of the relative width of the dental arches

sion or contraction. In the Class II patient with reduced or average LAFH, it may also be possible to gauge the progress in arch coordination by asking the patient to posture the mandible forward and observing the relative width of the dental arches (Fig. 10.16).

If preoperative maxillary arch expansion is required, a number of methods are available, including expanded archwires, removable appliances with expansion screws, auxiliary archwires, quadhelices, rapid maxillary expansion, and surgically assisted rapid maxillary expansion.

Elimination of occlusal interferences: Planning to prevent occlusal interferences begins before a single bracket is bonded. Additionally, during treatment the dental arches should be checked at every visit, in order to continue preventing the formation of potential interferences, and eliminating them when they occur.

It is important to check the patient's individual dental arches and their occlusion with keen observation and with interim 'snap models' when required, in order to detect potential occlusal interferences. The two most common potential interferences in orthognathic patients are lack of coordination of the intercanine width, usually due to a narrow maxillary intercanine width, and extrusion of maxillary second molar teeth, which will prevent good dental interdigitation. In addition, excessive buccal flaring of maxillary molars, inadvertent premolar extrusion (usually due to incorrect bracket positioning), overeruption of preoperatively unopposed teeth, dental substitutions, and prominent cusps may all lead to interferences, which should be identified and resolved prior to surgery.

10.7 Postoperative Orthodontics

Active orthodontic treatment is usually delayed for 2 weeks, until the patient feels up to having treatment. During this time the patient will usually be wearing light intermaxillary guiding elastics, which help to guide the patient into the planned dental occlusion. These should be worn full time, and the patient should be seen by the surgeon and orthodontist weekly for the first 2 weeks, for close observation of any changes to the dental occlusion. Some patients will have an obvious, well-interdigitated dental occlusal result postoperatively. However, others may need closer observation, with variations in the intermaxillary elastic vectors made as required during this time [10].

Repairs to the orthodontic appliance should be made as soon as practically possible during this initial period. If a bracket has debonded or a band is loose, it should be repaired or removed.

If full-thickness stainless steel archwires had been placed prior to surgery, i.e. 0.0215 × 0.025-in. archwire in a 0.022 × 0.028 bracket slot, then these stabilizing archwires will need to be replaced with working archwires. However, most orthognathic surgeons are happy to operate with a larger dimension stainless steel working archwire, e.g. 0.019 × 0.025-in. stainless steel archwire, so long as it has been placed for at least one visit and is considered passive, prior to the maxillofacial technologist's impressions or three-dimensional intraoral scans in preparation for surgery. If a working archwire is already in place, there is no requirement to change it at this stage.

The type of working archwire required in either the maxillary or mandibular arch depends on the tooth movements desired. Often the most important initial movement is to guide the teeth vertically into a better dental occlusion. The orthodontist must decide on the teeth they would like to extrude, and in which arch. For example, if the maxillary arch is level, the 0.019 × 0.025-in. stainless steel archwire may be maintained in position. If there are lateral open bites in the mandibular canine and premolar regions following a planned three-point landing, these teeth need to be extruded by elastic force; therefore, a flexible mandibular archwire is required. The dimensions and material of the flexible archwire depend on the other types of movement that may be required, e.g. torque control, but rectangular braided (multistrand) stainless steel, TMA (titanium-molybdenum alloy), or nickel-titanium (NiTi) are commonly used postoperatively.

The configurations and vectors of the working intermaxillary elastics depend on the type and direction of desired tooth movement. Incorrectly placed elastics will result in undesirable tooth movement; therefore, every effort must be made to ensure that patients do not incorrectly position them. A drawing demonstrating exactly which teeth should engage the elastics may be provided to the patient as a reminder or they may take a photograph of the elastics positioned whilst still in the clinic.

Vertical tooth movement in the buccal segments is usually facilitated with box elastics, maintaining a vertical vector as far as possible. Vertical intermaxillary elastics, whether box type or triangular in configuration, aim at extrusion of selected teeth to improve the interdigitation of the dental arches. Box elastics are required to level a mandibular curve of Spee. If necessary, a Class II or Class III vector may be advisable on one or both sides, depending on the desired tooth movements.

Short intermaxillary elastics, either Class II or Class III, may be useful, providing the Class II or III vector but limiting the potential detrimental vertical eruption of the maxillary or mandibular molars from routine Class II or III intermaxillary elastics. These may also be placed in a triangular configuration.

Persistent dental midline deviations may require a Class II elastic vector on one side and Class III on the contralateral side. Sometimes an anterior diagonal elastic may also be added (usually just night times). In such situations, care must be taken not to cause transverse canting of the maxillary occlusal plane by extruding the teeth attached to these elastics; theoretically temporary anchorage devices may be used in one arch as a means of elastic attachment instead of the teeth, though in practice this is rarely required.

Occasionally, the exact planned surgical result may not have been attained. Where the discrepancy with the planned result is relatively minor, and the facial aesthetic improvements are acceptable, the orthodontist and surgeon may decide if the case can be 'salvaged' by orthodontic treatment alone. This often involves some form of compensatory tooth movement, particularly in relation to incisor inclinations. For example, if a Class II mandibular advancement has been slightly over-advanced, with an edge-to-edge type incisor relationship, Class III elastics may be used, perhaps in conjunction with a round steel archwire in the mandibular arch, to improve the incisor relationship. Whatever the circumstances, the clinicians need to be aware that miracles are not possible, and significant problems resulting from surgical shortcomings may need further surgical modification.

Much of the active vertical orthodontic settling occurs with the intermaxillary working elastics. Intermaxillary elastic wear will be markedly reduced, if required at all, in the finishing stages of orthodontic treatment. Elastic wear should be completely stopped for at least 6 weeks prior to appliance removal, to ensure that a stable result has been achieved.

Minor variations in tooth crown morphology combined with minor variations in bracket position will mean that some tooth repositioning by 'artistic' wire bending is likely to be required in the finishing stages of treatment. Occasionally, first-order bends to vertically extrude specific teeth or second-order angulation bends for the incisor teeth may be required. Labial or lingual root torque (third-order bends) for specific teeth (usually maxillary lateral incisors) may also be required.

The postoperative phase of orthodontic treatment typically takes anything from 3 months to 6 months, depending mainly on the degree of postoperative tooth movement required.

10.8 Stability of Class II Correction

When considering the stability of correcting a Class II skeletal relationship, it is important to understand the difference in surgical approach based on the lower anterior face height (LAFH). Patients with a reduced or average LAFH may be treated with mandibular advancement alone. Patients with an increased LAFH and anterior open bite (AOB) are corrected in a more stable fashion with a bimaxillary procedure that impacts the maxilla (either total or posterior) and advances the mandible.

The data suggests that for Class II patients with a reduced or average LAFH, mandibular advancement is stable within the first year following surgery. In the long term (1–5 years post-treatment), approximately one-quarter of patients with mandibular advancement alone experience more than 2 mm relapse in mandibular length and ramus height. However, only 10% of these patients have an increase in overjet of 2–4 mm [14], i.e. the skeletal change is not mirrored by dental change. That means that as remodelling of the mandible occurs (primarily at the condyles), the dentition frequently compensates to maintain a more ideal sagittal dental-occlusal relationship, primarily by proclination of the mandibular incisors.

Class II patients with an increased LAFH and either total or posterior vertical maxillary excess are best treated with maxillary superior repositioning and forward mandibular autorotation, either with or without concurrent mandibular advancement. Isolated superior repositioning of the maxilla with rigid fixation is the most stable surgical procedure in the short term, as the maxilla essentially does not move in the first year after surgery [15]. At 5 years following surgery, 20% of patients experience 2–4 mm of change in the vertical position of the maxilla, and almost half as many have more than 4 mm of relapse. This long-term vertical change may be the result of unfavourable facial growth. Despite these skeletal changes, the overbite is usually maintained in these patients, primarily because of compensatory eruption of the incisors [16, 17].

There has been some concern that Class II patients with increased LAFH may be at greater risk for long-term condylar resorption when they undergo bimaxillary surgery. However, the data demonstrates that long-term resorption appears to be the same in patients who have isolated mandibular osteotomies and those who have bimaxillary surgery (10% for both) [18].

In specific circumstances, Class II patients with increased LAFH and an AOB may be treated with mandibular surgery alone [19]. Recently, data have become available regarding the long-term stability of correction using anticlockwise rotation of the mandible and rigid fixation. In a retrospective study, Fontes et al. [20] examined the records of 31 patients with an average of 4.5 years of follow-up data, and found that 60% of the skeletal anticlockwise rotation of the mandible was lost. Only 10% of these patients relapsed to clinical open bite. Again, dental compensation is seen for skeletal relapse. It is important to note that the average open bite for this sample was limited (−2.6 mm; SD, 1.1 mm).

10.9 Soft Tissue Changes with Mandibular Surgery

A systematic review on the profile changes after bilateral sagittal split osteotomy (BSSO) advancement concluded that there was poor evidence on the short- and long-term effects of advancement [21]. Studies tend to have small sample sizes, no power calculation and a mixture of surgical procedures performed on the study subjects [22].

With mandibular advancement alone, a downward and forward repositioning of soft tissue pogonion with a resultant reduction in facial convexity, increase in the LAFH and increase in submental length can be expected (Fig. 10.17) [23]. The increase in LAFH will be influenced by the maxillary occlusal plane inclination, with a steeper plane resulting in a greater increase in lower facial height. The reported short-term (<2 years) and long-term (>2 years) ratios with rigid fixation are summarized in Table 10.1 [21].

The figures in Table 10.1 generally suggest that a vertical gradient in effects exists with the greater proportional changes occurring at soft tissue pogonion with gradually reducing changes on moving up to the upper lip. In the short-term the upper lip can be affected by oedema and the upper lip may also follow the lower lip movement to some degree. Long-term changes to the upper lip may be related to relapse and the ageing process with gradual thinning and inferior movement of labrale superius [24]. The changes at soft tissue pogonion may be more predictable as there is close attachment of the facial muscles onto this bony region.

With mandibular advancement, one may also expect a reduction in facial convexity, an increase in submental length, reduction in any submental soft tissue sag and a reduction of the lower lip-chin-submental plane angle. There may also be an uncurling effect on the lower lip, particularly if the preoperative lower facial height was reduced [25]. Although mandibular advancement had no effect on absolute nasal dimensions, advancement of the chin point may reduce the relative perceived prominence of the nose in relation to the forehead and chin point [22].

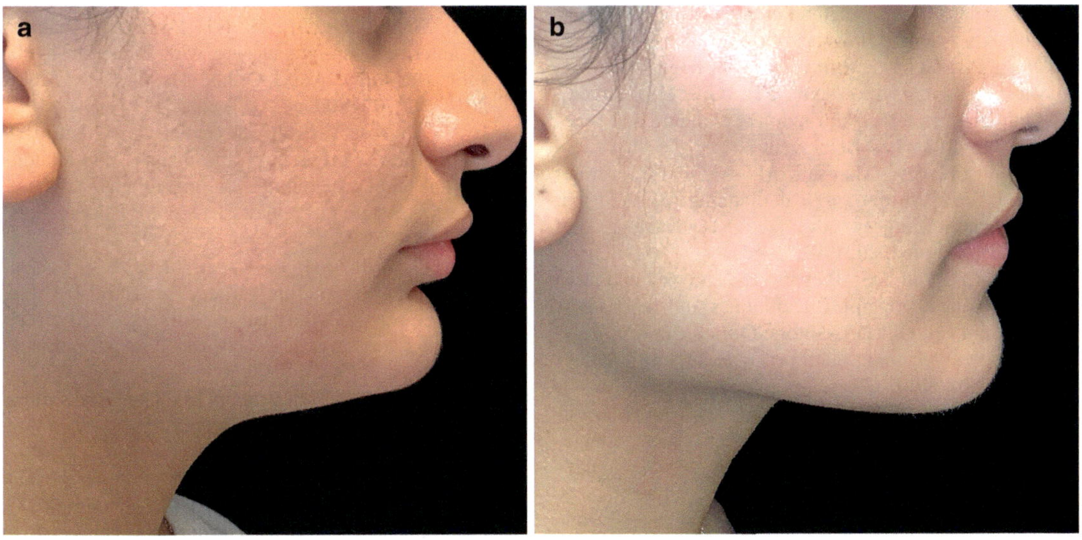

Fig. 10.17 (**a**) Preoperative profile of a Class II patient with mandibular retrognathia and reduced lower anterior face height (LAFH). (**b**) Following mandibular advancement to a three-point landing, there is downward and forward repositioning of soft tissue pogonion with a resultant reduction in facial convexity, increase in the LAFH, opening of the mentolabial angle and increase in the submental length

Table 10.1 Range of ratios for soft tissue to hard tissue movements for mandibular advancement, without genioplasty, with rigid internal fixation [21]

	Short-term (<2 years) ratios	Long-term (>2 years) ratios
Upper lip to incisor inferior	−2 to 29%	−10 to −67%
Lower lip to incisor inferior	35 to 108%	31 to 60%
Mentolabial fold to B-point	88 to 111%	86 to 111%
Soft tissue pogonion to hard tissue pogonion	90 to 124%	102 to 127%

References

1. Naini FB. Facial aesthetics: concepts and clinical diagnosis. Oxford: Wiley-Blackwell; 2011.
2. Naini FB, Gill DS, editors. Orthognathic surgery: principles, planning and practice. Wiley-Blackwell: Oxford; 2017.
3. Naini FB, Donaldson ANA, McDonald F, Cobourne MT. Influence of chin height on perceived attractiveness in the orthognathic patient, clinician and layperson. Angle Orthod. 2012;82:88–95.
4. Naini FB, Donaldson ANA, McDonald F, Cobourne MT. How does variation in lower anterior face height influence perceived attractiveness? A quantitative investigation. J Orthod. 2013;40:206–17.
5. Naini FB, Manouchehri S, Al-Bitar ZB, Gill DS, Garagiola U, Wertheim U. The maxillary incisor labial face tangent: clinical evaluation of maxillary incisor inclination in profile smiling view and idealized aesthetics. Maxillofac Plast Reconstr Surg. 2019;41:31–8.
6. Naini FB, Garagiola U, Wertheim D. Analysing chin prominence in relation to the lower lip: the lower lip-chin prominence angle. J Craniomaxillofac Surg. 2019;47(8):1310–6.
7. McNamara JA Jr. A method of cephalometric evaluation. Am J Orthod. 1984;86:449–69.
8. Naini FB, Gill DS. Principles of orthognathic treatment planning. In: Naini FB, Gill DS, editors. Orthognathic surgery: principles, planning and practice. Oxford: Wiley-Blackwell; 2017.
9. Donaldson CD, Manisali M, Naini FB. Three-dimensional virtual surgical planning (3D-VSP) in orthognathic surgery: advantages, disadvantages and pitfalls. J Orthod. 2021;48:52–63.
10. Naini FB, Gill DS. Preparatory and postoperative orthodontics: principles, techniques and mechanics. In: Naini FB, Gill DS, editors. Orthognathic surgery: principles, planning and practice. Oxford: Wiley-Blackwell; 2017.
11. Khamastha-Ledezma L. Archwires. In: Naini FB, Gill DS, editors. Preadjusted edgewise fixed orthodontic appliances: principles and practice. Oxford: Wiley-Blackwell; 2022.
12. Lee R, Kirschen R. Space planning for the dentition (space analysis). In: Gill DS, Naini FB, editors. Orthodontics: principles and practice. Oxford: Wiley-Blackwell; 2011.
13. Naini FB, Gill DS. Principles of treatment planning. In: Naini FB, Gill DS, editors. Preadjusted edgewise fixed orthodontic appliances: principles and practice. Oxford: Wiley-Blackwell; 2022.
14. Simmons KE, Turvey TA, Phillips C, Proffit WR. Surgical-orthodontic correction of mandibular deficiency: five-year follow-up. Int J Adult Orthodon Orthognath Surg. 1992;7:67–79.
15. Proffit WR, Phillips C, Turvey TA. Stability following superior repositioning of the maxilla by LeFort I osteotomy. Am J Orthod Dentofacial Orthop. 1987;92:151–61.
16. Bailey LJ, Phillips C, Proffit WR, Turvey TA. Stability following superior repositioning of the maxilla by Le Fort I osteotomy: five-year follow-up. Int J Adult Orthodon Orthognath Surg. 1994;9:163–73.
17. Proffit WR, Bailey LJ, Phillips C, Turvey TA. Long-term stability of surgical open-bite correction by Le Fort I osteotomy. Angle Orthod. 2000;70:112–7.
18. Jackson TH, Golden BA. Stability of orthognathic surgery. In: Naini FB, Gill DS, editors. Orthognathic surgery: principles, planning and practice. Oxford: Wiley-Blackwell; 2017.
19. Bloomquist D, Joondeph D. Surgical treatment of anterior open bite with mandibular osteotomies. In: Naini FB, Gill DS, editors. Orthognathic surgery: principles, planning and practice. Oxford: Wiley-Blackwell; 2017.
20. Fontes AM, Joondeph DR, Bloomquist DS, Greenlee GM, Wallen TR, Huang GJ. Long-term stability of anterior open-bite closure with bilateral sagittal split osteotomy. Am J Orthod Dentofacial Orthop. 2012;142:792–800.
21. Joss CU, Joss-Vassalli IM, Kiliaridis S, Kuijpers-Jagtman AM. Soft tissue profile changes after bilateral sagittal split osteotomy for mandibular advancement: a systematic review. J Oral Maxillofac Surg. 2010;68:1260–9.
22. Gill DS, Naini FB, Koudstaal M. The soft tissue effects of orthognathic surgery. In: Naini FB, Gill DS, editors. Orthognathic surgery: principles, planning and practice. Oxford: Wiley-Blackwell; 2017.
23. Gill DS, Lloyd T, East C, Naini FB. The facial soft tissue effects of orthognathic surgery. Facial Plast Surg. 2017;33:519–25.
24. Behrents RG. Growth in the aging craniofacial skeleton. In: McNamara JA, editor. Monograph 17, Craniofacial Growth Series. Ann Arbor: University of Michigan; 1985.
25. Maal TJJ, de Koning MJJ, Plooij JM, Verhamme LM, Rangel FA, Berge SJ, Borslap WA. One year postoperative hard and soft tissue volumetric changes after a BSSO mandibular advancement. Int J Oral Maxillofac Surg. 2012;41:1137–45.

GPSR Compliance

The European Union's (EU) General Product Safety Regulation (GPSR) is a set of rules that requires consumer products to be safe and our obligations to ensure this.

If you have any concerns about our products, you can contact us on ProductSafety@springernature.com

In case Publisher is established outside the EU, the EU authorized representative is:

Springer Nature Customer Service Center GmbH
Europaplatz 3
69115 Heidelberg, Germany

Batch number: 10732801

Printed by Printforce, the Netherlands